Contents

Contributors

Mark A. Williams, PhD, Editor-in-Chief

Writing Committee

Gary J. Balady, MD

Joseph J. Carlson, RD, PhD

Pat Comoss, RN, BS

Reed Humphrey, PhD, PT

Patricia F. Lounsbury, RN, MEd

Jeffrey L. Roitman, EdD

Douglas R. Southard, PhD, MPH, PA-C

Contributors

Philip A. Ades, MD

Dalynn T. Badenhop, PhD

Gary J. Balady, MD

Kathy A. Berra, MSN, ANP

Lawrence P. Cahalin, PT

Brian W. Carlin, MD

Pat Comoss, RN, BS

Mitzi Ekers, RN, MS

Christopher Gardner, PhD

Larry F. Hamm, PhD

Matthew L. Herridge, PhD

Reed Humphrey, PhD, PT

Janet B. Jaeger, RN

Marjorie L. King, MD

Thomas P. LaFontaine, PhD

Cindy Lamendola, MSN, ANP

Patricia F. Lounsbury, RN, MEd

Nancy Houston Miller, BSN

Fredric J. Pashkow, MD

Jane Z. Reardon, MSN, APRN

Barbara Southard, MS

Douglas R. Southard, PhD, MPH, PA-C

Ray W. Squires, PhD

Kerry J. Stewart, EdD

Mark A. Williams, PhD

Reviewers

Gary J. Balady, MD

Ann M. Gavic-Ott, MS

Karen K. Hardy, RN, BSN

Jody R. Heggestad Hereford, BSN, MS

Reed Humphrey, PhD, PT

Marjorie L. King, MD

Donald Mertens, MD, MS, MB, MSc

Jeffrey L. Roitman, EdD

F. Stuart Sanders, MD

Bonnie K. Sanderson, RN, PhD

Douglas R. Southard, PhD, MPH, PA-C

Mark A. Williams, PhD

We wish to acknowledge the contributions of Jan McNew in the preparation of the manuscript.

Thanks also to the Cardiac Center of Creighton University, Omaha, Nebraska, for assistance and cooperation.

Preface

The evolution of health care has produced changes in the way in which cardiac rehabilitation and secondary prevention connect to the larger continuum of care. In the past, cardiac rehabilitation too frequently operated in isolation from other cardiovascular services. Patient movement through the rehabilitation phases was segmental at best and often incomplete. In recent years, a number of models have allowed potential service gaps to be filled through cooperative partnerships with other departments or providers, and the flow of care has become more contiguous across the rehabilitation spectrum and more individualized for each rehabilitation participant. Thus, cardiac rehabilitation and secondary prevention are, and should continue to be, evolving processes for helping people change lifestyle behaviors while reducing risk factors for disease progression and thereby lessening the impact of the disease on quality of life, morbidity, and mortality.

As a result of this evolution, secondary prevention programs are assuming an exciting and potentially enormous role. At a time when chronic disease is at epidemic levels in this country, opportunities abound for providing these services. By definition, however, secondary prevention is a lifelong proposition. Thus, we must provide patients with low-cost programming that educates as well as motivates toward personal responsibility for disease prevention for years to come. Our challenge is to increase opportunities to provide risk interventions and promote positive lifestyle behavior patterns within the limit of finite resources. Management involves implementing more effective education, using risk-factor intervention, encouraging exercise, and urging symptom recognition before acute episodes occur to decrease cardiovascular disease morbidity and mortality.

At the same time, the proven efficacy of the secondary prevention model allows for a transition into the management of other chronic diseases. A variety of chronic disease states, including diabetes, chronic obstructive pulmonary disease, asthma, osteoporosis, and cancer, should also be affected by the preventive and rehabilitative aspects of this type of intervention. Much of the management of these non-cardiovascular diseases has been similar to that of cardiac rehabilitation programming for many years because at the center of the disease process and central to many chronic diseases are the four lifestyle-related risk factors—smoking, hypertension, inappropriate diet, and sedentary lifestyle. Additionally, the key to effective chronic-disease management is adherence to risk-factor reduction, healthy lifestyles, individualized diet modification, and medication recommendations. Thus, the cardiovascular disease secondary prevention program model can be expanded to serve in these settings as well.

New models of practice are changing the structure and delivery of cardiac rehabilitation services. Keeping up with the pace of change is a professional necessity. The fourth edition of the American Association of Cardiovascular and Pulmonary Rehabilitation (AACVPR) *Guidelines for Cardiac Rehabilitation and Secondary Prevention Programs* is one tool to help cardiovascular rehabilitation professionals meet that challenge and achieve the goal of securing a spot in the new continuum of care. By way of these guidelines, leaders in the field of cardiac rehabilitation and secondary prevention, cardiovascular risk reduction, reimbursement, and public policy have provided clinicians with the latest tools and information necessary for successfully starting new programs or updating existing ones. The fourth edition provides state-of-the-art methods of implementation of inpatient and outpatient cardiac rehabilitation and secondary prevention including risk stratification; risk-factor management; patient education and behavior modification; considerations for special patient populations; and program administration, including outcomes. In particular, the most recent guidelines for management of lipids, hypertension, exercise, and obesity are presented, along with the manner in which these recommendations interact with older patients, racially and culturally diverse populations, and people with heart failure as well as other patient groups. Also included for the first time in the AACVPR's guidelines is a careful review of dietary supplements and herbal medicines, which are frequently used by patients and thus warrant a thorough understanding by the program staff. As with the third edition, it is acknowledged that all programs may not have the personnel or resources to provide specific expertise in each area, and not all of the subcomponents will necessarily be appropriate for every program. The fourth edition of the guidelines provides a basis for all programs to address each of these essential components in a manner that is in keeping with the delivery of a comprehensive program of cardiac rehabilitation. The challenge to cardiac rehabilitation program professionals is to select, develop, and provide appropriate rehabilitative and secondary preventive services for individual patients and to tailor the method of delivery of these services to their individual needs. Determination of the best approach in each case should involve both health care provider recommendations and patient preferences. The strategy for success should reflect a desire for the patient's progressive independence in cardiac rehabilitation and long-term comprehensive care.

The AACVPR and these guidelines are critical links to keeping our profession and the services we provide recognized and valued by the scientific community; federal agencies; third-party payers; and, most importantly, the patients, families, and communities whose lives we touch. The fourth edition of the AACVPR *Guidelines* provides significant support to help us achieve our goals of continuing professional development and program excellence.

The Integration of Cardiac Rehabilitation and Secondary Prevention

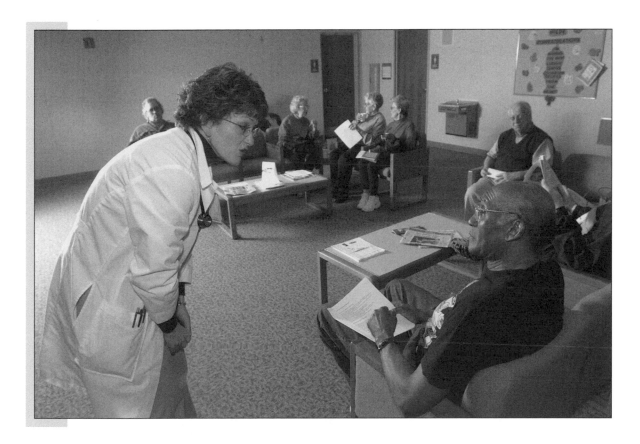

Cardiac rehabilitation (CR) programs provide patients, families, and communities with important resources in the battle against cardiovascular disease (CVD)—the leading cause of death and disability in the United States. The basis for CR began to take shape in the 1950s, with the major focus on the restoration of functional capacity. Restoration of functional capacity was critically important because of the prolonged bed rest required for patients hospitalized with acute myocardial infarction (AMI). Little was known about the causes of ischemic coronary disease, and few interventions were available. Thus the formidable rates of morbidity and mortality at that time associated with AMI should not be surprising. Over the past 50 years, major advances have been made in understanding pathophysiology, epidemiology, and interventions for coronary heart disease (CHD). Also during this period, CR has evolved as an accepted therapy.

OBJECTIVES

This chapter

■ discusses current status and future directions of CR and secondary prevention, both nationally and globally; and

■ identifies the challenges and opportunities that face those who work within the CR discipline.

National Perspective

In the twenty-first century, CR programs have become synonymous with health and wellness for persons with CHD. They are designed to decrease morbidity and mortality and improve a variety of clinical and behavioral outcomes, including quality of life. This is accomplished through medically supervised exercise as well as intensive lifestyle interventions and health education. In 1995, the Agency for Health Care Policy and Research (AHCPR) funded a broad scientific review of outcome data associated with the interventions provided by CR programs.[604] This document demonstrated that participation in CR programs resulted in a 20 to 25% reduction in mortality from CHD. In addition, this exhaustive review of the literature showed beneficial influences on functional capacity, coronary risk factors, and emotional health. The authors succinctly summarized the data by stating, "Cardiovascular disease is the leading cause of morbidity and mortality in the United States, accounting for over 50 percent of all deaths. Coronary heart disease, with its clinical manifestations of stable angina pectoris, unstable angina, acute myocardial infarction, and sudden cardiac death, affects 13.5 million Americans. The almost 1 million survivors of myocardial infarction (MI) and the 7 million patients with stable angina pectoris are candidates for cardiac rehabilitation, as are the 309,000 patients who undergo coronary artery bypass graft (CABG) surgery and the 362,000 patients who undergo percutaneous transluminal coronary angioplasty procedures each year."[604] The need for cardiac rehabilitation has not changed since these recommendations were written. Data published since 1995 have only confirmed earlier findings and in fact provided justification for broader inclusion criteria for CR, particularly for patients with chronic heart failure. CHD remains a societal epidemic and results in enormous social, medical, and economic burdens.

As noted, research has continued to demonstrate that the services CR programs provide remain critically important to the overall recovery and long-term

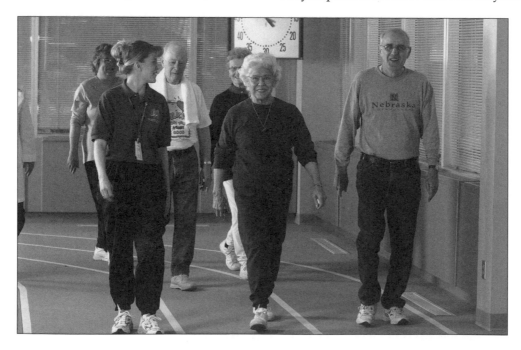

outcomes of people with CHD. Secondary-prevention research agendas of the 1990s focused on risk reduction through careful evaluation of medical and lifestyle interventions. This research further supported the importance of intensive management of dyslipidemia, diabetes, hypertension, cigarette smoking, physical inactivity, obesity, and psychological disorders.[140,263] Emerging risk factors have also been identified, and their role in the management of CHD is being carefully studied.[12,116,192,285,471,501,514] The inclusion of women's health issues, racial and cultural risk factors, genetic markers of risk, CVD risk factors in the young, and lifestyle interventions have become primary areas of research focus. Along with research, societal changes including tobacco legislation, healthy food choices in restaurants, employee wellness programs, and local and national emphasis on successful aging programs also provide great support of the CR message.

Cardiac rehabilitation professionals must maintain state-of-the-art programs that are responsive to evolving science while confronting the daily challenges of limitations in reimbursement, shortened hospital stays, an aging population, and costly medical services. The American Heart Association's 2003 Heart and Stroke Factors estimates that 650,000 Americans will have their first AMI in the year 2003, with 450,000 suffering a recurrent AMI. Along with these staggering statistics, consider the following:

- In 2003, 700,000 persons will have an acute stroke.
- More than 550,000 new cases of congestive heart failure (CHF) will be diagnosed each year, with hospital discharges for CHF having risen by 160% since 1979.

- Since 1979, the number of Americans discharged from short-stay hospitals with a primary diagnosis of CVD has increased by 28%.
- In 2003, CVD was listed as the first diagnosis in more than 6 million hospitalizations, with 65,843,000 physician office visits and 5,225,000 outpatient visits attributed to CVD.
- In 1999, payments totaling $26.3 billion were made to Medicare beneficiaries for hospital expenses resulting from a diagnosis of CVD.
- In 1998, costs related to CHD exceeded $351 billion.[31]

These data, combined with the nationwide epidemic of obesity and physical inactivity, further solidify the role of the CR program in identifying persons at risk and the importance of instituting programs to reduce CVD risk. With the increasing size and greater longevity of our population, these figures will continue to rise unless we implement intensive risk-reduction efforts. In light of the enormous personal and financial burdens associated with CHD, it is essential that patients be provided therapeutic services shown to improve the lives of those with CVD while positively affecting the medical costs associated with this disease. CR programs are positioned to deliver these important services.

Global Perspective

The prevalence of CHD continues to rise worldwide as well. It is estimated that by the year 2020, ischemic heart disease (IHD) will continue as the number-one cause of mortality and disability, with unipolar major depression rising to number two (figure 1.1).[399] Both

1990	2020
Ischemic heart disease	Ischemic heart disease
Cerebrovascular disease	Unipolar major depression
Lower respiratory disease	Road-traffic accidents
Diarrheal diseases	Cerebrovascular disease
Perinatal conditions	Chronic obstructive pulmonary disease (COPD)
Chronic obstructive pulmonary disease (COPD)	Lower respiratory infections
Tuberculosis	Tuberculosis
Measles	War injuries
Road-traffic accidents	Diarrheal diseases
Throat and lung cancers	Human immunodeficiency virus (HIV)

Figure 1.1 Global burden of disease study: Observed and projected leading causes of mortality, 1990 and 2002.[399]

of these projections affect the future of health care in general and CR in particular. We must continue to work with the international community to better understand global health issues.

Challenges and Opportunities

The prevalence of coronary risk factors mandates an intensive approach in both the identification and the treatment of all individuals at risk, particularly those at high risk. Determining and implementing successful methods for managing these risk factors provide challenges to those in clinical practice and research. Risk factors such as obesity, hypertension, dyslipidemia, cigarette smoking, physical inactivity, high levels of anger and hostility, and social isolation continue to rise in prevalence and remain difficult to treat effectively. Lack of effective treatment and rising prevalence are complex in their causality. Too frequently these risk factors are associated with lack of access to medical care, poverty, age, gender, ethnicity, culture, adherence to prescribed regimens, lack of efficacy of the interventions, and genetic relationships not yet well understood. CR programs provide a significant bridge to effectively address the rising need

for risk reduction. The application of effective models of risk reduction is essential to reduce morbidity and mortality from CHD. CR programs are challenged to provide leadership in designing and implementing these new models of care.

Cardiovascular risk reduction involves the integration of medical and psychosocial therapies with lifestyle changes. Over the past 40 years landmark scientific research has defined the pathophysiology and management of diseases of the vascular system. Vascular biology, percutaneous interventions, innovative surgeries, new and more effective medications, advances in understanding the role of genetics, improved noninvasive assessment techniques, and more effective lifestyle interventions have led the way in reducing death and disability from CHD and stroke. Through the systematic application of these advances and through continued scientific research, *evidence-based practice guidelines* have been developed. Medical care systems such as employee wellness programs, health maintenance organizations, group practice settings, individual physician associations, and hospital-based clinics can provide such applications. Of all the available medical care systems, CR programs are designed to specifically address the need for intensive risk reduction and are thereby positioned in a key leadership role to provide these services.

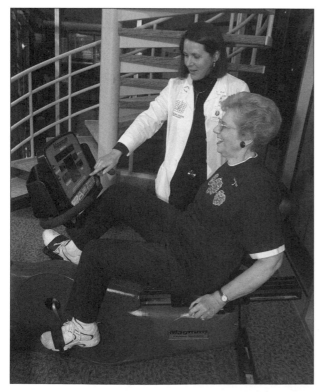

Summary

The worldwide epidemic of CHD has created an atmosphere where primary and secondary prevention have gained enormous attention. The future of these interventions lies in the effective implementation of evidence-based clinical practice guidelines. CVD risk factors demand an integrated approach to medical and lifestyle management because of their unique and complex interactions. Effective implementation relies heavily on a systematic approach to risk reduction. Case management through CR programming can be the cornerstone of multiple risk reduction and provides an excellent model for CVD management. The development and refinement of lifestyle skills will always remain at the foundation of risk factor interventions, providing both important metabolic and psychosocial benefits as well as the reduction of events of morbidity and mortality. CR programs including exercise and behavior modification not only are effective links in the implementation of case management but also provide successful ongoing lifestyle interventions and help patients attempt to reach risk-reduction goals.

The Cardiac Rehabilitation Continuum of Care

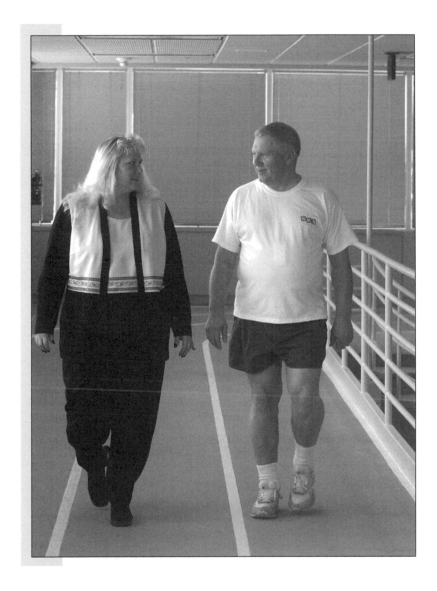

The Joint Commission on Accreditation of Healthcare Organizations (JCAHO) defines the continuum of care as a quality component of patient care consisting of the degree to which the care a patient needs is coordinated among practitioners and across organizations over time.[301,302,303] The continuum of care also includes the operational concepts and physical structures that exist to facilitate matching health care services to patients' needs. In CR, the continuum of care has been described and illustrated as a sequence of settings and services provided over weeks or months. This chapter reviews the CR continuum as it has evolved to date and suggests trends in its further evolution.

OBJECTIVES

This chapter

- provides an overview of the operational structure and sequence of CR programs in the past, present, and future;

- describes two practical tools that may be useful in the delivery of contemporary outpatient CR and that also help set the stage for future transformations; and

- identifies opportunities to redesign existing programs to optimize performance now while preparing for an evolving continuum.

A comprehensive review of the history and development of CR, from the early research of the 1950s through the turn of the new century, is beyond the scope of this text. The subject has been addressed in detail for those interested in exploring the roots of this still young specialty.[427] A brief overview is relevant, however, to provide perspective for later discussion.

Historically, CR predominantly consisted of the delivery of exercise services to postacute cardiac patients. In the 1960s, inpatient CR programs began delivering passive range-of-motion exercises to patients still confined to their beds in coronary care units (CCU). Days later, on step-down units, patients were cautiously walked in their rooms, still tethered by cables to bedside heart monitors. In the 1970s, outpatient services were initiated 8 to 12 weeks postevent. Maintenance programs became more prevalent in the 1980s in response to the growing volume of outpatient graduates and their desire to stay in a familiar, secure exercise environment. Because these exercise services were delivered in chronological sequence across settings, they became labeled as CR *phases* in numeric order. Although some programs still use phase labels, changes in both timeframes and settings in which rehabilitation occurs have made them less useful today. To avoid confusion and miscommunication about when and where a patient participates in CR services, the American Association of Cardiovascular and Pulmonary Rehabilitation (AACVPR) recommends the use of more explicit descriptors, such as *early outpatient* and *maintenance*, rather than the earlier phase label (see guideline 2.1). Early program structures were linear and one-dimensional. The operational focus was on building separate program components and then linking them together. Although CR coexisted with other cardiology services, few deliberate or consistent connections

were made to coordinate care. Outside services were engaged only episodically. The continuum of care was *program centered* and viewed from within CR as simply moving the patient from one phase to the next. From the outside, CR was viewed as a relatively isolated service entity. Most physicians remained skeptical as to the effectiveness and viability of CR and were seldom directly involved.

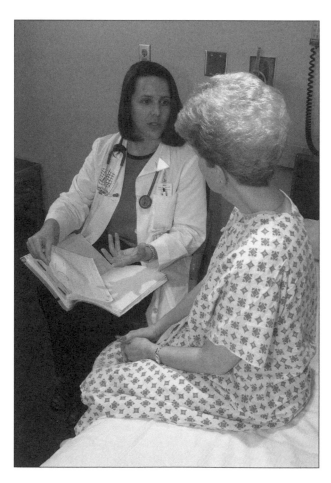

Guideline 2.1

To demonstrate its place in the continuum of care, each program should have available

■ an outline or illustration of the structure or sequence within which it operates, and

■ a written description of the scope of services provided to patients.

Contemporary Cardiac Rehabilitation: Secondary Prevention

In response to the economic pressures of the early 1990s and the movement toward evidence-based practice in the later half of that decade, CR programs began to be remodeled. The original sequence has remained, but the structure of phases has been substantially streamlined. Table 2.1 provides an example of one contemporary model. Most importantly, the current continuum of care has become *process centered*, characterized by service that is more continuous than it used to be across the rehabilitation spectrum and increasing professional partnerships for service delivery.

Length of Service Along the Continuum

In tandem with shorter lengths of stay for all health care services, duration of CR services, particularly inpatient and early-outpatient components, was also affected. Reduced service-delivery timeframes have necessitated simplified strategies. Individual patient-care priorities must be quickly identified and efficiently addressed. CR providers are compelled to responsibly integrate services. Figure 2.1 describes the current status of the CR continuum of care.

The need for such changes has produced challenges for many programs. The biggest of these challenges is to continue to deliver added services as budget and reimbursement limitations curb staffing and programming. Simultaneously, there is pressure to describe outcome data to demonstrate program efficacy, which tends to increase demands on staff and program components. However, working through problems associated with these challenges has generated opportunities that were previously unrecognized. Table 2.2 lists some examples that may be instructive.

Expanded Services Within the Continuum

Fulfillment of the secondary prevention mission of CR requires the delivery of risk factor intervention programs, education and counseling, and exercise training. The combination of these interventions has been shown to produce optimal reduction of cardiac risk.[604] Recognizing the need to shift from an exercise-dominated program to one that provides comprehensive risk reduction, optimal outpatient programming

Table 2.1 Cardiac Rehabilitation Circa 2003

Inpatient	TZ	Outpatient	TZ	Lifetime
• Aggressive ambulation • Survival education • Discharge planning	Refer to subacute facility, home recovery program, or early outpatient program	• Encourage early start • Adjust length of stay • Choose surveillance options	Offer short-term weaning program instead of ongoing maintenance involvement	• Self-management skills • Maintenance programming • Regular follow-up

TZ = transition zone.

Comoss PM. The new infrastructure for cardiac rehabilitation practice. In: NK Wenger, LK Smith, ES Froelicher, PM Comoss. *Cardiac Rehabilitation: A Guide to Practice in the 21st Century.* New York: Marcel Dekker, 1999, p. 319.

Inpatient Cardiac Rehabilitation

- Average length of stay = 3-4 days
- Progressive activity often integrated into clinical pathways or other protocol formats and performed by unit staff to ensure more timely, more aggressive delivery
- Education focused on predischarge priorities (survival teaching) such as recognition of signs and symptoms, dos and don'ts for home, medication instruction
- Posthospital follow-up arranged as part of discharge planning
  - Sicker patients may require transitional care.
  - Some patients may qualify for home health visits.
  - Healthier patients are referred to start outpatient programs within 1 to 2 weeks postevent.

Early Outpatient Cardiac Rehabilitation

- Starts sooner (1-2 weeks postevent) and shorter duration (average length of stay = 6-8 weeks) depending upon each patient's
  - level of risk, and
  - access to additional resources outside of formal CR program
- Emphasis on risk-factor reduction through focused interventions, education and counseling, and exercise
- Risk stratification to triage patients and optimize use of program resources
- Greater promotion of self-learning and self-monitoring among all patients
- Programming variations available to facilitate patient inclusion, such as elderly patients or those who have undergone transplants, heart failure, or vascular disease
- Increased collaboration with primary physicians as partners in secondary prevention
- Alternative settings or delivery systems in use or being explored for patients unable to participate onsite
- Measurement of selected patient outcomes and use of data to compile and monitor aggregate results

Maintenance and Follow-Up

- Begin within 2 to 3 months of event
- Continue long-term at hospital or clinic site, at home, or at community exercise facility (e.g., high school or college gym, hospital wellness center, YMCA or Jewish Community Center, commercial health/fitness club) under direction of rehabilitation staff as well as patient's self-direction
- Rehabilitation staff monitors compliance with lifestyle change through regularly scheduled follow-ups via one or all of the following:
  - Onsite checkups
  - Telephone calls or e-mail contacts
  - Mailed surveys
- Access to continuing education through
  - Hospital or community health classes
  - Video/Internet programs

Figure 2.1 The changing continuum of care: Characteristics of contemporary CR.

based on an operating structure defined in the 1995 clinical practice guideline (CPG) on CR is recommended (see figure 2.2).

As shown in the CPG model, exercise training and education and counseling for risk reduction are the essential services that constitute contemporary outpatient CR. However, because each CR patient has different problems and needs, successful implementation of this model is aided by the use of additional tools.[123] Services must be individualized, but standardizing how this is accomplished establishes credibility, improves communication, and ensures consistency across settings and among providers (guideline 2.2).

Table 2.2 Examples of Challenges and Opportunities Across the Cardiac Rehabilitation Continuum

	Challenges	Opportunities
Inpatient cardiac rehabilitation	• Budget cuts in cardiac rehabilitation = less staff to cover inpatient & outpatient programs • Shortened length of stay minimizes the amount of activity and teaching that can be completed	• Shared responsibility: Form a performance improvement team to explore how delivery of simplified exercise & education services can be shared between rehabilitation staff and other caregivers • Professional alliance: Offer to instruct home health nurses and/or staff within transitional care units to continue basic rehabilitation progression after patient transfer to their care
Outpatient cardiac rehabilitation	• Budget cuts limit the routine use of multi-disciplinary resources (e.g. dietitian, psychologist) to assess and advise individual patient behavior change • Patients' health plans only cover a few exercise visits, enough to set up a home exercise plan, but patients' needs require more time to learn how to manage risk factors	• Risk factor triage: Implement the use of self-assessment tools for patient's risk factors; based on scores, assign 1:1 expert time to highest risk patients; encourage class or self-learning options for others • Internet supplements: Explore appropriate self-learning modules available on the Internet; some are interactive and will provide feedback to patient; schedule rehabilitation telephone follow-up for questions
Maintenance programs and follow-up	Out-of-pocket expenses, logistic issues, and general inability to continue face-to-face programming has limited participation in long-term efforts to maintain physical activity and risk factor modification programming	Rehabilitation checkup day: Reserve one day every 2-3 months (depending on volume) for checkups; all visits on that day are scheduled for graduates to return for monitored exercise and risk factor update; current patients are given a day "off" to exercise at home and report doing so

Guideline 2.2

To help organize and standardize service delivery, each program should develop the following:
- A menu of rehabilitative services, including exercise, risk intervention, and education and counseling
- Standards of care that outline how each service will be delivered and evaluated

Menu of Rehabilitation Services

Program staff should develop a list of available exercise, risk factor intervention, and education and counseling services. Figure 2.3 illustrates an example of a service menu. The purpose of such a menu is to aid in prioritization of care delivery. Based on each patient's assessed needs, appropriate services can be selected from the menu and corresponding care delivered following a protocol or action plan (a standard of care).

Standards of Patient Care

Standards of patient care are internally developed protocols outlining how each item on the rehabilitation service menu will be addressed in CR practice. These prewritten treatment plans specify the services to be delivered and the expected results (outcomes). For example, a standard of care should be available outlining how each risk factor will be monitored and managed. Each standard needs to be based on current scientific

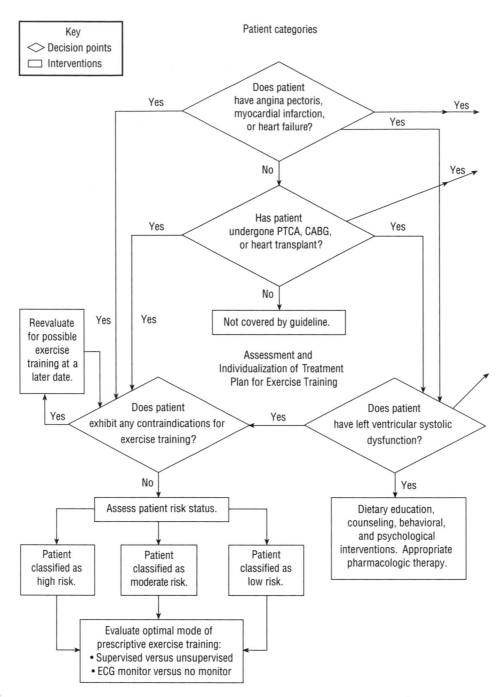

Figure 2.2 Clinical practice guideline: Decision tree for CR services. PTCA = percutaneous transluminal coronary angioplasty.

Wenger NK, Froelicher ES, Smith LK, and expert panel. *Cardiac Rehabilitation*. Clinical Practice Guideline No. 17. Rockville, MD: U.S. Department of Health and Human Services, Public Health Agency for Health Care Policy and Research for the National Heart, Lung, and Blood Institute. AHCPR Publication No. 96-0672 October 1995, pp. 22-23.

evidence and national guideline documents. An example of such a standard is the document cowritten by the American Heart Association (AHA) and the AACVPR, "Core Components of Cardiac Rehabilitation/Secondary Prevention Programs" (figure 2.4).[55] This document serves as a single-source, quick-start guideline for standard-of-care development. Program administrators should consider modifying such sources to reflect program-specific practices and implementing them upon recommendation from local and regional practitioners and governing bodies.

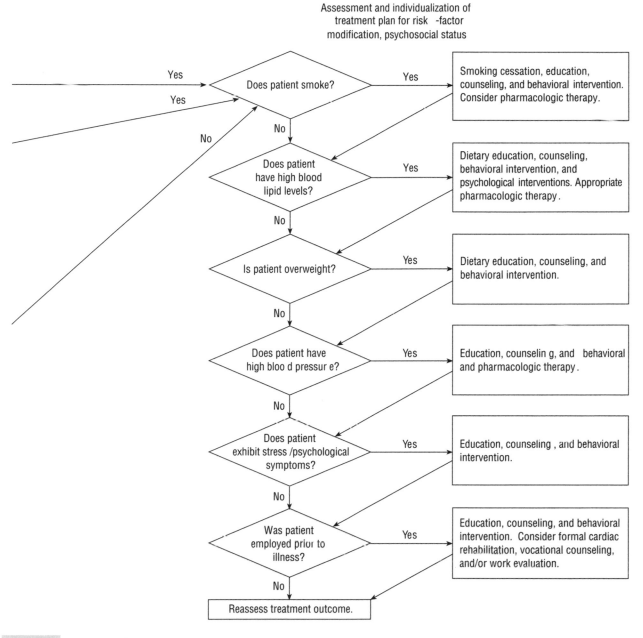

Assessment and individualization of
treatment plan for risk -factor
modification, psychosocial status

Figure 2.2 *(continued)*

Describing a menu of rehabilitative services and developing standards of patient care are very effective approaches to individualizing and prioritizing rehabilitation efforts.[573] From program admission to discharge, providing services directly or arranging for others to provide these services allows rehabilitation staff to address each patient's needs. Menus of rehabilitative services and standards of patient care help ensure quality and consistency in the management of CR and secondary prevention.

The Future of Cardiac Rehabilitation and Secondary Prevention

The rate of change of both practice and programming within health care continues to accelerate. Patients as well as providers are affected. Keeping pace is the challenge.

Exercise services	Education, counseling, and behavioral services
Emphasis on risk stratification	Emphasis on risk reduction
<ul><li>Periodic exercise checkups</li><li>Prescription or instruction for independent maintenance</li><li>Prescription or instruction for unsupervised training</li><li>Pretraining exercise orientation</li><li>Professionally supervised exercise training</li><li>Resistance/strength training</li><li>Submaximal fitness testing</li><li>Symptom-limited exercise stress testing</li><li>Stress management class</li><li>Telemetry-monitored exercise training</li><li>Telephone follow-up of home-based exercise</li><li>Transtelephonic ECG monitoring of home-based exercise</li><li>Transition program</li></ul>	<ul><li>Blood pressure monitoring and management</li><li>Complementary therapies</li><li>Diabetes education</li><li>Lipid monitoring and management</li><li>Medication teaching and compliance monitoring</li><li>Periodic risk factor checkups</li><li>Psychological referrals</li><li>Self-monitoring skills</li><li>Smoking cessation program</li><li>Support groups (patients, spouses)</li><li>Vocational counseling</li><li>Weight loss program</li></ul>

Figure 2.3 Sample menu of services: Outpatient CR.

Comoss PM. The new infrastructure for CR practice. In: NK Wenger, LK Smith, ES Froelicher, PM Comoss. *Cardiac rehabilitation: A guide to practice in the 21st century.* New York: Marcel Dekker, 1999. p. 322.

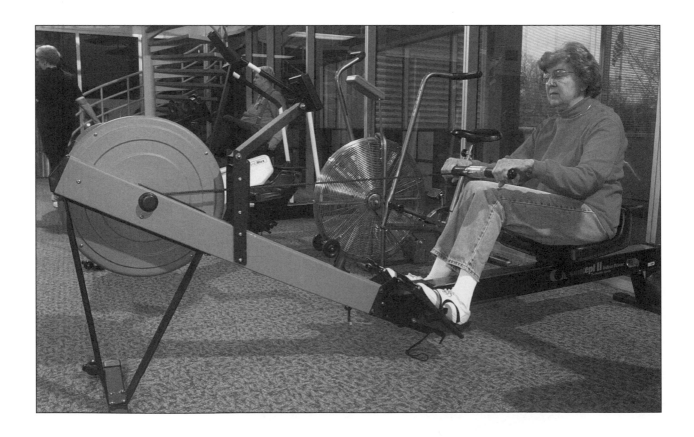

Core Components of Cardiac Rehabilitation/Secondary Prevention Programs

Patient Assessment

Evaluation
- Medical history: include cardiovascular (including peripheral vascular and cerebro-vascular) diagnoses and prior cardiovascular procedures (including assessment of left ventricular function); comorbidities; symptoms of cardiovascular disease; risk factors for atherosclerotic disease progression; and medications and medication compliance. (See below for physical activity and psychosocial assessment.)
- Physical examination: include vital signs; cardiovascular and pulmonary examination; postprocedure wound sites; and joint and neuromuscular examination. (See below for specified examination for hypertension, weight, and diabetes.)
- Testing: obtain resting ECG; assess quality of life using standard questionnaires (e.g., MOS SF-36). (See below for specified tests for exercise, lipids, and diabetes.)

Interventions
- Compose written records that reflect the patient evaluation and contain a patient care plan with detailed priorities for risk reduction and rehabilitation.
- Actively communicate this plan to the patient and the primary health care provider.

Expected Outcomes
- Development and implementation of short-term (i.e., weeks or months) and long-term (i.e., years) goals and strategies to reduce disability and subsequent cardiovascular disease risk.
- Improvement in quality of life as identified by positive changes on follow-up questionnaire.
- Generation of a written summary of patient outcomes upon completion of the program that is provided to the patient and to the primary and referring health care providers. Written summaries should identify specific areas that require further intervention and monitoring.

Nutritional Counseling

Evaluation
- Obtain estimates of total daily caloric intake and dietary content of fat, saturated fat, cholesterol, sodium, and other nutrients.
- Assess eating habits, including number of meals, snacks, frequency of dining out, and alcohol consumption.
- Assess target areas for nutrition intervention as outlined in the core components of weight, hypertension, and diabetes, as well as heart failure, kidney disease, and other comorbidities.

Interventions
- Prescribe specific dietary modifications aimed to at least attain the saturated fat and cholesterol content limits of the AHA Step II diet
- Individualize diet plan according to specific target areas as outlined in the core components of weight, hypertension, and diabetes (as outlined in this table), as well as heart failure and other comorbidities.
- Educate and counsel patient (and family members) regarding dietary goals and how to attain them.
- Incorporate behavior-change models and compliance strategies in counseling sessions.

Expected Outcomes
- Patient adherence to prescribed diet.
- Patient understanding of basic principles regarding dietary content of calories, saturated fat, cholesterol, and other nutrients.
- Plan in place to address eating-behavior problems.

Lipid Management

Evaluation
- Obtain fasting measures of total cholesterol, HDL, LDL, and triglycerides. In those with abnormal levels, as per NCEP, obtain a detailed history to determine whether diet, drug use, and/or other conditions that may affect lipid levels can be altered.
- Assess current treatment and compliance.
- Repeat lipid profiles at 4–6 weeks after hospitalization and at 2 months after initiation of or change in lipid-lowering medications.

(continued)

Figure 2.4 Core components of cardiac rehabilitation/secondary prevention programs.

Reprinted, by permission, from G.J. Balady et al., 2000, "Core components of cardiac rehabilitation/secondary prevention: A statement for healthcare professionals from the American Heart Association and the American Association of Cardiovascular and Pulmonary Rehabilitation," *Circulation* 102: 1069-1073.

(continued)

Interventions	• Provide nutritional counseling and weight management aiming for at least an AHA Step II diet in those patients with LDL ≥100 mg/dL; consider adding drug treatment in those with LDL >130 mg/dL.
	• Provide interventions to increase HDL to >35 mg/dL. These include exercise, smoking cessation, and consideration of targeted drug therapy.
	• Provide interventions to reduce triglycerides to <200 md/dL. These include nutritional counseling and weight management, exercise, alcohol moderation, and drug therapy as per NCEP.
	• Provide and/or monitor drug treatment in concert with primary health care provider.
Expected Outcomes	• Short term: continued assessment and modification of intervention until LDL <100 mg/dL.
	• Long term: LDL <100 mg/dL Secondary goals include HDL >35 mg/dL and triglycerides <200 mg/dL.

Hypertension Management

Evaluation	• Measurement of resting BP on ≥2 visits.
	• Assess current treatment and compliance.
Interventions	• If BP 130–139 mmHg systolic or 85–90 mmHg diastolic:
	- Provide lifestyle modifications including exercise, weight management, moderate sodium restriction, alcohol moderation, and smoking cessation.
	- Drug therapy in patients with heart failure, diabetes, or renal failure.
	• If BP ≥140 mmHg systolic or ≥90 mmHg diastolic:
	- Provide lifestyle modification and drug therapy.
	- Provide and/or monitor drug treatment in concert with primary health care provider.
Expected Outcomes	• Short term: Continued assessment and modification of intervention until BP <130 mmHg systolic and <85 mmHg diastolic.
	• Long term: BP <130 mmHg systolic and <85 mmHg diastolic.

Smoking Cessation

Evaluation	• Document smoking status as never smoked, former smoker, or current smoker (which, because of the high rate of relapse, includes those who have quit in the last 6 months); specify both the amount of smoking (packs per day) and duration of smoking (number of years). Assess use of cigar smoking, pipe smoking, and chewing tobacco, as well as exposure to secondhand smoke.
	• Assess for confounding psychosocial issues.
	• Determine readiness to change by asking every smoker if he/she has considered quitting in the last 6 months.
	- If no (precontemplation), firmly advise that he/she give it some thought; plan to ask again at future visits.
	- If yes (contemplation stage), proceed with interventions below.
	• Ongoing contact: update status at each visit during first 2 weeks of cessation, periodically thereafter for at least 6 months.
Interventions	• When readiness to change is confirmed, help the smoker set a quit date and select appropriate treatment strategies (preparation):
	Minimal
	• Provide individual education and counseling by program staff, supplemented by self-learning materials.
	• Encourage physician, staff, and family support.
	• Provide relapse prevention.
	Optimal
	• Provide formal smoking cessation program using group and/or individual counseling.

	• Provide and/or monitor pharmacological support as needed in concert with primary physician.
	• Offer supplemental strategies if desired (e.g., acupuncture, hypnosis).
	• Arrange follow-up by return visits or telephone contact for at least 6-12 months.
Expected Outcomes	• Short term: patient will demonstrate readiness to change by initially expressing decision to quit (contemplation) not selecting a quit date (preparation). Subsequently, patient will quit smoking and use of all tobacco products (action); adhere to pharmacotherapy, if prescribed; practice strategies as recommended; and resume cessation plan as quickly as possible when relapse occurs.
	• Long term: complete abstinence from smoking and use of all tobacco products at 12 months from quit date.

Weight Management

Evaluation	• Measure weight, height, and waist circumference. Calculate body mass index.
Interventions	• In patients with BMI >25 kg/m^2 and/or waist >40 inches in men (102 cm) and >35 inches (88 cm) in women:
	- Establish reasonable short-term and long-term weight goals individualized to patient and associated risk factors (e.g., reduce body weight by at least 10% at a rate of 1–2 lb/wk over a period of time up to 6 months).
	- Develop a combined diet, exercise, and behavioral program designed to reduce total caloric intake, maintain appropriate intake of nutrients and fiber, and increase energy expenditure.
	- Aim for an energy deficit of 500–1000 kcal/d.
Expected Outcomes	• Short term: Continued assessment and modification of interventions until progressive weight loss is achieved. Provide referral to specialized, validated nutrition weight loss programs if weight goals are not achieved.
	• Long term: adherence to diet and exercise program aimed toward attainment of established weight goal.

Diabetes Management

Evaluation	• Identify patients with diabetes by initial history. Note medication type, dose, and regimen; type and frequency of glucose monitoring; and history of hypoglycemic reactions.
	• Obtain fasting plasma glucose measurement in all patients and HbA1c in patients with diabetes to monitor therapy.
Interventions	• Develop a regimen of dietary adherence and weight control that includes exercise, oral hypoglycemic agents, insulin therapy, and optimal control of other risk factors. Drug therapy should be provided and/or monitored in concert with primary health care provider.
	• Monitor glucose levels before and/or after exercise sessions; instruct patient regarding identification and treatment of postexercise hypoglycemia. Limit or prohibit exercise if blood glucose ≥300 mg/dL.
	• Refer patients without known diabetes whose fasting glucose is >110 mg/dL to their primary health care provider for further evaluation and treatment.
Expected Outcome	• Normalization of fasting plasma glucose (80–110 mg/dL or HbA1c <7.0), minimization of diabetic complications, and control of associated obesity, hypertension (BP <130/85 mmHg), and hyperlipidemia.

Psychosocial Management

Evaluation	• Using interview and/or standardized measurement tools, identify psychological distress as indicated by clinically significant levels of depression, anxiety, and anger or hostility; social isolation; sexual dysfunction/maladjustment; and substance abuse (alcohol or other psychotropics).
Interventions	• Offer individual and/or small group education and counseling regarding adjustment to CHD, stress management, and health-related lifestyle change. When possible, include family members and significant others in such sessions.

(continued)

- Develop supportive rehabilitation environment and community resources to enhance patient's and family's level of social support.

- Teach and support self-help strategies.

- In concert with primary health care provider, refer patients experiencing clinically significant psychological distress to appropriate mental health specialists for further evaluation and treatment.

Expected Outcomes
- Evidence of emotional well-being indicated by the absence of clinically significant psychological distress, social isolation, or drug dependency.

- Demonstration of self-responsibility for health-related behavior change; relaxation and other stress management skills; ability to obtain effective social support; compliance with use of psychotropic medication, if prescribed; and reduction or elimination of alcohol, tobacco, caffeine, or other nonprescription psychoactive drugs.

- Develop a plan for ongoing management if important psychosocial issues are present.

Physical Activity Counseling

Evaluation
- Assess current physical activity level and determine domestic, occupational, and recreational needs.

- Question activities relevant to age, gender, and daily life, including driving, sexual activity, and social support in making positive changes.

Interventions
- Provide advice, support, and counseling about physical activity needs on initial evaluation and in follow-up. Target exercise program to meet individual needs (see "Exercise Training": section of table). Provide educational materials as part of counseling efforts. Consider simulated work testing for patients with heavy labor jobs.

- Set goals to increase physical activity that include 30 minutes per day of moderate physical activity on 5 days per week. Explore daily schedules to suggest how to incorporate increased activity into usual routine (e.g., parking farther away from entrances, walking up 2 or more flights of stairs, walking for 15 minutes during lunch break).

- Advise low-impact aerobic activity to minimize risk of injury. Recommend gradual increases in intensity over weeks.

Expected Outcomes
- Increased participation in domestic, occupational, and recreational activities.

- Improved psychosocial well-being, reduction in stress, facilitation of functional independence, prevention of disability, and enhancement of opportunities for independent self-care to achieve recommended goals.

Exercise Training

Evaluation
- Obtain an exercise test (or other standard measure of exercise capacity) before participation which is repeated as changes in clinical condition warrant. Test should include assessment of heart rate and rhythm, signs, symptoms, ST-segment changes, and exercise capacity.

Interventions
- Develop a documented individualized exercise prescription for aerobic and resistance training that is based on evaluation finding, risk stratification, patient and program goals, and resources. Exercise prescription should specify frequency (F), intensity (I), duration (D), and modalities (M).
  - For aerobic exercise: F = 3–5d/wk; I = 50%–80% of exercise capacity; D = 30–60 min; and M = walking, treadmill, cycling, rowing, stair climbing, arm ergometry, and others.
  - For resistance exercise: F = 2–3d/wk; I = 8–15 repetitions maximum for each muscle group (where repetition maximum is maximum number of times a load can be lifted before fatigue); D = 1–3 sets of 8–10 different upper- and lower-body exercises (20–30 min); and M = elastic bands, cuff/hand weights, dumbbells, free weights, wall pulleys, or weight machines.

- Include warm-up, cool-down, and flexibility exercises in each exercise session. Provide updates to the exercise prescription routinely and when patient condition warrants.

Structured outpatient or home-based programs are appropriate and may include ECG monitoring as deemed necessary. Regardless of program site, supplement the formal exercise regimen with at-home activity guidelines as outlined in the "Physical Activity Section" of this table. Caloric expenditure of at least 1000 kcal/wk should be a specific exercise program objective.

Expected Outcomes
- As a component of an overall program of cardiac rehabilitation/secondary prevention, exercise will assist in lowering cardiovascular risk and improve overall outcomes. Improved functional capacity through enhanced muscular endurance and strength, flexibility, and weight management will improve symptoms and physiological responses to physical challenges and should assist in the modification of various unhealthy behavior and psychosocial characteristics.
- Patient understanding of safety issues during exercise.

ECG indicates electrocardiogram; MOS SF-36, Medical Outcomes Study Short Form 36; AHA, American Heart Association; HDL, high-density lipoprotein; LDL, low-density lipoprotein; NCEP, National Cholesterol Education Program; BP, blood pressure; HbA1c, major fraction of glycosylated hemoglobin; and CHD, coronary heart disease. This statement was also published in the September/October 2000 issue of the Journal of Cardiopulmonary Rehabilitation (*Circulation*, 2000;102:1069-1073.)

Patient Options

Statistics document that only 11-38% of patients needing CR services receive them.[604] Results from another nationally conducted survey conclude that the vast majority of individuals with cardiovascular disease do not receive CR services.[558] These findings most likely reflect issues related to

- logistics, such as when a patient has returned to work and is unable to attend scheduled sessions, there is no local program, the distance to the facility is too great, or there is a lack of transportation;

- lack of physician referral or positive reinforcement;

- lack of a personal support system, (i.e., absence or lack of support from spouse, family, or significant others);

- inadequate financial resources, such as a lack of adequate insurance or an inability or unwillingness to pay for the program out of pocket; and

- a patient's personal preference not to exercise or participate in risk intervention and education and counseling programs.

The limited number of alternatives to traditional cardiac services often leaves many patients without suitable options. Even for those receiving traditional services, the duration of therapy (i.e., the number of sessions) and the therapeutic emphasis (e.g., diet, exercise, smoking cessation, psychosocial interventions) are often dictated by financial constraint—that is, patient resources and reimbursement policies—more than by patient need.

Formats other than the traditional hour-long sessions occurring three times a week have been developed to provide secondary prevention services, and these have proven to be effective. They include

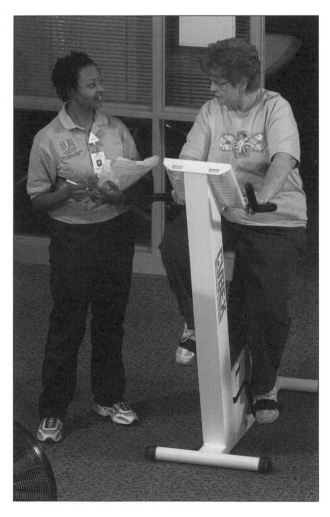

- nurse case-management systems using telephone calls as the primary intervention modality,[141,391]

- interventions in which intensive diet therapy and psychosocial counseling and support are heavily emphasized,[237,420]

- home exercise programs in which exercise is monitored through transtelephonic transmission of electrocardiograms,[5] and

- computer-guided risk-factor programs that supplement or serve as an alternative for facility-based secondary prevention efforts.[289]

In addition, Internet-based case-management systems are being developed that provide education, professional assistance with lifestyle modification, graphical feedback, and social support.[128,265,289] The use of telecommunications and the Internet also facilitates the development of online medical records and outcome assessments (with appropriate security to protect patient confidentiality) that primary care providers, CR professionals, physicians, and patients can access. These systems offer tremendous opportunities to enhance communication and facilitate a coordinated treatment plan. Internet-based services also integrate well with Web-enabled blood pressure monitors, digital scales, glucose monitors, and other devices that provide ongoing feedback to both patient and practitioner about risk-factor control in the home environment.[80]

Unfortunately, these interventions are generally not reimbursable under current guidelines from the Centers for Medicare/Medicaid Services (CMS), formerly the Health Care Financing Administration (HCFA). CMS guidelines for CR services focus on payment for supervised exercise conducted under physician supervision in hospital-based programs or physician-directed clinics. The availability of the alternative intervention modalities noted earlier, along with the need to provide patient-focused services in the most cost-effective manner possible, may eventually lead to a reassessment of reimbursement strategies. Early evidence of this is illustrated by private payers' starting to reimburse for cardiac disease management services and by the CMS demonstration projects in which patients are being reimbursed for Ornish-type interventions.[128, 264] Reimbursement for both traditional and alternative intervention modes would finally give clinicians the flexibility they need to provide services that are individually tailored to

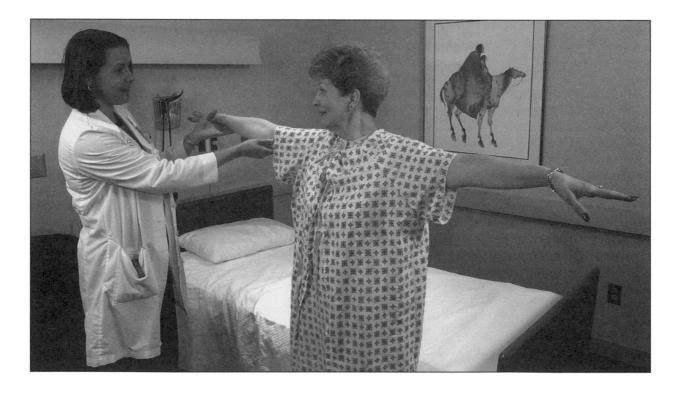

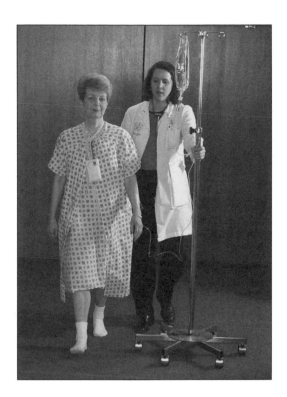

To serve the needs of the majority of patients with cardiovascular disease, more research is needed to assess the cost-effectiveness of alternative methods of providing secondary prevention services and to determine the optimum mix of services, such as supervised exercise, home-based risk-factor case management, and community support for various patient needs. Based on this research, policy makers, clinical researchers, and health care providers must collaborate in the development of clinical practice guidelines and financial policies that are flexible and optimize utilization of, and reimbursement for, the most cost-effective integration of services.

Emerging Provider Opportunities

As a result of the emerging pathways of service delivery previously described, it is expected that future CR and secondary prevention program models will provide a number of opportunities for CR practitioners to break out of the program "box." Imaginative new models are beginning to emerge that redefine the continuum of care, perhaps beyond the linear concept of a chronological sequence. Figure 2.5 suggests one such innovative structure.

specific patient needs and the opportunity to provide services to people who are unwilling or unable to participate in onsite programs.

Internal Impact

The model depicted in figure 2.4 is patient centered and involves active collaboration and interaction

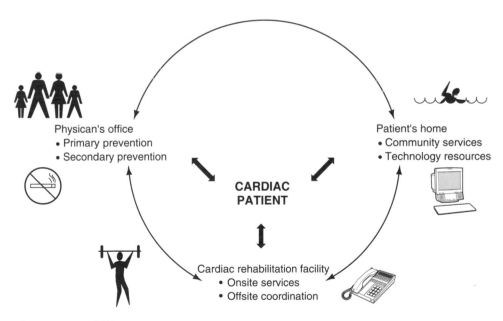

Figure 2.5 A future vision of CR.

among the key parties involved in the provision of CR: the patient, the physician, and the CR staff. Together, these individuals identify the secondary prevention services that are needed and those to be provided, including the specifics of the patient-individualized process. Some services will continue at the rehabilitation facility if the patient is willing and able to utilize them. Other services may not require frequent face-to-face interaction, and still others may take place in the home using technical support ranging from simple telephone monitoring to sophisticated interactive computer programs. Thus, the primary function of the rehabilitation program will be the coordination of services and delivery options that will individualize each program to a patient's specific needs and preferences while optimizing outcomes.

External Expansion

Newer CR and secondary prevention models may not only increase the number of cardiac patients who will have access to services but may also position practitioners to extend these services to additional populations. Newly developed standardized risk-reduction services can be applied directly onsite or through emerging technologies to populations to whom the more traditional models were previously inaccessible. In essence, such alternative models may provide an opportunity for CR to position itself securely within the larger continuum of cardiovascular care. Figure 2.6 describes how CR-based secondary prevention services might be extended to primary prevention as well as long-term disease management.

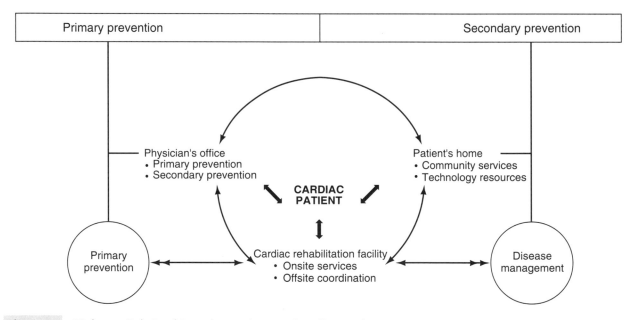

Figure 2.6   CR future: Relationship to the continuum of cardiovascular care.

Summary

To prepare for an exciting future, clinicians must optimize what is taking place today to ensure that programs meet national expectations, deliver quality services efficiently, and demonstrate the effectiveness of secondary prevention services through sound outcome measurement. This must also include the evaluation of potential opportunities for program expansion and the consideration of alternative programming. The result of today's work will be the acceptance of secondary prevention services not only for the management of cardiovascular disease but also as an integral part of tomorrow's wider continuum of care for a variety of diseases.

3

The Emergence of Nutrition and Plant-Based Diets in the Treatment and Prevention of Cardiovascular Disease

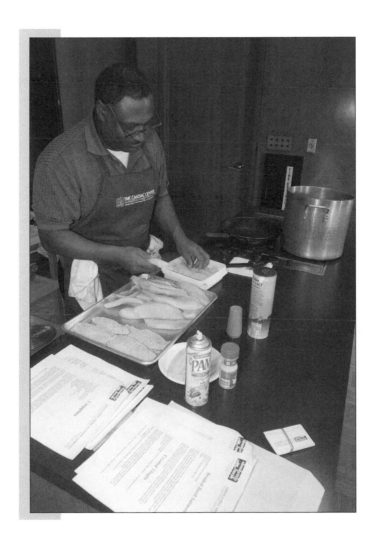

The impact of nutrition on CVD and cardiovascular health includes effects on serum lipids, blood pressure, body mass, blood glucose, antioxidant status, homocysteine, endothelial function, and fibrinolytic activity. A long and growing list of dietary components, with varying levels of supportive evidence, is thought to affect these CVD risk factors. Historically, a shorter list of these dietary components would have included some specific fatty acids, fiber, cholesterol, sodium, and antioxidants such as vitamins E and C. [296,374,384,442,508,581] A more current list, however, includes isoflavones from soybeans; allicin from garlic; plant sterols from vegetable and seed oils; specific amino acids such as arginine; B-vitamins such as folate, B, and B12; minerals such as selenium, potassium, and magnesium; and an expanded group of antioxidants such as flavonoids and carotenoids.[20,100,126,273,354,385,451,468,475,505,563] Each of these lists of specific CVD risk factors and dietary components is not intended to be exhaustive but underscores that the effect of nutrition on CVD is complex. Consequently, advising CVD patients and the general public about the practical implementation of nutrition in the treatment and prevention of heart disease can be challenging. In apparent response to this challenge, nutrition professionals are now using the term *plant-based diets* with increasing frequency as a means of unifying and simplifying much of the complexity in the area of nutrition and CVD.

OBJECTIVES

This chapter includes a discussion of

- plant-based diets and the role of phytochemicals;
- the epidemiologic and clinical evidence of the benefits of such interventions;
- the use of dietary supplements and herbs; and
- practical considerations for such interventions, including changing the paradigm from a program of avoidance to one of inclusion.

Plant-Based Diets and Phytochemicals

Simplistically and literally, the term *plant-based diet* refers to a pattern of food selections derived in greater proportion from vegetables, grains, legumes, nuts, seeds, and fruits than from meats, poultry, fish, dairy products, and eggs. This simple dichotomization of food groups is helpful in drawing several distinctions. Plant foods contain no cholesterol. Animal foods contain no fiber. With few exceptions, the saturated fat content of most plant foods is low to negligible. Furthermore, the best food sources of vitamins E and C, isoflavones, allicin, plant sterols, arginine, folate, potassium, magnesium, flavonoids, and carotenoids are all plant foods. Therefore, the overall pattern of dietary components in plant foods is consistent with what has been either established or suggested to be optimal nutrition for cardiovascular health.

The term *plant-based diet* can therefore be useful in helping to combine what is known about many separate dietary components into an overall dietary pattern. However, despite the potential usefulness of its simplicity and brevity, the term also has inherent limitations due to its lack of specificity. To avoid misuse and misinterpretation, it should be understood that promoting a plant-based diet implies several important qualifications. First, a diet with a foundation in jellybeans, french fries, and high-fructose corn syrup beverages would technically qualify as plant based but would be contrary to the intention of its use. Second, to follow a plant-based diet, a person could but would not have to be a vegetarian or vegan. With the important concept of moderation in mind, there is room for virtually all foods in a plant-based diet. Third, promoting plant-based diets does not exclude the value of non-plant-based nutrients or dietary components, such as the long-chain, highly unsaturated fatty acids found in fish oils.[246] The primary intention is that a plant-based diet has a foundation of nutrient-dense, phytochemical-rich foods that are good sources of cardioprotective fats, fiber, vitamins, minerals, and phytochemicals and provide low levels of saturated fat and cholesterol.

Several of the dietary components mentioned previously that may be protective of heart disease, such as isoflavones, allicin, plant sterols, flavonoids, and carotenoids, can be considered phytochemicals. The prefix *phyto* refers to plants, and *phytochemicals* simply means chemicals and compounds found in plant foods that are not vitamins or minerals and do not have a recommended daily allowance (RDA) or daily recommended intake (DRI) but may confer health benefits. A rapidly growing number of studies provides substantial evidence for the potential benefits of these phytochemicals with regard to CVD, CVD risk factors, or both.[273,327,385,563] Overall, however, these data are preliminary; several examples of inconsistencies exist.[9,131,216-218,327] More studies are needed to establish the benefits of the phytochemicals in specific doses, for specific populations, and in the treatment of specific CVD risk factors (e.g., serum cholesterol, blood pressure). Until these data are available, it would be practical to consider that the food sources of these potentially protective phytochemicals are typically foods that are good sources of fiber, vitamins, and minerals and are low in saturated fat, cholesterol, and sodium, such as vegetables, whole grains and cereals, legumes and beans, nuts, seeds, and fruits.

Epidemiological Evidence for Benefits of Plant-Based Diets

Four recent prospective cohort studies reported findings consistent with the hypothesis that a dietary pattern rich in plant-based foods is protective of CVD outcomes. In the Women's Health Study, some 40,000 female health professionals were followed for 5 yr, during which time researchers documented 418 CVD events. Results indicated a 32% lower relative risk of CVD among the highest versus the lowest quintile of fruit and vegetable intake.[352] In the Iowa Women's Health Study, investigators followed approximately 35,000 postmenopausal women for 9 yr, during which time 438 IHD deaths occurred. Results found that adjusted relative risk of IHD was lowest among those with the greatest whole-grain intake.[292] The third investigation, the Nurses' Health Study, followed approximately 85,000 nurses for 14 yr and documented 1,255 major coronary disease events. Results suggested that women who consumed about 5 oz of nuts per week had a 35% lower relative risk of total coronary heart disease compared to women who consumed less than 1 oz of nuts per week.[283] Lastly, among approximately 45,000 men from the Health Professionals Follow-up Study, 1,089 CHD events were documented during 8 yr of follow-up. This study noted a 30% lower relative risk of CHD for those who consumed a prudent dietary pattern, such as higher intake of vegetables, fruits, legumes, whole grains, fish, and poultry.[282] Each of these studies is consistent with increased protection from CVD with increased intakes of plant-based foods.

Clinical Trial Evidence for Benefits of Plant-Based Diets

There are only a few good examples of clinical trials that have investigated the effect of plant-based diets on CVD. Among this small set of clinical trials, several merit further discussion.

In the Dietary Approaches to Stop Hypertension (DASH) study, investigators attempted to lower participants' blood pressure through dietary interventions that focused on eating patterns rather than on isolated nutrients.[45] In this study, 459 adults with systolic blood pressures of less than 160 mmHg and diastolic blood pressures of 80-95 mmHg were provided with all of their meals for 11 weeks and were randomly assigned to one of three different eating patterns: (1) control, (2) high fruit and vegetable intake, and (3) a combination of high fruit and vegetable intake and low-fat dairy. Notably, the combination diet also contained less beef, pork, and ham and more grains and vegetables than the other diets. By design, sodium and alcohol intake and weight were kept similar in all three treatment groups. Relative to the control diet, the combination diet significantly reduced systolic and diastolic blood pressure by 5.5 and 3.0 mmHg, respectively. Among the subset of 133 participants with hypertension, the combination diet reduced systolic and diastolic blood pressure by 11.4 and 5.5 mmHg, respectively, more than the control diet (p <.001). The high fruit and vegetable diet had intermediate effects. Ancillary analyses of serum lipid changes revealed that the combination diet also reduced low-density-lipoprotein cholesterol (LDL-C) by 11 mg/dL, or 9%, relative to the control diet.[412]

The Lyon Heart Study evaluated post–myocardial infarction (MI) patients consuming a 33% fat "Mediterranean" diet (n = 302) compared to a "typical" diet (n = 302) and evaluated rates of coronary artery disease (CAD) morbidity and mortality.[144] Some of the primary differences between the two diets were more bread, fruits, vegetables, legumes, oleic acid, linolenic acid, and vitamin C and less meat, butter, cream, deli food, saturated fat, and cholesterol for the Mediterranean versus the typical diet group. The Mediterranean diet group exhibited a 67% risk reduction in combined primary and secondary CVD outcomes compared to the typical diet group after 46 months.

Singh and colleagues randomized 406 patients with definite or possible acute MI and unstable angina to diet group A or B.[513] Both groups were advised to follow a reduced-fat diet, but group A was additionally advised to eat more vegetables, nuts, grain products, fruits, and fish. After 1 yr, the researchers reported a significant reduction in events for group A for both cardiac events and total mortality.

A unifying theme in the interpretation of results from all three of the studies just cited was that there was no single nutrient or dietary component to which the outcome benefits could be attributed. Rather, it was assumed that multiple dietary differences existed between the study groups, working additively or synergistically on potentially multiple steps along the etiological path of CAD.

Two other studies that used nutrient-dense, phytochemical-rich plant-based diets were the Pritikin program and the Lifestyle Heart Trial.[65,421] In both these studies, however, the impact of the diet component alone cannot be separated from the potential confounding effects of other lifestyle changes that took place simultaneously, including increased physical activity and stress reduction. Overall, the results of these clinical trials are consistent with a beneficial effect of plant-based diet patterns on CAD risk and outcomes.

Paradigm Shift: From Avoidance to Inclusion

The growing interest in plant-based diets and phytochemicals has led to an important paradigm shift in the field of nutrition and cardiovascular disease. That shift involves movement away from the traditional approach of recommending particular foods to avoid toward a more practical approach of recommending foods to include. A historical review of dietary recommendations made by a number of national organizations (National Cholesterol Education Program [NCEP], American Diabetes Association, National High Blood Pressure Education Program, National Research Council, American Heart Association [AHA]) reveals a consistent pattern of recommendations for specific dietary components to limit, restrict, or avoid.[28,115,403,406] At the top of these lists are saturated fat, cholesterol, and sodium, and for each of these, long lists of clinical trials and epidemiological studies support the recommendations. The science behind these recommendations is sound, and the intentions are appropriately targeted toward controlling and improving proven risk factors for CVD such as plasma lipids and blood pressure. In practice, however, this approach has two major limitations. First, patients may know the dietary components they should be avoiding but do not realize that some of the foods they consume are high in these very components. Second, with the primary emphasis given to what patients should avoid, it has not been particularly clear what it is that they should include. Therefore, one of the benefits of the growing interest in plant-based diets and phytochemicals has been a shift in the emphasis of nutrition recommendations to a new focus on what to include. Perhaps the best example of this shift is evident in a comparison of the AHA's Revised Dietary Guidelines 2000 with previous versions of the AHA Dietary Guidelines (figure 3.1).

Dietary Supplements and Herbal Medicines

A large proportion of the U.S. population reports taking multivitamins or dietary supplements regularly, and more than a third take either of the antioxidant vitamins, E and C.[165,194] This high prevalence of usage reflects the mass circulation of evidence from large epidemiological studies suggesting that vitamins can prevent CVD and decrease mortality.[153] More and more people are also using various nutritional supplements such as fish oil, garlic, and L-carnitine, to name a few, that are not classified in terms of any recommended daily allowances and have yet to undergo rigorous studies regarding their effectiveness and toxicity levels. Program staff will face an increasing number of questions from patients and the public regarding this significant trend. In this chapter we summarize some of the important current clinical evidence.

People can obtain nutrients and other dietary components from both foods and dietary supplements. However, if food has already provided adequate and optimal levels of intake, then additional intake from dietary supplements is unlikely to confer additional health benefits. In the case of inadequate or suboptimal intake from foods, however, supplements have the potential to offer health benefits. Thus, it is reasonable to consider that dietary supplements can be used appropriately to augment (not replace) a healthy diet. Whether a specific dietary supplement will confer actual health benefits for a particular person remains a challenging unanswered question.

Currently, the dietary supplement industry is a multibillion-dollar business. There exist not only hundreds of products and product combinations, but also multiple manufacturers and brands for many of these products. In order to recommend these to patients, or to respond to patient-initiated questions about products, program staff would optimally know the evidence establishing the presence or absence of beneficial effects. However, in most cases data regarding efficacy and safety for patients with cardiovascular disease who may also be taking various cardiovascular medications are simply not available. Even within the subset of dietary supplements for which decades of research findings are available, it is rare to find a particular dietary supplement for which an established consensus exists as to the appropriate dose a patient should take to improve a specific CVD risk factor or outcome.

It may be of practical value to be familiar with a set of dietary supplements that have been shown to elicit a range of responses from beneficial to harm-

2000 Revised AHA Dietary Guidelines for Healthy American Adults[331]

1. Healthy Eating Pattern

   Consume 5 or more servings of vegetables and fruits per day.

   Consume 6 or more servings of a variety of grain products, including whole grains, per day.

2. Healthy Body Weight

   Match energy intake and needs.

   Be physically active at level that meets or exceeds intake.

3. Desirable Lipid Profile

   Limit sources of saturated and trans fat and cholesterol.

   Substitute grains, fish, vegetables, legumes, and nuts.

4. Normal Blood Pressure

   Limit salt/sodium chloride and alcohol.

   Maintain healthy weight.

   Maintain dietary pattern that emphasizes vegetables, fruits, and low-fat dairy.

1988, 1993 AHA Dietary Guidelines and Rationale for Healthy American Adults [33,115]

1. Limit total fat to 30% of energy.
2. Limit saturated fat to 8-10% of energy (step 1), or 7% of energy (step 2).
3. Polyunsaturated fat should not exceed 10%.
4. Limit cholesterol to 300 mg/d (step 1), or 200 mg/d (step 2).
5. Carbohydrate intake should be >50% of energy, with emphasis on complex carbohydrate (CHO).
6. Limit sodium to 3 g/d.
7. Alcohol intake should not exceed 2 drinks per day.
8. Maintain recommended body weight.
9. Consume a wide variety of foods.

Figure 3.1 Comparison of AHA dietary guidelines.

ful. The following examples are offered for the sake of helping practitioners communicate to patients that many factors are important in establishing the potential benefits of supplements, and each must be considered on an individual basis.

Plant Sterols

The plant sterol type of supplement is an example of a plant component that has been shown to effectively lower cholesterol levels and is now being marketed in various commercial forms, such as margarines.[385] The potential benefits of this phytochemical must be considered in the context of how it is taken. For example, simply adding margarine to your diet will increase energy intake, lead to weight gain, and eventually cause more problems than benefits. In several studies, doses ranging from 1.5 to 3.3 g/d of sterol intake incorporated into study margarines lowered LDL-C by an average of 8 to 14% relative to control

margarines that did not contain plant sterols.[254,385,608] On the other hand, if these margarines replace an equivalent amount of butter, there is a good likelihood of a net benefit. The potential benefit, therefore, depends on the context.

Antioxidants

Epidemiological studies have provided evidence of an inverse relation between antioxidant intake and CAD. The hypothesis is that reduced peroxidation of low-density lipoprotein (LDL) modifies atherosclerosis development, and its use should result in more-favorable clinical outcomes. Several other important mechanisms may account for antioxidants' prevention of the clinical manifestations of CAD. For example, there is evidence that plaque stability, vasomotor function, and thrombotic tendency are subject to modification by specific antioxidants. Specifically, cellular antioxidants inhibit monocyte adhesion, protect against the cytotoxic effects of oxidized LDL, and inhibit platelet activation. Furthermore, cellular antioxidants protect against the endothelial dysfunction associated with atherosclerosis by preserving endothelium-derived nitric oxide activity.

Vitamin E

Vitamin E is an antioxidant that has been studied extensively for over 20 yr, and the potential of vitamin E supplements to increase antioxidant status is very promising. However, several recently completed randomized clinical trials examining the effects of vitamin E supplementation on cardiovascular mortality outcomes have yielded disappointing results. The CHAOS study reported significant reductions in rates of cardiovascular events, but the effects were restricted to nonfatal myocardial infarction.[539] Neither the GISSI prevention trial nor the HOPE study reported any significant benefits of vitamin E supplementation on cardiovascular events.[246,634] In the ATBC study, a slightly lower CAD death rate was reported for the vitamin E group, but the effect was modest and was offset by higher mortality rates from cancer and hemorrhagic stroke.[20] Adding confusion to this disappointing set of results were substantial differences between the four trials that included differences in study populations, such as primary versus secondary prevention, dose of vitamin E (75-800 IU/d), and type of vitamin E (synthetic or natural). Therefore, although important research questions remain to be addressed and scientific interest in plausible beneficial effects of vitamin E intake continues to exist, the results of these four clinical trials have substantially dampened the claims made previously for vitamin E supplementation.

Beta-Carotene

Twenty years of scientific investigation have pointed to the antioxidant properties of the compound beta-carotene and its strong association with lower rates of heart disease as well as some cancers. However, randomized clinical trials with beta-carotene supplements have reported no benefits and some adverse results.[20,269,420] No one has questioned or challenged the safety and potential benefit of foods rich in beta-carotene, but supplements with isolated beta-carotene do not appear to provide additional risk reduction and could even be harmful for individuals with a specific profile. Subgroup analyses of the trials that reported excess lung cancer among those taking beta-carotene versus placebo suggested that the cancer occurred in those who were heavy smokers (≥20 vs. <20 cigarettes/d) and consumed larger amounts of alcohol (≥11 g ethanol/d [~1 drink/d]

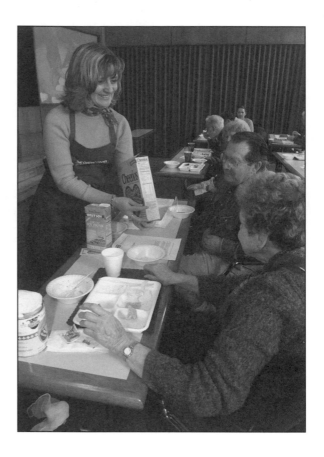

compared with lower intakes). Therefore, some have suggested that long-term, heavy smokers, and particularly those heavy smokers who consume larger amounts of alcohol, should be advised not to ingest pharmacologic doses of beta-carotene.[11,451]

B Vitamins (B6, B12, Folate)

Studies conducted more than 40 years ago first suggested that extremely high levels of homocysteine in the blood led to coronary artery disease. Evidence from large-population studies indicates that in many patients with elevated homocysteine levels, B vitamin deficiencies occur and suggest that B vitamin supplementation could protect against heart disease.[164] The Nurse's Health Study followed the dietary intake of more than 80,000 women over 14 yr. Results from this study show that women consuming the most folate and B6 had a 45% decrease in CAD after 14 yr of follow-up.[475] This protective effect was even more dramatic for those women drinking at least one alcoholic drink daily (~70% reduction in CAD). B6 deficiencies are found in 20% of patients with atherosclerosis, and the estimate that 88% of the U.S. population consumes less than 400 µg/d of folate points to the potential therapeutic role of folate, B6, and B12 supplementation.[368]

A meta-analysis of 12 clinical trials found that daily supplementation with 0.5-5.0 mg folate decreased blood homocysteine levels 25% and 0.5 mg B12 by an additional 7%.[278] The RDA for folic acid has been increased to at least 600 µg/d for pregnant women, and some medical professionals urge co-supplementation of folic acid with at least 1 mg of B12.[54] However, there are few data suggesting that a reduction in homocysteine will result in improved cardiovascular outcomes. A combination of folic acid (1 mg), vitamin B (400 µg), and pyridoxine (10 mg) in patients following PTCA decreased the rate of restenosis and the need for revascularization of the target lesion.[494a]

Homocysteine is now recognized as an important CVD risk factor, and increased folate intake can lower homocysteine levels. There are at least three distinct sources of dietary folate: multivitamins or B-complex vitamins; fortified foods (e.g., many breakfast cereals); and natural foods, including beans and leafy greens. Among these, it is evident that not all sources are created equal. The folate in vitamin supplements and fortified foods is found in a monoglutamated form (folic acid), whereas that found in beans and greens is a polyglutamated form (folate). The monoglutamated form appears to be more bioavailable than the polyglutamated form, and so a patient may improve folate status and subsequently lower homocysteine more easily with supplements and fortified foods than with other food sources.[100,468]

Fish Oils

Evidence to support benefits from the daily intake of fish is more compelling than that for garlic or vitamin E.[592] Fish contains a class of polyunsaturated fatty acids known as n-3 fatty acids and these have been studied for their ability to lower LDL and triglycerides, raise high-density lipoprotein (HDL), prevent cardiac arrest and arrhythmias, and retard the growth of the plaques leading to atherosclerosis. The Chicago Western Electric Study found a reduction in death from CHD with increased fish consumption, whereas the Physicians' Health Study found no such association.[138a,246a] The GISSI-Prevenzione trial indicated that the benefit of the 875-mg fish oil capsules was reducing mortality, not reducing nonfatal MI.[226]

This conflicting data have led the AHA to refrain from recommending fish intake beyond 1-2 servings per day for the prevention of CAD. There are also unresolved issues related to pesticide and mercury content as well as the cost of fish oil capsules as compared to that of dietary consumption of fish.

These issues will require large-scale clinical trials for clarification. It is safe to say, however, that fish oil via diet or nutritional supplementation is appropriate for inclusion in secondary prevention programs for patients with CHD.

Selenium and Zinc

Some have suggested that the minerals selenium and zinc, for which RDA values exist, possess antioxidant or cell-protective activity. Selenium is an antioxidant that some believe plays a role in protection against cancer and heart disease.[544] Another demonstrated that patients suffering from AMI exhibit lower levels of selenium than the controls.[87] The actual value of selenium supplementation to achieve antioxidant activity remains unclear.

Zinc is important in cell growth and healing and is generally included in multivitamin preparations, and some clinical trials of multivitamin preparations are currently in progress.[271] Currently little evidence suggests that zinc provides any long-term protection from cell death.

The dietary supplements briefly described here were selected with the intent of providing specific examples of the range of potential effects that have been observed; many other specific dietary supplements might also warrant discussion. Gathering the necessary evidence to distinguish the beneficial from the benign or even harmful dietary supplements is a slow process that requires addressing several challenges, including the following:

- Establishing the appropriate doses
- Establishing the appropriate sources (e.g., natural vs. synthetic vitamin E)
- Limited standardization and regulation of commercial products
- Effects on overall health versus specific disease or health outcomes
- Potentially different reactions from different population subgroups
- Interactions of dietary supplements with one another and with medications

Until this evidence is available, the appropriate approach to dietary supplements remains a simple message: Supplements can potentially augment but should not be used to replace a healthy diet.

Herbal Medicines

Herbal medicines are currently of intense interest to the public. This reflects, in part, the erroneous assumption many people make that because they are "natural," herbal medicines are intrinsically benign. In fact, the amount of active ingredients in allegedly comparable preparations often differs vastly. "Medicine is medicine," points out Marcia Angell, former editor of the *New England Journal of Medicine,* and the same rules that apply to demonstration of efficacy and safety for other medications should apply to these substances as well.[39] For an outstanding source on herbal medicines, we recommend *The Complete German Commission E Monographs.*[86]

Garlic

Garlic supplements contain the active ingredient *allium,* which in at least one meta-analysis was shown to decrease total cholesterol by 9% with one-half to one clove/d (1 clove = 900 mg).[598] However, the majority of garlic studies, small in size and inconsistent in garlic capsule standardization, suggest only modest, if any, benefits with supplemental intake.[216,290,345,346,506,599] The most recent meta-analysis confirms that though garlic is superior to placebo in reducing total cholesterol levels, the size of the effect is modest, and the robustness of the effect is debatable.[540] A recent study further suggests that garlic therapy has no impact on HDL subclasses, lipoprotein (a) (Lp(a)), apolipoprotein B, postprandial triglycerides, or LDL subclass distribution.[546] The use of garlic for hypercholesterolemia is therefore of questionable value, particularly when compared to the robust effect of statins or even the more moderate reductions seen with psyllium[36] or Chinese red-yeast-rice supplement.[266]

Ginkgo Biloba

Ginkgo biloba has proven efficacy in the treatment of memory deficit and other manifestations of dementia, but its usefulness in the treatment of cardiovascular disorders is less clear. A recent meta-analysis that looked at its use for the treatment of claudication suggests that ginkgo biloba extract is superior to placebo in the symptomatic treatment of intermittent claudication.[441] However, the size of the overall treatment effect is modest and of uncertain clinical relevance.

Hawthorn

The herbal hawthorn has been used for cardiovascular problems for centuries. For example, it was used in 17th-century England for the treatment of edema.[248] Today, it is commonly prescribed for hypertension, angina, palpitation, and heart failure, particularly in Germany, where processed tincture is standardized for potency. Observational studies using surrogate endpoints such as subjective symptoms and exercise tolerance (not mortality or hospital admissions)

report improvement.[277,550] A large, randomized, multicenter clinical trial is in progress. Until then, usage of this agent for heart failure therapy is not recommended.

Soy-Derived Isoflavone Phytoestrogens

The final nutrition topic in this overview is that of soy and soy-derived isoflavones. Interest in the potential health benefits of soy isoflavones for CAD and other chronic diseases has grown exponentially in the past 10 years. A 1995 meta-analysis of 38 clinical trials reported that a mean intake of 47g/d of soy protein was associated with a 13% reduction in LDL-C concentration.[37] Investigators have speculated that the hypocholesterolemic effect of the soy protein preparations used in these trials might have been largely attributable to estrogenic activities of soy isoflavones. Several investigators have now examined this possibility. Crouse reported a significant LDL-C-lowering effect of soy isoflavones among adults with LDL-C levels of 140-200 mg/dL.[131]

Ancillary analyses, however, revealed that the effect was restricted to those with baseline LDL-C concentrations above the median (mean LDL-C = 185 mg/dL). Two separate trials with monkeys reported a greater LDL-C concentration–lowering effect of isoflavone-rich soy supplements versus supplements with isoflavones mostly extracted.[42,43] In both these studies, though, the average LDL-C plus very low density lipoprotein–cholesterol (VLDL-C) concentrations of the monkeys were in the range that would be considered very high in humans (225-430 mg/dL). A fourth study reported a modest LDL-C concentration reduction from soy protein isolate isoflavones during two of four menstrual cycle phases among 13 normocholesterolemic, premenopausal women.[376] Despite these reports of statistically significant hypocholesterolemic effects, it remains unclear or unsubstantiated from these studies that isoflavones could meaningfully improve serum lipid profiles among adults with mild to moderate dyslipidemias, the specific population most likely to receive counsel to use dietary approaches for lipid management.

In contrast to these findings, at least five randomized trials, four with humans and one with cynomolgus monkeys, recently reported that neither isoflavones from soy protein nor isoflavone supplements or extracts significantly improved serum lipid profiles.[68,217,241,407,510] The inconsistencies in this research area are likely attributable in large part to the different doses and sources of isoflavones used and the different study populations examined.

At this time, the evidence is insufficient to clearly support the use of soy isoflavones—particularly in the form of supplements or extracts—for improving serum lipid profiles.

Beyond serum lipids, there is considerable interest in soy isoflavones and other aspects of cardiovascular health, including beneficial effects on vascular reactivity and systemic arterial compliance.[279,407,564] All of these areas of research require further study, but they are consistent with putative cardiovascular benefits of soy isoflavones. Many of these studies, as well as some in vitro work done with isoflavones and atherosclerotic plaque formation, are discussed in greater detail in a recent review,[563] and the potential mechanisms of action related to atherosclerosis have also been reviewed.[44]

The studies cited provide exciting preliminary evidence for the potential health benefits of soy-derived isoflavone phytoestrogens, but the sum total of evidence at this time remains insufficient to substantiate any clear health claims for improving clinical outcomes. Given the need for further research into issues of dose, interactions, contraindications, and so on, it is therefore disturbing to find that isoflavone extracts are already available to the public through some manufacturers of nutritional supplements. The estrogenic activity of these phytoestrogens has been clearly established, and the potential exists for pharmacological abuse of these dietary components when consumed in tablet or extract form in unregulated doses.[636]

It is important to distinguish between the use of isolated isoflavone extracts for the elucidation of their metabolism under the closely controlled conditions of scientific investigation, and the use of these extracts as nutritional supplements to be sold to the general public. This is one particularly clear example where food sources, as part of a plant-based diet containing a variety of foods, offer several advantages over supplemental sources. First, the long history of soy consumption in certain cultures suggests that isoflavone doses achieved from food sources are unlikely to be toxic or deleterious. Second, the food sources of isoflavones, soybeans and soy products such as tofu, tempeh, soy milk, and edamame, are also important sources of other cardioprotective dietary components such as arginine, soy protein, unsaturated fat, folate, fiber, and plant sterols.[37,126,310,475,582] Third, when these plant-based sources of high-quality protein are incorporated into the diet, they often displace other high-protein sources that can typically be animal products with relatively high saturated fat and cholesterol content. Lastly, when soybeans and soy products such as tofu and tempeh are included in the diet, they are often incorporated into the types of dishes and menus that are heart healthy even without the soy (e.g., stir-fries, soups), an important point that can easily be overlooked.

Practical Suggestions

We offer several practical tips for those trying to help patients make a transition to a more plant-based diet. The first is to consult a registered dietitian or a professional trained in the science of food and nutrition. The second is to allow the patients to transition at their own paces; some people do better with big, rapid changes, whereas others prefer smaller, slower changes. The third is to encourage patients to look for menu suggestions from the many different cultural cuisines around the world that have historically been plant based. Examples include Latin American enchiladas, tacos, and burritos that use beans, rice, tortillas, and salsas as staples; Asian vegetable- and rice-based stir-fry dishes with a variety of spices and flavorings; Asian-Indian lentil- and vegetable-based curry dishes and chutneys; Middle Eastern dishes such as hummus, tabouleh, and falafel; and salads and pastas from Mediterranean regions. A fourth suggestion, building on the third, is to keep in mind that a heart-healthy approach to eating needs to be one that can be maintained for life, and therefore it cannot simply be healthy but should also be colorful, aromatic, and flavorful.

Finally, for people trying to make alterations in their diets, additional important considerations include finding food and meal selections that fit comfortably with such practical needs as convenience, economics, and social situations. These final considerations are often a matter of being open-minded and patient with initial attempts that may be less successful than later ones. Taken together, these tips can help to maximize the enjoyment of meals, and the enjoyment of life.

Summary

A diet rich in whole grains, vegetables, nuts, seeds, and fruits and limited in animal products maximizes nutrient, fiber, and phytochemical content and minimizes saturated fat and cholesterol intakes. A broad spectrum of research provides evidence for the cardiovascular disease benefits of this plant-based dietary pattern. Supplements that provide these plant-based nutrients and phytochemicals can be useful in augmenting, not replacing, a diet of healthy food choices, but for most popular nutritional supplements the claims for health benefits remain unsubstantiated, and in a few cases there is evidence of potential harm.

4

Cardiac Rehabilitation in the Inpatient and Transitional Settings

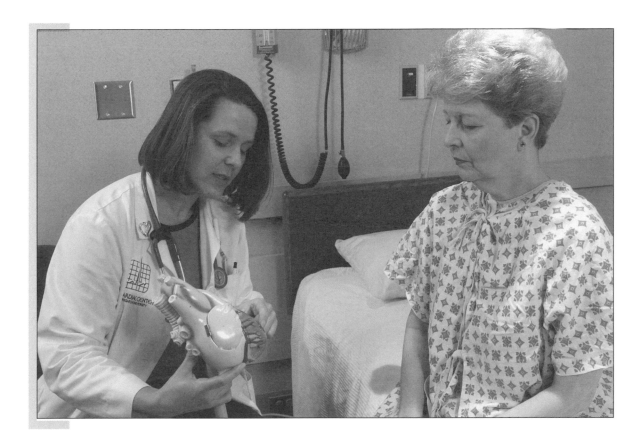

Levine and Lown in the 1950s and Wenger and colleagues in the 1960s laid the foundation for what is now recognized as a specialty practice. A number of textbooks provide extensive detail regarding the current practice of inpatient CR.[38,75,122,468,476,605] This chapter provides recommendations regarding the structure and process of inpatient and transitional CR while recognizing emerging trends in the field and continuing change in the overall health care arena.

The most obvious change to the provision of inpatient care is the decreasing length of hospitalization for most cardiac patients, resulting in a greater need for follow-up resources. Consequently, a variety of postacute or transitional settings are addressing this new challenge by providing CR services. Because the patient-oriented goal is to provide a continuum of care between inpatient and transitional settings and beyond (see figure 4.1), this chapter addresses various programming considerations.

OBJECTIVES

This chapter addresses programming considerations for

- the inpatient setting, including clinical pathways and staffing considerations;
- transitional facilities; and
- home programming.

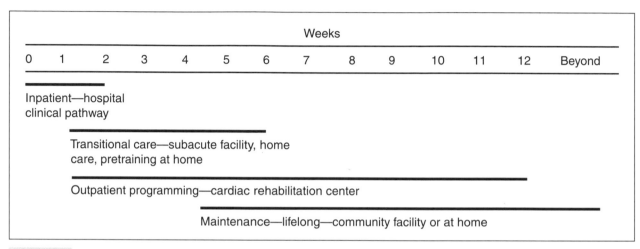

Figure 4.1 Recommended continuum of care for CR services.

Early Assessment, Mobilization, and Risk-Factor Management

Inpatient CR commences once a referral is made, either directly for each patient or via standing orders (guideline 4.1). Assessment of each patient referred for inpatient cardiac rehabilitation services involves both a thorough chart review and a brief patient interview (guideline 4.2). The purpose of the chart review is to

- verify cardiac diagnosis and current medical status (figure 4.2),
- identify cardiovascular disease risk factors to begin planning interventions (figure 4.3), and
- determine the existence of any conditions or complications that may increase the risk of recurrent cardiac event (see chapter 5, table 5.2 on page 59).

Guideline 4.1 | Cardiac Rehabilitation Within the Inpatient and Transitional Settings

Following a documented physician referral, patients hospitalized for an event or procedure associated with CAD, valvular disease, or cardiac muscle dysfunction should be provided with a program of CR consisting of

- early assessment and mobilization, identification, and information regarding cardiovascular disease risk factors and self-care; and
- a comprehensive discharge-planning session that includes a discussion of follow-up options for transitional care, home programming, and formal outpatient CR.

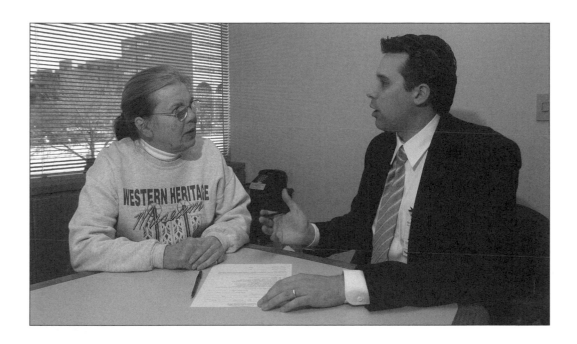

Guideline 4.2 Early Assessment

An initial patient interview will focus on assessment of the patient's readiness for activity and education.

Check all that apply.

Present illness(es):
___ post-AMI
___ post-CABG surgery
___ acute episode of heart failure
___ post–sudden death syndrome
___ unstable angina
___ post-transcatheter procedure
___ post-pacemaker/ICD implant
___ COPD
___ PAD
___ orthopedic limitations
___ stroke
___ other: _____

Present sign(s)
___ atrial arrhythmias
___ ventricular arrhythmias
___ hypotension
___ hypertension
___ other: _____
___ none

Present symptom(s)
___ typical angina
___ atypical angina
___ dyspnea/SOB
___ dizziness
___ other: _____
___ none

Past medical history:
___ previous MI
___ CABGS
___ heart failure
___ pacemaker/ICD
___ none
___ history of angina
___ transcatheter procedure
___ sudden death
___ other: _____

Pertinent social history:
Marital status:
___ single
___ married
___ divorced
___ widowed

Family status: In town
___ children   ____
___ siblings   ____
___ parents   ____
___ significant other(s)____

Employment status:
___ currently working outside of
    the home
___ currently working inside the
    home
___ not working due to illness
___ unemployed
___ retired
___ caregiver for family member

Figure 4.2 Sample assessment/interview checklist. COPD = chronic obstructive pulmonary disease; ICD = implantable cardioverter defibrillator; PAD = peripheral arterial disease; SOB = shortness of breath.

Response is required in each category.

Smoking	Dyslipidemia	Hypertension
__ Current smoker at time of hospitalization; # packs/day = _____ __ Quit at time of hospitalization __ Former smoker (not smoking >6 months prior to hospitalization) __ Never smoked __Uses other tobacco products (identify) _____	__ Told of abnormal lipid levels prior to hospitalization __ Previous lipid values or lipids drawn within 24 hr of admission Chol_____ LDL_____ HDL_____ TRIG _____ __ Unknown __ History of normal lipid levels	__ Told of high blood pressure prior to hospitalization values = _____ __ Taking medication to control blood pressure at time of hospitalization __ Stopped taking/sporadically taking medication __ Unknown __ History of normal blood pressure
Physical inactivity __ Has not exercised ≥3 times/week for ≥20 min in ≥3 months prior to hospitalization __ Reports to be a regular exerciser	**Stress/psychological concerns** __Reports history of high stress levels __ History of prior psychological/ psychiatric treatment __ No history of perceived high stress or prior problem __ Appears or acts ❑ angry ❑ depressed ❑ hostile ❑ lonely	**Overweight** Current height = _____ Current weight = _____ Body mass index (BMI) = _____ ____ Healthy weight, BMI <25 ____ Overweight, BMI 25-29 ____ Obese, BMI 30-40 ____ Very obese, BMI >40
Diabetes __ History of elevated blood sugar levels/diabetes; fasting BS = _____ __ History of normal blood sugar levels	**Alcohol/substance abuse** __Reports history of alcohol/ substance abuse at time of hospitalization __ Denies history but initial presentation suggestive __ No evidence of alcohol/substance abuse	**Other** _____ _____ _____ _____

Figure 4.3 Cardiovascular disease risk-factor checklist.

The personal interview is essential in that documentation in the chart may not provide comprehensive information as to personal, family, or social history. Management of a variety of parameters not limited to cardiovascular disease risk factors is critical to the success of the rehabilitation program, and staff must be thorough with the patient's chart as well as the personal interview. In addition, a description of symptoms in the patient's own words gives the rehabilitation professional the specific terminology to use when actively assessing symptoms (e.g., noting the patient's description of angina as "burning"). Emphasis during this initial encounter, however, should be on assessing the patient's

- readiness for activity (figure 4.4), and
- readiness to learn (figure 4.5).

The CR professional should assess whether patient goals are reasonable and realistic (guideline 4.3). Early recognition of unrealistic goals (e.g., return to work as soon as discharged or unrealistic activity expectations) will allow staff to determine the need for intervention.

Generally, activity performance progresses from supine through sitting and standing to ambulation and includes an assessment of activities of daily living (ADL), such as brushing the teeth or hair, dressing, or bathing (showering). If no adverse responses are noted (see figure 4.6), patients may proceed with ambulation to their level of tolerance. Adverse responses to activities, including sitting or standing, may require termination of the session.[219] When abnormal responses are noted with ADL or ambulation, recommendations may involve a request for assistance when performing ADL until normal responses are observed. In some instances the patient may require medical intervention before resuming any upright activity.

To begin rehabilitation
Patient is considered "stable" under the following conditions:

- No new/recurrent chest pain in past 8 hr
- CK and/or troponin levels are not rising
- No new signs of uncompensated failure (dyspnea at rest with bibasilar rales)
- No new significant, abnormal rhythm or ECG changes in past 8 hr

Progression of rehabilitation
Patient may be considered for activity progression when activity responses include the following:

- Adequate HR increase
- Adequate systolic BP rise to within 10-40 mmHg from rest
- No new rhythm or ST changes are identified on telemetry rhythm strip
- No cardiac symptoms such as palpitations, dyspnea, excessive fatigue, or chest pain are observed

Figure 4.4   Assessment parameters for inpatient/transitional CR activity program.

I. To proceed with any teaching encounter
Confirm readiness to learn.

Is the patient physically able to learn now?

___ stable physical condition
(as per activity parameters)

___ adequate energy level/alertness
(not too fatigued or overmedicated)

___ absence of brain injury with event
such as anoxia

Is the patient psychologically willing to learn now?

___ appropriate emotional state
(not too anxious or too depressed)

___ awareness of cardiac problem
(informed of diagnosis; not in denial)

II. To determine teaching sequence
Ask patient to complete a learning assessment tool (see example in figure 4.8); proceed to teach topics identified by patient as priorities.

Figure 4.5   Assessment parameters for inpatient/transitional CR education program. Note, if assessment indicates that patient is not ready to learn at this time, *do not proceed with teaching;* instead, document assessment and document that teaching was deferred due to patient's lack of readiness.

Guideline 4.3   Assessment of Patient's Goals for Cardiac Rehabilitation

The patient's personal goals for rehabilitation should be assessed to facilitate compliance and post-event adjustment. As appropriate, goals should be developed for such areas as

- physical function,
- return to work,
- risk factor reduction,
- psychological well-being, and
- family and social adjustment.

Progression of activity depends on the initial assessment as well as the daily assessment, the latter including both chart notes and the physical assessment (heart or lung sounds, rhythm, heart rate [HR], and blood pressure [BP] (guideline 4.4 and appendix A). Progression may vary from a more rapid increase in activity tolerance in the low-risk patient (uncomplicated MI or a patient without left ventricular dysfunc-tion) to a slower progression in higher-risk or more debilitated patients, such as those with congestive heart failure (CHF) or abnormal BP response (e.g., failure of systolic BP to rise with moderate activity). Table 4.1 and figure 4.7 are examples of progression models that staff may adapt as needed. (See page 63 in chapter 5 for risk-stratification models.)

Management of risk factors may begin immediately with the assessment of the patient's readiness to learn about and capacity to understand the disease process. Educating the patient as well as his or her family is an integral component in the management of risk factors.[66,135,595] However, with the reduced length of hospital stays, time constraints may allow the rehabilitation staff to address only the most pressing concerns, such as survival skills and smoking cessation (guideline 4.5). A number of successful inpatient smoking-cessation interventions have been reported in the literature,[371,389,507] and detailed strategies are described beginning on page 96 in chapter 8.

- Diastolic BP ≥110 mmHg
- Decrease in systolic BP >10 mmHg
- Significant ventricular or atrial arrhythmias
- Second- or third-degree heart block
- Signs/symptoms of exercise intolerance, including pectoris, marked dyspnea, and electrocardiogram changes suggestive of ischemia

Figure 4.6 Adverse responses to inpatient exercise leading to exercise discontinuation.

Guideline 4.4 | Physical Assessment and Mobilization

- Before activity begins, a CR staff member with appropriate skills and competencies should perform a baseline physical assessment.

- This assessment should include listening to heart and lung sounds, palpating peripheral pulses, evaluating gross musculoskeletal strength and flexibility, and assessing the patient's self-care capability.

- Results of this assessment should be documented along with baseline HR, BP, and cardiac rhythm strip data.

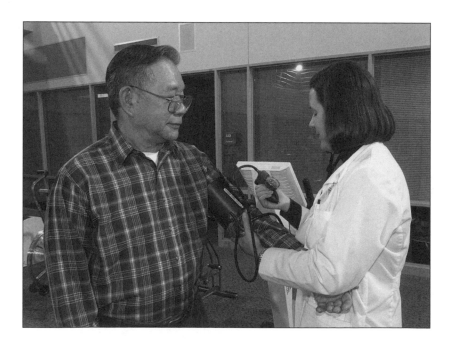

Table 4.1 Types of Activities Commonly Used in Early Cardiac Rehabilitation

Activity	Method	METs	Average HR response
Toileting	Bedpan	1-2	5-15 beats ≠ from RHR
	Commode	1-2	
	Urinal (in bed)	1-2	
	Urinal (standing	1-2	
Bathing	Bed bath	2-3	10-20 beats ≠ from RHR
	Tub bath	2-3	
	Shower	2-3	
Walking	Flat surface		5-15 beats ≠ from RHR
	2 mph	2-2.5	
	2.5 mph	2.5-2.9	
	3 mph	3-3.3	
Upper body exercise	While standing		10-20 beats ≠ from RHR
	Arms	2.6-3.1	
	Trunk	2-2.2	
Leg calisthenics		2.5-4.5	15-25 beats ≠ from RHR
Stair climbing	1 flight = 12 steps		
	Down 1 flight	2.5	10 beats ≠ from RHR
	Up 1-2 flights	4.0	10-25 beats ≠ from RHR

Data from Comoss PM. The new infrastructure for cardiac rehabilitation practice. In: *Cardiac rehabilitation: A guide to practice in the 21st century.* NK Wenger, et al. (eds.). New York: Marcel Dekker, 1999, pp. 315-326.

	MET Level	Activity
Day 1: Critical care unit (CCU)	1-2	• Bed rest until stable • Then OOB in chair • Bedside commode
Day 2: Transfer to step-down unit	2-3	• Routine CCU activities, with emphasis on self-care • Sitting warm-ups • Walking in room
Day 3	2-3	• OOB as tolerated • Standing warm-ups • Walking 5-10 min in hall 2-3 times (first time with supervision)
Day 4	3-4	• Shower with seat • Standing warm-ups • Walking 5-10 min in hall 3-4 times; walking up one flight of stairs or treadmill walking

Figure 4.7 Sample progressive activity plan for 4-day length of stay. MET = metabolic equivalent; OOB = out of bed.

Adult learning theory provides the foundation for effective in-hospital patient education (see page 88 in chapter 7). To help staff members apply the principles of adult learning, figure 4.5 outlined checkpoints to assess readiness and priorities for learning, and figure 4.8 provides a sample learning-assessment tool. A growing body of evidence supports the idea that patients can identify what is important for them to know, and teaching to those patient priorities results in the most effective education, especially in short lengths of stay.[70,96]

CR education programs are patient driven based on individually selected learning priorities, with only one exception—the universal need for safety-related information (see *Discharge Planning* on page 42 in this chapter). Handouts, pamphlets, videos, and the like can be used to supplement the patient's learning experience. Staff must choose those materials that best reinforce topics of importance, giving special attention to the reading level of selected teaching aids. Materials appropriate to a sixth- to ninth-grade reading level are recommended to help ensure that the majority of patients understand them. Figures 4.9 and 4.10 are examples of teaching plans.

Guideline 4.5 Importance of Smoking-Cessation Intervention

- The smoking status of each hospitalized cardiac patient must be identified.
- Educational and behavioral interventions should help patients through the period when they are not smoking in the hospital, assess their readiness to continue smoking cessation after discharge, and provide advice on how to maintain smoking cessation if patients are ready to do so.

Dear Patient:

Like most people with heart problems, you probably have many questions. During the next few days we want to address these concerns that are uppermost in your mind. So, to help plan our discussions, please check the three topics for which you would like more information:

___ heart machines and treatments	___ stress and your heart
___ heart structure and function	___ smoking and your heart*
___ heart arteries, normal/abnormal	___ alcohol and your heart
___ activity progression during hospital stay	___ guidelines for activities at home*
___ what to do for chest pain	___ activity/exercise precautions*
___ emergency planning for home*	___ heart catheter procedure
___ heart attack and healing	___ bypass graft surgery
___ your risk factors	___ heart balloon procedure
___ how to take your pulse	___ stent placement
___ high blood pressure	___ heart failure
___ high blood cholesterol	___ internal cardiac defibrillator
___ your medications	___ cardiac rehabilitation program*
___ fitness and health	___ treadmill exercise test
___ eating for a healthy heart	___ effects of heart problems on families
___ sexual activity and your heart	___ return-to-work questions*
___ emotional changes after heart problems	___ heart rhythms
___ development of heart disease	

Other questions you would like to have answered:

* These topics will be discussed by the cardiac rehabilitation staff before you go home.

Figure 4.8 Example of a learning-assessment tool.

Adapted from *Critical care nursing*, J.M. Clochesy, et al., p. 1413, Copyright 1993, with permission from Elsevier.

Teaching Plan

How to handle a sudden heart problem

(Emergency planning)

Purpose

To prepare patients to have a plan of action
in the event of a cardiac emergency at home
(length of lesson is 20 minutes)

When to use

1. As requested by patient and/or family member
2. For inpatients, required with discharge planning

Expected Learning Outcomes

The cardiac patient/family will

1. recall and compare his or her own presentation of heart attack to common signs and symptoms,
2. describe the proper sequence of steps to be taken should similar/suspicious symptoms occur,
3. state the importance of not wasting time waiting and wondering, and
4. choose some form of emergency identification.

Content Outline

I. Purpose

II. Symptom Recognition

   A. Ask the patient to describe his or her own symptoms with the acute event.

   B. Review common signs/symptoms of heart attack, relating to the patient's own experience.

   C. Focus on chest pain/discomfort features since recurrence of pain is a common concern (if, when, and so on).

   D. Reassure the patient that another event is unlikely, but that "what-if" planning is wise for everyone.

III. Plan of Action

   A. Instruct the patient that should he or she experience signs/symptoms of another heart attack, he or she should take the following steps:

   1. Stop whatever he or she is doing.

   2. Quickly sit or lie down.

   3. If the symptom does not begin to lessen in 1 to 2 min, then

      IF NITROGLYCERINE PRESCRIBED:

         - Place one tablet under the tongue.

         - Expect relief in 3 to 5 min.

         - If discomfort persists or worsens, place a second tablet under the tongue.

         - Wait another 5 min, repeat nitroglycerine a third time if necessary.

      OR IF NITROGLYCERIN NOT PRESCRIBED:

         - Summon help immediately, shout for anyone nearby, and have them call 911.

         - Request emergency transport to the nearest hospital emergency room.

         - Time is of the essence to minimize heart damage.

         - Do not waste time trying to get through to the physician office.

         - Do not attempt to drive yourself to the hospital.

         - Do not worry that it may be a false alarm and you will unnecessarily bother the hospital staff.

IV. Means of Identification

   A. Show patient emergency ID items (e.g., Medic Alert bracelet, Nitro pendant, mini EKG).

   B. Suggest that the patients consider purchasing one of their choice (provide information once choice is made).

V. Questions and Answers

(continued)

Figure 4.9 Example of a teaching plan.

Adapted from *Rehabilitation of the coronary patient,* 3d ed., N.K. Wenger and H.K. Hellerstein, eds., Copyright 1992, with permission from Elsevier.

(continued)

Teaching methods:

1-to-1 discussion with patient and/or family

Teaching aids:

1. AHA brochure—"Heart Attack & Stroke: Signals and Action"
2. Hospital instruction sheet on nitroglycerin (if applicable and not already given)
3. Medic Alert order form

Learning evaluation:

WHEN: Decided by instructor

____ upon completion of the session

____ the next day (inpatient)

____ at the next visit (outpatient)

WHAT: Expected outcomes

1. Ask patient to verbally respond to #I-III
2. Ask patient to make choice of #IV

Figure 4.9 *(continued)*

Purpose

To provide specific guidelines for at-home activity in the first few weeks of recovery.

When to Use

1. As requested by patient or family
2. Required with discharge

Expected Learning Outcomes

The cardiac patient or family will

1. describe those daily activities of interest that the patient can do and those that should be avoided for now;
2. outline a home walking plan to be carried out daily and state related safety guidelines;
3. discuss when specific activities may be resumed, including driving, sex, and work; and
4. identify professional resources to contact for additional questions that might arise.

Content Outline

I. Daily Capabilities

   A. Review activity progress in hospital, including performance of ADLs and ambulation.

   B. Ask patient to describe his or her usual "leisure day" routine; get description of home environment (e.g. stairs, hills).

   C. Compare and contrast current capabilities to the patient's usual routine.

   D. Advise the patient as to which activities to resume and which to avoid for now.

   E. Recommend balancing activities with rest and relaxation (including light hobbies and family social time).

II. Walking Program

   A. Give the patient a written copy of the home walking program and review instructions in detail, including how to progressively increase.

   B. Emphasize safety preparations:

      1. Review the lesson on how to handle a sudden heart problem if necessary.

      2. Verify the prescription for nitroglycerin, and discuss how the patient intends to carry it; advise using a Nitropendant or other carrier.

      3. Recommend that the patient walk with a buddy and carry a cell phone.

(continued)

Figure 4.10 Teaching plan: Guidelines for activities at home.

(continued)

4. Provide individualized guidelines for the patient to use for self-monitoring.

❐ heart rate limit = _____ bpm   ❐ RPE = _____

❐ other _____

5. Get a commitment from the patient regarding the exercise plan:

When patient will walk (time of day) _____

Where _____ With whom _____

6. Suggest that the patient keep a walking diary or journal (provide a sample) and that he or she take the journal to doctor office visits, CR visits, etc., for review and discussion.

III. Specific Concerns

  A. Advise that most patients have questions about driving, sex, and work; and offer to address any of these issues that concern this patient.

  B. Confirm what the doctor has already told the patient about these concerns.

  C. Driving for short distances, during off-hours, is usually allowed to resume as follows:

    1. Medical patients = 2 weeks

    2. Surgical patients = 4 weeks

  D. The patient can resume his or her usual pattern of sexual activity with a familiar partner when the patient has demonstrated physical capacity near 5 METs (brisk walk or walking up 2 flights of stairs); discuss with patient in light of current functional capacity (for many, the first week or two after hospitalization is appropriate, as long as the patient is rested and not stressed about sexual performance).

  E. Work is the least predictable of these concerns.

    1. Ask the patient about plans and options (i.e., issues regarding return to work, sick leave, and retirement).

    2. Urge the patient to discuss work issues further with the doctor at follow-up office visits.

IV. Follow-Up Plans and Resources

  A. Doctor office visit scheduled for _____

  B. Phone number of cardiac case manager to call with questions: _____

  C. Outpatient CR referral or alternate home-based plan:

    1. Provide contact information for the program nearest the patient's home.

    2. Urge the patient to call the program or another rehabilitation provider within the first 2 weeks he or she is at home to make an appointment and get started.

V. Questions and Answers

Figure 4.10 *(continued)*

Item	Provider of service	Responsible for follow-up	Date of appt.
Transitional care/home health			
Physician follow-up • Cardiologist • Surgeon • Primary care physician			
Outpatient cardiac rehabilitation			
CVD risk factor follow-up • Smoking-cessation program • Lipid management • Hypertension management • Stress-management/psychosocial counseling • Weight management • Diabetes management • Medication management			
Insurance/reimbursement issues • Indigent programs			
Transportation			
Additional therapies • Physical therapy • Occupational therapy			

Figure 4.11 Example of discharge instructions and intervention follow-up checklist.

Management of CVD risk factors requires behavior counseling along with patient education. Chapters 7, 8, and 9 describe risk-factor management in greater detail. Reduced hospital stays often preclude specific interventions for modifying risk factors. Consequently, the role of inpatient staff is to identify risk factors (where possible); inform patients of these risk factors' implications; provide information about how they may obtain additional risk interventions following hospital discharge; and document the levels of responsibility for follow-up, including patient responsibilities, primary care physician responsibilities, and transitional or outpatient program staff responsibilities to ensure the continuum of care and increase patient compliance (see figure 4.11). Early family involvement in the management of risk factors—for example, getting other smokers to quit or, at a minimum, to facilitate the patient's ability to quit, or participating in the exercise program—is also critical to the success of the interventions and must be encouraged.

Discharge Planning

Discharge planning has taken on greater significance with decreased lengths of hospital stays (guideline 4.6). No longer can an inpatient program be viewed as a phase that the patient will finish before being discharged. Therefore, discharge planning should focus on making appropriate connections for the continuation of rehabilitation—for example, referral to an outpatient program prior to hospital discharge.

Regardless of where the patient will continue rehabilitation, addressing safety issues is the highest priority for discharge planning. Essential to patient safety are survival skills (recognition of signs and symptoms, nitroglycerin use, emergency assistance) and recommendations and limitations during recovery (with regard to the walking program and other activities). Rehabilitation professionals should be active participants in the discharge-planning team, providing the patient assistance in evaluating options for both formal and informal continuation of CR.

Guideline 4.6 | Discharge Planning Design

The process of discharge planning should consider two basic tenets: patient safety and program continuity.

Figure 4.1 illustrates major tracks for CR continuity (see page 32). Formal program options (transitional programs) that would precede entrance into a more typical outpatient program are discussed in the next section of this chapter.

Implementation Strategies

Just as there are checkpoints to assess readiness for exercise and readiness to learn, criteria have been identified for discharge-readiness assessment.[565] These include

- physiological stability and functional ability,
- competency (cognitive and psychomotor) to carry out self-care,
- perceived self-efficacy,
- availability of social support, and
- access to health care resources.

Objective assessment of each patient's functional activity level and tolerance for activity should be documented on a daily basis. Predischarge exercise testing or a 6-min walk test can provide exercise response data that is useful for setting home activity guidelines and formal outpatient programming. Areas of question and concern for cardiac patients during the first month after discharge include

- return to work,
- driving,
- household activity,
- stair climbing,
- lifting,
- sexual activity,
- walking, and
- socializing.

Anticipating questions will allow the staff to provide individualized, objective advice regarding HR and symptoms (e.g., the rating of perceived exertion [RPE] and angina or angina equivalent) where appropriate before discharge.

Clinical Pathways

The CR service components (exercise, education, and behavior counseling) have traditionally been provided to patients within the construct of a structured and sequenced inpatient CR program. Historically, such programs were frequently separate from routine daily patient care. However, the current health care environment necessitates increased interdepartmental cooperation for quality improvement and cost containment.[379] The use of the clinical pathway allows for the provision of a framework for the overall care of cardiac patients and integrates CR services into the comprehensive plan.[163]

Clinical pathways provide a description of the typical course of treatment for patients with a particular diagnosis such as postacute MI or post-CABGS. As a case-management tool, the purpose of a pathway is to standardize care so that length of stay is predictable for the majority of patients in the respective diagnostic groups. However, pathways need to be individually tailored to each facility. As clinical guides, pathways provide a protocol of how to progress patients through the hospital stay. Furthermore, they serve as tools for evaluating both the process and the outcomes of patient care.[132] Clinical pathways are intended to be comprehensive and multidisciplinary. Categories of patient care typically mapped out on the path include

- activity,
- consultations,
- diagnostics,
- discharge planning,
- education,
- medications,
- nutrition, and
- treatments.

The grid format (see table 4.2) of the clinical pathway allows easy visualization of the overall plan of care. Read vertically, it outlines the care to be given each day. Read horizontally, it identifies how services are to proceed through the treatment timeframe. Because activity progression and education are core elements of the inpatient CR program, these services are inserted under the "Activity" and "Education" headings.[462] Additionally, special visits by the CR staff for such things as the initial assessment for CR and predischarge instructions may be included under "Consults." To ensure optimal integration of rehabilitation services as well as to clarify roles and responsibilities, staff members, including those from CR, should participate in the multidisciplinary committee that designs each cardiac-related clinical pathway.

Once pathways for cardiac patients are developed and implemented, most patients progress accord-

ingly. Variations from the pathway do occur, however, caused by either comorbidities or complications such as those listed in figure 4.12.[256] Although such problems may disrupt the treatment timeline, they usually do not eliminate the need for rehabilitation services. The CR specialist may make case-by-case adjustments, documenting those adjustments so that other members of the rehabilitation team are aware of the variance and can implement changes accordingly. Variance tracking is a part of the data-collection requirements of clinical pathways.

Table 4.2 Sample Clinical Pathway for Rehabilitation Services: Uncomplicated

	Day 1	Day 2	Day 3	Day 4
Consults		CR to assess: • Readiness for activity • Readiness to learn		
Activity	Bed rest until stable, then OOB in chair; bedside commode	Routine CCU activities; sitting warm-ups, walk in room	Up in room; standing warm-ups; walk 5-10 min in hall 2-3 times/d (first time with supervision)	Up in room; standing warm-ups; walk 5-10 min in hall 3-4 times/d; walk down & up 1 flight of stairs with supervision
Education	Orient to CCU; basic explanation of event and treatment plan	Assess readiness to learn; when ready, teach survival lesson—signs/symptoms recognition, nitroglycerine use, emergency plan	Assess readiness to learn; when ready, teach survival lesson—safety factors, precautions for home	Review survival lessons; discuss postdischarge plans: 1. Phone number to call with questions 2. CR f/u: where, when 3. MD office visit
Discharge planning				CR predischarge visit and evaluation for follow-up services: home, transitional, outpatient

MI length of stay = 4 d; f/u = follow-up.

Preexisting conditions	CV complications
• General frailty	• Postoperative bleeding
• Chronic renal insufficiency	• Arrhythmia
• Cerebrovascular accident	• Pulmonary infections
• Orthopedic problems	• Perioperative MI
• Cognitive impairment	• Reduced left ventricular function
	• Cerebrovascular accident
	• Postoperative wound infections

Figure 4.12 Variations in the pathway.

Staffing

Considerations for staffing include defining responsibility, competency, and productivity (guideline 4.7). CR specialists, including specially trained exercise specialists, physical therapists, and nurses, have been the traditional providers of inpatient CR services. The integration of rehabilitation into clinical pathways, however, often includes a reevaluation and reallocation of staff resources. Table 4.3 provides an example of such delineations. The particular role assigned depends on the needs, expectations, and resources of each facility.

Cardiac Rehabilitation Specialist

Even within the dedicated CR specialist role, variations in practice patterns exist (guideline 4.8). Responsibilities range from daily delivery of exercise and education services to a focused predischarge visit only. Figure 4.13 contrasts these variations.

Guideline 4.7 Staff Responsibilities

Specific decisions should be made regarding how personnel will function within the rehabilitation setting and the role expectations for each staff member.

Table 4.3 General Cardiac Rehabilitation Role Expectations in the Inpatient Setting

Role	Focus	Function
Cardiac educator (RN, exercise physiologist, PT, other allied health staff)	All cardiac patients in hospital	Responsible for teaching regarding diagnostic procedures, preventive strategies, and recovery from medical/surgical interventions
Rehabilitation specialist (RN, exercise physiologist, PT, other allied health staff)	Postacute recovery	Responsible for evaluation exercise and education of patients eligible for rehabilitation
Nurse or licensed practical nurse	Postacute recovery and postsurgery nursing care	Responsible for assisting with daily care (e.g., getting patients OOB, inspecting incision sites, doing medication teaching, assisting with transfer) as well as providing rehabilitation exercise and education
Cardiovascular clinical nurse specialist, nurse practitioner, or case manager	Selected or all cardiac patients	Role is defined by institution; may include implementation of teaching, activity progression, and discharge planning; or may include the direction of the bedside staff to do so

---

Guideline 4.8 Staff Competencies

To meet inpatient CR expectations, all personnel must be adequately prepared for their rehabilitation-related roles.

Minimum	Moderate	Maximum
Predischarge visit only for: • Education—emergency plan, precautions for home • Exercise—activity evaluation (e.g., stair climbing, 6-min walk test), treadmill demonstration, and home program • Discuss need for outpatient or transitional follow-up; seek referral	Shared responsibility with unit nursing staff for daily services: • Responsible for education or exercise • Responsible for a selected combination of risk-factor topics and exercise • Discuss need for outpatient or transitional follow-up; seek referral	All day-to-day rehabilitation services: • Education—daily lessons based on individual patient priorities • Exercise—daily assessment and activity advancement based on protocol/clinical pathways • Discuss need for outpatient rehabilitation or transitional care follow-up; provide referral to the outpatient program

Figure 4.13 CR specialist role variations in the inpatient setting.

Other Health Professionals

By their nature, clinical pathways encourage the involvement of many disciplines in the cardiac recovery process. To optimize results, cardiac staff nurses or other health care professionals may share responsibility with the CR specialists for activity progression (figure 4.7) and patient teaching.[122] The American Association of Critical Care Nurses (AACN) has published clinical practice protocols outlining role expectations of acute care nurses in providing inpatient CR services.[21] Once the extent of the involvement of rehabilitation specialists and other staff is clarified, respective job descriptions must be revised to reflect roles and responsibilities. CR specialists are expected to meet the AACVPR core competencies and to be working toward specialty certification.[524]

Other staff members will require in-service education to prepare for rehabilitation applications. Programs combining classroom instruction with supervised clinical practice are recommended. Such training not only improves the quality of the inpatient program but also helps fulfill the expectation for specialty training that ensures staff competence.[302]

Regardless of which staff members are assigned to deliver inpatient rehabilitation services, it is important to determine how long each encounter takes (guideline 4.9). This information facilitates the computation of how many staff members (within the selected role or responsibility) are needed to cover the volume of CR patients and the development of departmental productivity standards. Figure 4.14 provides a typical time breakdown.

Service	Time
Assessment to determine stability for exercise and readiness to learn*	10-15 min
Education: One new session per day	20-30 min
Exercise: First time each day**	15-45 min
Total per patient per day	45-90 min
Average rehabilitation service time per patient per day	55 min

Figure 4.14 Time requirements for inpatient CR services.
* Initial assessment will require an additional 30-60 minutes. ** Exercise may be indicated more frequently each day and should be applied each day.

Guideline 4.9 Staff Productivity

Within the given responsibilities, determine the time required for each staff position to deliver the service.

Space and Equipment

The most common physical site for the delivery of inpatient CR services is the patient's room. Bedside activity and patient and family education can take place there while more progressive ambulation can be carried out in adjacent hallways. Telemetry monitoring is recommended to assess response to activity progression.

Some hospitals with high volumes of surgical or interventional patients may use an inpatient exercise room specially equipped with treadmills and bicycle ergometers to limit hallway traffic and further advance exercise performance before discharge. In others, patients are transported to the outpatient CR center (time and space permitting) for treadmill walking once or twice before discharge. The outpatient center visit has the added advantage of introducing patients to the outpatient program and encouraging early patient entry into it. However, patients appear to benefit from progressive activity with or without the use of exercise equipment.

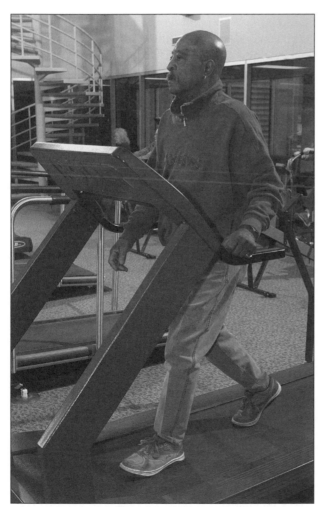

Funds must be budgeted for education equipment and supplies. A portable VCR and CD system and a collection of educational videotapes or discs are recommended, along with a quantity of pamphlets and other handouts designed for use in education sessions. Office space is recommended for storage of these educational materials and to serve as a work area and contact point for inpatient CR staff. Access to a conference room or small classroom is also helpful for group teaching.

Transitional Programming

Patients should leave the hospital with a clear plan for follow-up. They must continue and progress with activities initiated in the hospital. Unfortunately, shortened hospital stays and patient limitations in readiness to learn often reduce opportunities for effective patient teaching in the hospital. This results in added responsibility for the outpatient program. When patients do not move directly from the inpatient to the outpatient setting, the immediate postdischarge (transition) period may provide an opportunity for participation in a transitional program, depending on the needs and capabilities of the individual patient as well as the options available in the area (guideline 4.10). Figure 4.15 illustrates admission criteria for three of the most current transitional tracks.

Because of cardiac complications, comorbidities, or age-related frailty, some patients will leave the hospital without the ability to perform ADL. Others may require physical therapy or other services in addition to CR. These types of patients may be temporarily referred to a subacute inpatient facility or transitional care unit such as a skilled nursing facility or rehabilitation hospital.

Skilled Nursing Facility

Skilled nursing units may be available within the acute care hospital or as independent centers. Such facilities have specific admission criteria centered around a patient's ability to carry out ADL. Patients who require assistance with basic ADL such as eating, dressing, elimination, or personal hygiene during cardiac recovery may qualify to be admitted to a skilled nursing facility.

Rehabilitation Hospital

Over the past several decades, inpatient rehabilitation programs have been developed as a bridge between the acute-care facility and independent home living. Utilizing a multidisciplinary approach that includes

Guideline 4.10 | Transitional Programming

As a part of the inpatient clinical pathway, discharge-planning efforts include making arrangements for continuation of CR after hospital discharge.

Skilled nursing facility	Rehabilitation hospital	Home health care
Patients are temporarily unable to carry out some activities of daily living.	Patients require specific rehabilitation therapies; patients should be capable of participating in at least 3 hr of combined rehabilitation per day.	Patients are homebound and in need of skilled nursing care.

Figure 4.15 Admission criteria for transitional programs.

physical, occupational, vocational, and recreational therapy; speech pathology; nutrition; psychology and psychiatry; and continued medical and nursing management, these programs prepare patients for a safe and independent return to home. Particularly in postsurgical cardiac patients, such a team approach has been documented to reduce fragmentation of care; improve patient outcomes; and enhance patient, family, staff, and physician satisfaction.[110]

Admission criteria to acute rehabilitation programs generally include a greater need for skilled nursing and rehabilitation care compared to subacute or skilled nursing facilities. This can include management of medical issues such as fluid status; dysrhythmia; tracheotomy care; oxygen and bronchodilator therapy; wound care; intravenous therapy; and adjustments of medications for comorbidities such as depression, postoperative confusion, diabetes, and hypertension. The frequency and intensity of therapy sessions are also increased and include individual and group education, gait retraining, strength, endurance, and range-of-motion exercise, ADL evaluation and retraining, cognitive evaluation and retraining, and therapy specific to any preexisting or postoperative neurological or musculoskeletal disabilities that interfere with recovery. Those with permanent disabilities (e.g., paraplegia, amputation, neuromuscular disorders) who have had acute cardiac problems may also benefit from the multidisciplinary assistance that an acute rehabilitation hospital can provide. Rehabilitation goals are set by the patient, family, and the multidisciplinary team and generally include return to independent community function, with referral to home care or outpatient CR as appropriate.

Home Health Care

Many patients leave the hospital after short stays in need of follow-up nursing care that a few years ago would have been provided in the hospital. Nursing care such as wound care, medication instruction and administration, blood pressure or blood sugar surveillance, and anticoagulation may be more than the patient or the home caregiver can manage, prompting home health care follow-up. In fact, the availability of home health nursing services, especially for the postsurgical and CHF populations, provides an alternative for managing cardiac recovery that is attractive to patients, physicians, and payers alike. Home health care facilitates early hospital discharge.[243]

To receive home health services under Medicare, patients must be "homebound," meaning they are unable to leave their homes unassisted.[478] A number of cardiac patients are likely to qualify for several weeks of home care due to either actual physical-mobility problems or temporary restrictions imposed by their physicians (e.g., no driving). A patient being transported by another person to day care or any other circumstance other than medical appointments, however, is not considered homebound. The maximum length of time for insurance coverage is determined individually. Payers may cover home follow-up care for a fixed number of visits or weeks as a routine component of total case management.

Figure 4.15 summarizes the admission criteria for the transitional settings discussed. When exploring patient options for any of the three transitional programs mentioned, CR professionals must address two major issues: who provides CR care, and the level of reimbursement.

Nurses, physical therapists, and others who typically staff skilled nursing facilities and home care agencies may not have the expertise to provide CR services. Therefore, these individuals should develop competencies through in-service training, or CR specialists may be hired to staff these programs. Successful programs recommend between 4.5 and 20 hr of training (classroom plus clinical) for home care nurses assuming CR roles, depending on the extent of their cardiac background.[199,472] Physical assessment skills need to be strong in that telemetry monitoring equipment is usually not available in transitional settings. Although these transitional settings may provide CR exercise and education services, generally these services are not reimbursable through Medicare. Medicare reimburses only for skilled nursing visits or specific therapy visits such as physical or occupational therapy, which points to the need to emphasize the training and experience of these providers in the effective delivery of CR in these settings.

The mechanism for service delivery in transitional settings, similar to that in inpatient settings, is the clinical pathway. Transitional pathways can build on the inpatient programming results by gradually increasing ambulation time and introducing upper-body exercises. Because transition is still considered a low-level period of rehabilitation, the same performance parameters used with inpatient programs apply. Additionally, the same education assessments, curriculums, and teaching aids are used to address each patient's learning priorities.

In an attempt to provide continuity of CR service from one setting to the next, some programs have developed pathways that span the entire rehabilitation continuum: inpatient, transitional, outpatient, and maintenance. Two major advantages have been documented with this approach: (1) downtime between CR settings is minimized, and (2) referrals from tertiary treatment centers to community rehabilitation programs are maximized.[155]

The continuity provided is as helpful to the uncomplicated patient who is discharged quickly as it is to the more complicated patient who needs transitional care. Ironically, those patients considered uncomplicated may have the fewest options for post-hospitalization care; transitional care tends to be provided most often to patients at higher levels of illness and incapacitation. Additionally, because uncomplicated patients often have shortened inpatient stays, less time in the hospital is available for education and physical activity. Unfortunately, some of these patients, although uncomplicated, may not be able to enter an outpatient program immediately. Therefore, traditional outpatient CR program staff should consider developing transitional programs.

Current national guidelines recommend early initiation of outpatient CR, that is, within 1 to 3 weeks postevent.[604] The innovative transitional programs discussed here, including subacute facilities, rehabilitation hospitals, home care, and specifically designed transitional programs within traditional outpatient settings, meet the expectation of a quality continuum of rehabilitation care.

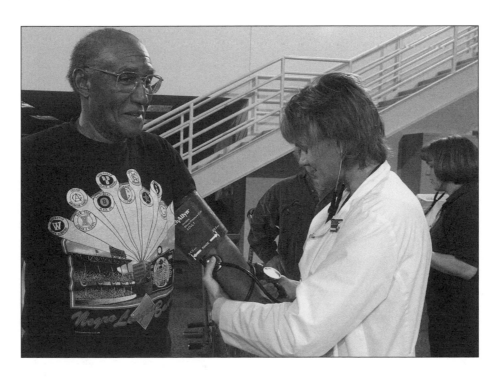

Summary

Inpatient CR has become streamlined, and simplified inpatient services serve as the foundation of CR interventions. In keeping with today's collaborative practice efforts, these services are integrated into clinical pathways and include a wide range of delivery options. The paradox is that inpatient activity efforts contribute to a shortened length of stay, while shorter stays eliminate the time required for adequate patient teaching. Therefore, the need for post-hospitalization follow-up or transitional programs has become increasingly urgent in recent years, particularly for medically complex patients. Several versions of transitional programs have emerged to provide rehabilitation continuity for different levels of patient need and capability.

Given the diversity of sites, facilities, and personnel, CR professionals must ensure patient safety and program effectiveness. At the very least, CR professionals need to be part of the quality team that designs both types of programs. Additionally, they may be called on to instruct other health professionals who provide rehabilitation services while continuing to function as direct providers of inpatient CR professionals.

As a result of these inpatient and transitional efforts, expected patient outcomes include

- decreased length of hospital stay;
- more rapid, more complete resumption of usual activities;
- confident, competent self-management;
- less psychological distress; and
- fewer readmissions.

Most importantly, patients are provided with a continuum of cardiac rehabilitative care that begins in the hospital, continues in the immediate postdischarge period, and connects with the traditional outpatient CR program for intensive risk reduction. Figures 4.16 and 4.17 summarize program structure and process recommendations.

Exercise

1. Design and implementation should be based on physiological principles that can be used by a variety of health professionals
   - within either an inpatient or a transitional setting, and
   - integrated into a cooperative clinical pathway.
2. Opportunities should exist to modify the activity plan or develop an individualized alternative for patients who do not fit the pathway.
3. Criteria should be specific for initiating and advancing inpatient activities.

Education

4. A standardized collection of cardiac teaching plans (see figures 4.9 and 4.10) should be available that outline the content area topics.
5. Appropriate and readable teaching aids should be selected to reinforce lesson content.
6. Patients should be involved in identifying their own high-priority learning needs.
7. A patient's readiness to learn should be assessed before every potential teaching encounter.
8. The teaching encounter should be evaluated; this evaluation includes patient comprehension.

Discharge planning

9. At a minimum, one predischarge visit for every CR patient should
   - address survival skills and postdischarge dos and don'ts,
   - evaluate and estimate predischarge functional ability, and
   - provide information about outpatient programming.

Figure 4.16 Summary of structure recommendations—CR in the inpatient and transitional settings.

Mechanism

1. The purpose and goals of the inpatient/transitional CR program should be defined.
2. CR expectations between rehabilitation specialists and other health care professionals should be clarified.

Resources

3. The extent of responsibility rehabilitation specialists have (minimum, shared, and maximum) should be specified.
4. The time required for delivery of rehabilitation services should be documented.
5. The complete scope of practice statement for all professionals involved in rehabilitation service delivery that is to be inserted into respective job descriptions should be completed.
6. Inservice training for other health care professionals assuming some rehabilitation responsibilities should be developed and presented.
7. The location of patient activities and education should be identified.
8. Standards clarifying the educational and exercise therapy criteria of the inpatient program should be developed.

Continuity

9. CR staff should participate in discharge planning to facilitate CR follow-up.
10. Potential transitional resources and respective patient qualifications should be identified, including
    - subacute facilities,
    - acute rehabilitation hospitals, and
    - home care follow-up.
11. Advisory and/or educational assistance to transitional sites should be made available.
12. The redesign of transitional outpatient programs to include a transition/pretraining period should be considered.
13. Outpatient CR continuation after transition is complete is strongly recommended.

Figure 4.17 Summary of process recommendations—CR in the inpatient and transitional settings.

5

Outpatient Cardiac Rehabilitation and Secondary Prevention

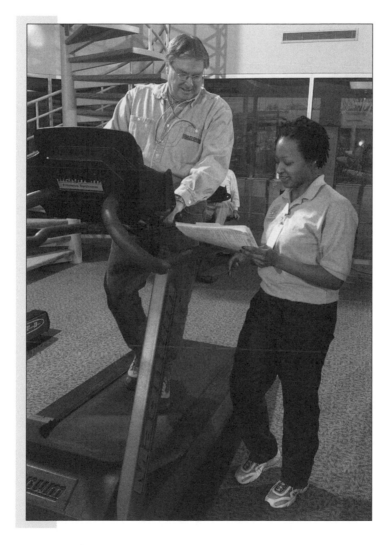

The changing nature of medical strategies, interventional techniques, and advancing research on the beneficial effects of lifestyle intervention in CHD has led to increased awareness of the importance of comprehensive risk reduction in the therapeutic management and prevention of CHD. As a result, it is important to review and, in some cases, redefine program structure. Models for risk assessment; eligible patient populations; supervision of the exercise portion of secondary prevention programs, including monitoring; and the rationale for delivering secondary prevention services are included in this redefinition of CR. Changes in risk-factor status, therapeutic efficacy and regimens, and knowledge of pathophysiology require that professionals stay abreast of the knowledge base and changing practices that can positively affect patient outcomes.

OBJECTIVES

This chapter focuses on

- assessment and management of risk factors for CVD progression,
- stratification of risk for events during exercise and appropriate supervision, and
- implementation of secondary prevention programming.

The AHCPR, in *Clinical Practice Guideline: Cardiac Rehabilitation*, published in 1995, and the American College of Cardiology (ACC) and AHA have developed documents that address secondary prevention.[22,24,55,58,187,517] These documents present the basis for the utilization of a CR model to provide a multifaceted program of secondary prevention of CHD. This program is an aggressive therapeutic regimen addressing risk factors amenable to change and thus becomes the basis for admitting patients to CR and secondary prevention programs.[331] A broad array of assessments, therapeutic modalities, and follow-up is necessary for secondary prevention to be successful. Finally, tracking and reporting outcomes to patients, physicians, and payers is critical to the ongoing success and acceptance of secondary prevention.

Case-management models for delivering services are ideal for implementing secondary prevention in CR.[140,233,263] Clinical pathways and the decreasing length of hospital stays provide the opportunity for an expanded role for outpatient care. Inclusion of CR and secondary prevention in the clinical pathway beginning in the acute-care phase and continuing in the outpatient phase are important components of quality secondary prevention and patient care.

Unfortunately, however, it is apparent that effective secondary prevention efforts are not as widespread. Recent reports from Europe confirm that risk factors such as smoking, obesity, and diabetes are frequently more prevalent four years after surgery. Hypertension is poorly managed in the population of people with CHD, and, although lipid-lowering drugs are widely available, the majority of patients remain above recommended levels for both cholesterol and LDL.[629,630] Similar findings have been reported in North America.[209,338] Only 11 to 37% of eligible patients are referred to outpatient CR programs. Thus, it might be concluded that despite widespread acknowledgment of the efficacy of secondary prevention and the considerable emphasis aimed at the medical community to actively and aggressively implement this therapy with drugs as well as lifestyle intervention, secondary prevention is being neither widely utilized nor effectively implemented.[338,409,629]

Structure of Secondary Prevention

Restoration of physical function has always been the cornerstone of CR. However, exercise training, while the most visible focus of CR, must be considered as only one of several components of secondary prevention programs aimed at reducing the risk of morbidity and mortality as well as improving function and quality of life. A patient accomplishes this by changing behaviors that lead to disease progression, specifically targeting those behaviors related to tobacco use; nutrition; exercise; stress; psychological health; and control of metabolic disorders such as diabetes and insulin-resistance syndrome, dyslipidemia, and obesity. Extensive evidence exists that optimal management of these lifestyle behaviors and metabolic disorders results in stabilization and possibly regression of the atherosclerotic process.[150,203,338,497] In fact, some have strongly suggested that so-called conventional medical therapy may have to be reconsidered in light of its lack of success in preventing coronary events and that comprehensive risk-factor intervention be considered a primary intervention.[178] Thus, a paradigm focusing on aggressive risk-factor reduction through medical therapy and lifestyle change should receive increasing emphasis as the primary aim of CR and secondary prevention programs (guideline 5.1).

Optimal secondary prevention requires a team of health care professionals to function in close partnership with physicians to assist and guide patients toward safe and efficacious therapy. Helping patients progress toward the stated outcomes of risk reduction aimed at having a significant impact on morbidity and mortality is a primary goal of secondary preven-

Guideline 5.1 Structure of Secondary Prevention Programming

- All patients should be assessed for the presence and extent of modifiable CVD risk factors, including smoking, hypertension, abnormal lipid profile, diabetes, obesity, psychosocial dysfunction, and inactivity.

- Depending on their medical history and physiological and psychological status, the majority of patients are able to and should begin aggressive secondary prevention and CR while still in the hospital and continue after discharge. Appropriate pharmacologic therapy, including beta blocker therapy, aspirin, and angiotensin-converting enzyme (ACE) inhibitors, should also begin while patients are in the hospital. Exercise training should begin within 1 to 3 weeks of discharge from the hospital. Most patients, including those with uncomplicated percutaneous transluminal coronary angioplasty (PTCA)/stent, can and should begin within 1 week of hospital discharge.

- Outcomes should include the complete cessation of smoking, improved lipid profiles, controlled hypertension, recognition and treatment of psychosocial dysfunction, and improved nutritional and physical activity habits.

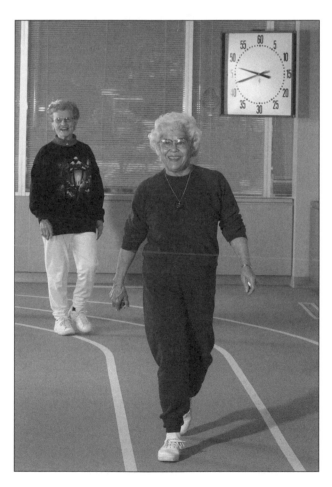

Case Management

Case management is an integrated disease-state management approach for providing specific risk-factor intervention strategies. It is necessary that therapies be coordinated between the primary care physician (cardiologist or other physician specialist) and other health care professionals. The patient is the center of the process and should take an active role in disease management. Case-management techniques have proved successful in risk-factor reduction programs, resulting in lowered morbidity and mortality from CHD.[140,233]

Case management in the context of secondary prevention and CR consists of three primary steps:

1. assessing all risk factors for disease progression and subsequently instructing patients in how to reduce or change the behaviors associated with each risk factor—for example, providing resources for smoking cessation to smokers;

2. establishing rapport and maintaining extensive contact with patients and physicians (by telephone or other correspondence or clinic visit) to provide necessary ongoing support for behavior change; and

3. providing regular follow-up regarding progress in meeting outcome goals and resetting goals for specific risk factors, as well as continued support for changing health behaviors that increase the risk of disease progression and recurrent events.

tion programs. If secondary prevention programs are to be held responsible for outcomes, then such programs must foster close partnerships with primary care and specialty physicians. These positive relationships, based on optimal patient outcomes, are critical to the success of secondary prevention programs.

Although the ultimate goal for each risk factor is to fall within the lowest levels of risk, the patient, physician, and CR staff should confer and agree on intermediate goals. The application of this type of treatment regimen allows for the individualization of therapeutic modalities as well as the implementation of predetermined algorithms for each risk factor.[29,304,403,537]

Contemporary secondary prevention programs provide tangible patient support that is critically important for success in changing behavior. Establishing a rapport with the patient through planned, consistent contact gives CR staff the opportunity to obtain feedback regarding the effectiveness of these changes.[390,465] Contact may take many forms, including exercise and education sessions, telephone calls, e-mails, letters or other written correspondence, or visits to the facility for follow-up counseling and testing.

Assessment of Risk Factors for Disease Progression

Contemporary secondary prevention programs optimally manage each patient's disease state to maximize reduction of subsequent event risk. Risk assessment allows for the development of therapeutic objectives designed to help stabilize vulnerable plaque. A discussion of plaque vulnerability and other factors associated with the atherosclerotic process appears in appendix B. The risk factors are those typically assessed in either primary or secondary prevention programs and that are established, independent risk factors for CVD morbidity and mortality.

There is cumulative and added risk in patients who have multiple risk factors.[136,210,235,362] Factors such as diabetes and low levels of HDL may significantly increase risk for recurrent events, especially in the presence of other risk factors.[29,136,496,537,591] Additionally, specific combinations of risk factors, such as high LDL, high triglycerides, and impaired glucose metabolism (insulin-resistance syndrome or diabetes), may also increase risk in patients with CHD.[309,436] Finally, several risk factors are emerging for which the relationship to atherogenesis and endothelial function has not been fully described, nor has the risk of some of these factors been completely quantified. Some of these emerging risk factors increase risk whereas others may simply be markers of CAD or atherogenesis.[136,253,276,287,591,629,630] The use and assessment of these risk factors is discussed in chapter 8 (see page 95).

The basic entities of risk-factor management presented in table 5.1 should be assessed as soon as a patient enters a secondary prevention program.

Table 5.1 AHA/ACC Secondary Prevention for Patients With Coronary and Other Vascular Disease: 2001 Update	
Goals	**Intervention recommendations**
Smoking: Complete cessation	Assess tobacco use. Strongly encourage patient and family to stop smoking and to avoid secondhand smoke. Provide counseling; pharmacological therapy, including nicotine replacement and buproprion; and formal smoking-cessation programs as appropriate.
BP control: <140/90 mmHg or <130/85 mmHg if heart failure <130/80 mmHg if diabetes or renal insufficiency	• Initiate lifestyle modification (weight control, physical activity, alcohol moderation; moderate sodium restriction; and emphasis on fruits, vegetables, and low-fat dairy products) in all patients with BP ≥130 mmHg systolic or 80 mmHg diastolic. • Add BP medication, individualized to other patient requirements and characteristics (i.e., age, race, need for drugs with specific benefits) if BP is not <140 mmHg systolic or 90 mmHg diastolic *or* if BP is not <130 mmHg systolic or 85 mmHg diastolic for individuals with heart failure (<80 mmHg diastolic for individuals with diabetes or renal insufficiency).
β-blockers	Start in all post-MI and acute ischemic syndrome patients. Continue indefinitely. Observe usual contraindications. Use as needed to manage angina, rhythm, or blood pressure in all other patients.
Lipid management (primary goal): LDL <100 mg/dL	Start dietary therapy in all patients (<7% saturated fat and <200 mg/d cholesterol) and promote physical activity and weight management. Encourage increased consumption of omega-3 fatty acids. Assess fasting lipid profile in all patients, and within 24 hr of hospitalization for those with an acute event. If patients

Goals	Intervention recommendations
Lipid management (primary goal): LDL <100 mg/dL *(cont'd)*	are hospitalized, consider adding drug therapy on discharge. Add drug therapy according to the following guide:

• LDL <100 mg/dL (baseline or on-treatment) • Further LDL-lowering therapy not required. • Consider fibrate or niacin (if low HDL or high TG).	• LDL 100-129 mg/dL (baseline or on-treatment) • Therapeutic options - Intensify LDL-lowering therapy (statin or resin*). - Fibrate or niacin (if low HDL or high TG). - Consider combined drug therapy (statin + fibrate or niacin) (if low HDL or high TG).	• LDL ≥130 mg/dL (baseline or on-treatment) • Intensify LDL-lowering therapy (statin or resin*). • Add or increase drug therapy with lifestyle therapies.

Goals	Intervention recommendations
Lipid management (secondary goal): If TG >200 mg/dL, then non-HDL should be <130 mg/dL**	• If TG ≥150 mg/dL or HDL <40 mg/dL: Emphasize weight management and physical activity. Advise smoking cessation. • If TG 200-499 mg/dL: Consider fibrate or niacin *after* LDL-lowering therapy*. • If TG ≥500 mg/dL: Consider fibrate or niacin *before* LDL-lowering therapy. • Consider omega-3 fatty acids as adjunct for high TG.
Physical activity: Minimal goal: 30 min, 3 to 4 d/week Optimal goal: Daily	• Assess risk, preferably with exercise test to guide prescription. • Encourage minimum of 30-60 min of activity, preferably daily, or at least 3 or 4 times weekly (walking, jogging, cycling, or other aerobic activity) supplemented by an increase in daily lifestyle activities (e.g., walking breaks at work, gardening, household work). Advise medically supervised programs for moderate- to high-risk patients.
Weight management: BMI 18.5-24.9 kg/m²	• Calculate BMI and measure waist circumference as part of evaluation. Monitor response of BMI and waist circumference to therapy. • Start weight management and physical activity as appropriate. Desirable BMI range is 18.5-24.9 kg/m². • When BMI ≥25 kg/m², goal for waist circumference is 40 inches in men and 35 inches in women.
Diabetes management: HbA1c <7%	• Appropriate hypoglycemic therapy to achieve near-normal fasting plasma glucose, as indicated by HbA1c. • Treatment of other risks (e.g., physical activity, weight management, BP, and cholesterol management).
Antiplatelet angets/ anticoagulants	Start and continue aspirin 75-325 mg/d if not contraindicated. Consider clopidogrel 75 mg/d or warfarin if aspirin contraindicated. Manage warfarin to international normalized ration = 2.0 to 3.0 in post-MI patients when clinically indicated or for those not able to take aspirin or clopidogrel.
ACE inhibitors	Treat all patients indefinitely post-MI; start early in stable high-risk patients (anterior MI, previous MI, Killip class II [S3 gallop, rales, radiographic CHF]). Consider chronic therapy for all other patients with coronary or other vascular disease unless contraindicated.

BP = blood pressure; TG = triglycerides; BMI = body mass index; HbA1c = major fraction of adult hemoglobin; MI = myocardial infarction; CHF = congestive heart failure.

* The use of resin is relatively contraindicated when TG >200 mg/dL.

** Non-HLD cholesterol = total cholesterol – HDL cholesterol.

Reprinted, by permission, from S.C. Smith Jr, et al., 2001, "Guidelines for preventing heart attack and death in patients with atherosclerotic cardiovascular disease: 2001 update: A statement for healthcare professionals from the AHA/ACC," *Circulation* 104:1577-1579.

Guideline 5.2

At the time of program entrance, all patients should undergo the following screening and assessments:

- Current medical history—medical or surgical profile (or both), including complications, comorbidities, and other pertinent medical history
- Physical examination—cardiopulmonary systems assessment and musculoskeletal assessment, particularly upper and lower extremities and lower back
- Resting 12-lead ECG
- Current medications, including dose and frequency
- CVD risk profile, including
  - identification of age and gender and menopausal status if female;
  - use of tobacco products;
  - history of hypertension;
  - lipid profile, including total cholesterol, HDL, LDL, and triglycerides (prior to event or more than 6-8 weeks postevent);
  - nutritional status, especially dietary fat, saturated fat, cholesterol, and calories;
  - body composition analysis (weight, height, BMI, waist-to-hip ratio, relative body fatness, waist circumference);
  - fasting blood glucose or hemoglobin A1c and history of diabetes;
  - physical activity status;
  - level of anger and hostility;
  - psychosocial history, particularly evidence of depression; and
  - family history.

Programming structured around affecting these risk factors is critical to both short- and long-term success in decreasing morbidity and mortality. Screening and assessment requirements for entry into a secondary prevention program are outlined in guideline 5.2 and discussed further in chapter 6.

Candidates for secondary prevention should be considered based on potential for rehabilitation and disease management and the presence of factors amenable to change, thereby ameliorating the disease process. The AHCPR clinical practice guideline also recommends a broadened range of indications for CR and specifies secondary prevention as the basis for outpatient CR.[604]

Assessment of risk for progression of CHD is beneficial to help establish length and intensity of therapy as well as for prioritizing risk-factor intervention and measuring outcomes in secondary prevention. After the assessment, establishing goals with the patient according to readiness and self-efficacy is another step in secondary prevention. Goals should be both achievable and mutually acceptable to the patient and clinician. It is advisable to establish both short-term and long-term goals in writing.

Smoking

The Surgeon General's report on the health hazards of smoking concludes that smoking increases CV mortality by 50% and increases the risk of subsequent events. Smoking negatively affects outcomes of CABGS and increases the risk of restenosis following angioplasty. Both active and passive smoking cause acute endothelial dysfunction persistently throughout exposure.[284,545,628] Smoking cessation produces a significant reduction in mortality (range 20-90%) over a 2- to 4-yr timeframe and has particular efficacy after MI. Smoking status can be assessed easily, and there are effective pharmacological and behavioral approaches to smoking cessation (table 5.2).[579]

Dyslipidemia

Because dyslipidemia—that is, elevated levels of total cholesterol or LDL, a decreased level of HDL, or an elevated triglyceride level—is associated with the progression of atherosclerosis as well as endothelial dysfunction, treating dyslipidemia should be a high priority.[41,101,235,403,538,603] Lowering LDL as quickly as possible through medication and diet has been shown to decrease cardiac events, probably through plaque stabilization and improved endothelial function.[284,518] Oxidized LDL at the vascular wall causes endothelial dysfunction as well as vascular remodeling and plaque formation. Assessing lipids soon after an acute event usually results in falsely low values. Quantification of dietary fat, saturated fat, and cholesterol provides for a minimum assessment of nutritional habits. Optimally, dietary content of omega-3 and monounsaturated fat, fiber, sodium, and refined carbohydrates should also be assessed. The CR staff should discuss pre-event lipids indicating dyslipidemia and the results of a nutritional assessment with the patient's physician to provide recommendations for lipid-lowering therapy. The NCEP guidelines (NCEP-III) recommend diet therapy as the first step in lipid management.[403] LDL level less than 100 mg/dL is an established target in patients with CHD (table 5.3). This level of LDL increases the likelihood of regression and stabilizes vulnerable plaque in patients with CHD.[403] Lowering LDL in patients with CHD can prevent recurrent clinical events.[479,518] Therefore, nutrition education should begin as early as possible, including specific recommendations and suggestions from the registered dietitian and other secondary prevention specialists regarding ways to immediately decrease fat and saturated fat in the diet as well as dietary cholesterol, refined carbohydrates, and sodium.

Though reduction in dietary fat is important, it is becoming apparent that the type of dietary fat consumed is important in secondary prevention. Thus, reduced fat alone is not sufficient for maximum dietary efficacy in secondary prevention programs. The so-called Mediterranean diet appears to be associated with lower rates of subsequent events, including MI and stroke in patients with CHD.[332,333] This diet is rich in monounsaturated fats (although canola oil may actually be superior to olive oil in its effects on CHD), omega-3 fatty acids, and fiber. Recommendations for dietary modification in lipid-lowering therapy should include changing the type of fat in the diet as well as increasing omega-3 fatty acids and fiber and decreasing refined sugars.[143,287,291,588]

Table 5.2 Risk Stratification Guidelines for Smoking

Risk factor	Lowest Risk	Moderate Risk	Highest Risk
Smoking	NONE If quit ≥6 months at time of event	SMOKER if quit <6 months	SMOKER

Table 5.3 Risk Stratification for Dyslipidemia/Inappropriate Dietary Fat Intake

Risk factor	Lowest risk	Moderate risk	Highest risk
Dyslipidemia/ Inappropriate dietary fat intake	**Diet** ❑ 15-25% fat <7% sat fat <150 mg chol or **Lipids** ❑ LDL <100 Chol/HDL ratio: <5.0 or Triglycerides <100	**Diet** ❑ 25.1-29% fat 7-9% sat fat 150-299 mg chol or **Lipids** ❑ LDL = 100-129 Chol/HDL ratio: 5.0-6.0 or Triglycerides 100-149	**Diet** ❑ ≥30% fat >9% sat fat ≥300 mg chol or **Lipids** ❑ LDL ≥130 Chol/HDL ratio: >6.0 or Triglycerides ≥150

Diabetes Mellitus

Eighty percent of diabetic mortality is due to occlusive artery disease.[221] Many people with diabetes have multiple risk factors, including hypertension, abnormal blood lipids, impaired fibrinolysis, increased inflammation, and central obesity related to insulin resistance. Evidence suggests that improved control of blood glucose reduces vascular disease (microvascular and macrovascular) in type 1 and type 2 diabetes.[151] Not only are people with diabetes more prone to mortality (and morbidity) from CHD, but the presence of multiple risk factors also seems to increase their risk compared to people without diabetes, and NCEP-III guidelines consider persons with diabetes to be at equivalent risk as persons with CHD (table 5.4).[338,403] Assessing and addressing risk factors in people with diabetes therefore becomes even more critical to secondary prevention efforts. Aggressive treatment of the risk factors and the lifestyle behaviors that contribute to and exacerbate them is very important in reducing the increased mortality and morbidity from CHD in people with diabetes.[29,151,152,363,496] This includes the use of statins in aggressively treating dyslipidemia associated with both diabetes and CHD.[203,537]

Obesity

Obesity is related to CHD and all-cause mortality and is associated with increased blood pressure, dyslipidemia, glucose intolerance, and other risk factors for CHD. Established levels of obesity classify individuals in risk categories.[195] Modest weight loss (5-10% of body weight) can significantly benefit various risk factors, including lipids, hypertension, and hyperglycemia (table 5.5).[479]

Hypertension

Evidence that systolic and diastolic BP is directly and linearly related to risk for CVD is clear.[304] End organ damage occurs at relatively modest levels of hypertension. Hypertension increases CVD risk through an increase in sheer stress on the arterial wall and by increasing myocardial oxygen demand. Excessive turbulent shear stress on vulnerable plaque increases endothelial and vascular wall dysfunction, thus increasing risk of plaque rupture and thrombus formation.[177,208,272] Reducing BP decreases risk for CVD, including MI, CHF, and cerebrovascular accident (table 5.6).[304]

Table 5.4	Risk Stratification for Diabetes Mellitus		
	Lowest risk	Moderate risk	Highest risk
Diabetes mellitus	HbA1c<6.5% or FBG <120	HbA1c = 6.6-7.9% or FBG = 120-180	HbA1c ≥8% or FBG >180

FBG = fasting blood glucose.

Table 5.5	Risk Stratification for Obesity		
	Lowest risk	Moderate risk	Highest risk
Obesity	BMI <25.0	BMI = 25-29.9	BMI ≥30

Table 5.6	Risk Stratification for Hypertension		
	Lowest risk	Moderate risk	Highest risk
Hypertension	<120 <80	120-139 80-89	≥140 ≥90

Sedentary Lifestyle

A sedentary lifestyle is the most prevalent risk factor (approaching 70% or greater in subgroups over age 50 and in minorities).[479] Low levels of physical activity are associated with increased risk of CHD (table 5.7). Highly active men and women with risk factors (hypertension, high cholesterol, diabetes, obesity) have lower mortality rates than low-activity men and women without risk factors.[82,83] Levels of activity in excess of 1,500–2,000 kcal/week are associated with significantly decreased incidence of CHD.[425] A similar level of caloric expenditure is associated with atherosclerotic regression or reduction of other risk factors.[560] Reduced mortality has been reported in patients participating in exercise-based CR programs.[414,418] Though these thresholds are important, it is also important to realize that in studies of primary prevention that assess activity and exercise, decreased risk is inherent in a continuum of increased activity. It is clear that regular activity produces benefits to both those with and those without CHD and that moderately to highly fit, physically active persons with CHD have decreased morbidity and mortality.[402]

It appears that moderate-intensity, regular exercise training also enhances endothelial function.[257] These effects may account for some of the decreased mortality shown in long-term studies of exercise, as well as for the continuum of activity that seems related to this decreased mortality. The specifics of intensity and duration as well as the duration of the effect are unknown; however, the use of moderate and frequent physical activity (6-7 d/week) may be the most effective exercise prescription for secondary prevention.[195]

Initiation of an exercise program at entry is routine in secondary prevention programs. Program staff should assess the patient's pre-event exercise habits at entry and assess functional capacity by exercise testing. Quantifying exercise habits by weekly caloric expenditure is important in establishing risk level and may be helpful in designing a program.

Depression/Psychosocial Dysfunction

Psychosocial dysfunction is associated with increased mortality and morbidity in people diagnosed with CHD (table 5.8).[62,200] Significantly increased risk of mortality has been reported in post-MI patients who are depressed. Some literature suggests a link between psychosocial factors and sudden death. Depression, social isolation and lack of social support, and acute and chronic life stress have all been associated with increased mortality, morbidity, and endothelial dysfunction in patients with CHD.[222,482] Consequently, secondary prevention programs should screen for psychosocial dysfunction. Assessment is recommended at entry, although implementing appropriate and acceptable techniques for management is sometimes difficult.[62,200,479,482] However, effective policies and procedures for referral to mental health professionals should be in place and implemented as indicated.

Stratification of Risk for Events During Exercise

The goal of an exercise program within a secondary prevention program is for patients to achieve physiological, symptomatic, psychological, and vocational benefits of physical activity at an acceptably low risk level. Accomplishing this goal requires careful patient evaluation, education, and supervision. A key element of exercise safety is stratification of patients

Table 5.7 Risk Stratification for Sedentary Lifestyle

	Lowest risk	Moderate risk	Highest risk
Sedentary lifestyle	≥1,500 kcal/week	700-1,499 kcal/week	<700 kcal/week

Table 5.8 Risk Stratification for Depression

	Lowest risk	Moderate risk	Highest risk
Depression	Not clinically depressed	Mildly depressed	Clinically depressed

according to risk for acute CV complications during exercise, as well as overall prognosis (guideline 5.3). Risk-stratification criteria for events during exercise or activity are derived from research concerning factors associated with increased risk of morbidity and mortality in general.[433,434] It is not clear, however, whether risk for exercise-related events is related to exercise itself or to the overall morbidity and mortality risk related to the person's clinical status.[584] Furthermore, established models for risk stratification may not clearly stratify patients into a single risk category because patients can have risk factors in more than one category, making classification using such tools difficult.[189,195] Nonetheless, despite these potential limitations in the process, risk stratification is another clinical tool that can help the exercise pro-

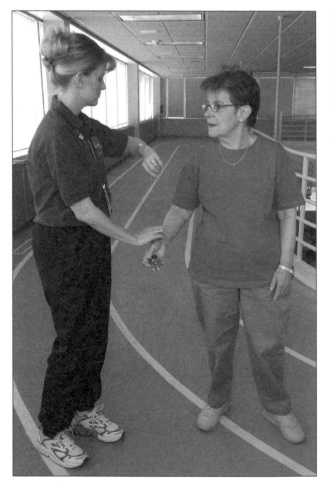

fessional determine the appropriate level of supervision for individual patients.

The risk of cardiac events during exercise appears to be greatest in those patients with poor left ventricular function, significant ventricular dysrhythmias, or a non-Q-wave MI because of an increased risk of later ischemic events.[195] Additionally, research indicates that noncompliance with the exercise prescription increases risk of mortality.[479] Specifically, exercising above an appropriately prescribed intensity is a significant risk factor for exercise-related complications. Although this factor may be difficult to assess prior to participation, secondary prevention programs should offer both sensible exercise prescriptions and adequate supervision of exercise in structured settings. The model presented in figure 5.1 uses variables common to those established models and allows categorization to a single risk class. It is helpful to identify the lowest-risk, moderate-risk, and the highest-risk patients for exercise participation. The lowest-risk patients have all of the characteristics listed. The highest-risk patients have any one of the characteristics listed. Those who do not fit either classification are considered to be at moderate risk.

Patients who have not undergone exercise testing before entering a program or those with nondiagnostic exercise tests may be inadequately categorized using criteria from figure 5.1. Such patients may receive a more cautious approach to risk stratification at program entry and an accompanying conservative methodology for the prescription of exercise. Patients with nondiagnostic exercise tests include

- those with abnormal resting electrocardiograms (ECG), including left bundle branch block, left ventricular hypertrophy with or without resting ST-T changes, nonspecific intraventricular conduction delays, Wolff-Parkinson-White ECG pattern, and ventricular paced rhythms;

- those on digitalis therapy;

- those who test negative for ischemia but who fail to achieve 85% of maximal predicted heart rate; and

- those with significant additional medical problems (comorbidities) that limit exercise capacity.

Guideline 5.3 Stratification of Risk for Exercise Events

All cardiac patients entering exercise rehabilitation should be stratified according to risk for the occurrence of cardiac events during exercise.

Characteristics of patients at lowest risk for exercise participation (all characteristics listed must be present for patient to remain at lowest risk)

- Absence of complex ventricular arrhythmias during exercise testing and recovery
- Absence of angina or other significant symptoms (e.g., unusual shortness of breath, light-headedness, or dizziness, during exercise testing and recovery)
- Presence of normal hemodynamics during exercise testing and recovery (i.e., appropriate increases and decreases in heart rate and systolic blood pressure with increasing workloads and recovery)
- Functional capacity ≥7 METs

Non–exercise testing findings:

- Rest ejection fraction ≥50%
- Uncomplicated MI or revascularization procedure
- Absence of complicated ventricular arrhythmias at rest
- Absence of CHF
- Absence of signs or symptoms of postevent/postprocedure ischemia
- Absence of clinical depression

Characteristics of patients at moderate risk for exercise participation (any one or combination of these findings places a patient at moderate risk)

- Presence of angina or other significant symptoms (e.g., unusual shortness of breath, light-headedness, or dizziness occurring only at high levels of exertion [≥7 METs])
- Mild to moderate level of silent ischemia during exercise testing or recovery (ST-segment depression <2 mm from baseline)
- Functional capacity <5 METs

Non–exercise testing findings:

- Rest ejection fraction = 40-49%

Characteristics of patients at high risk for exercise participation (any one or combination of these findings places a patient at high risk)

- Presence of complex ventricular arrhythmias during exercise testing or recovery
- Presence of angina or other significant symptoms (e.g., unusual shortness of breath, light-headedness, or dizziness at low levels of exertion [<5 METs] or during recovery)
- High level of silent ischemia (ST-segment depression ≥2 mm from baseline) during exercise testing or recovery
- Presence of abnormal hemodynamics with exercise testing (i.e., chronotropic incompetence or flat or decreasing systolic BP with increasing workloads) or recovery (i.e., severe postexercise hypotension)

Non–exercise testing findings:

- Rest ejection fraction <40%
- History of cardiac arrest, or sudden death
- Complex dysrhythmias at rest
- Complicated MI or revascularization procedure
- Presence of CHF
- Presence of signs or symptoms of postevent/postprocedure ischemia
- Presence of clinical depression

Figure 5.1 Stratification of risk for cardiac events during exercise participation.

Reprinted from *Cardiology Clinics,* Vol. 19, M.A. Williams, "Exercise testing in cardiac rehabilitation: Exercise prescription and beyond," p. 415-431, Copyright 2001, with permission from Elsevier.

Medical Supervision and Electrocardiogram Monitoring of Patients During Exercise

Guidelines concerning clinical supervision of patients exercising in secondary prevention programs remains an area of discussion.[189] Decisions regarding the intensity of medical supervision of the exercise program, including necessary personnel and the type and duration of supervision and frequency of ECG monitoring (continuous and intermittent), should be made by the CR program medical director, considering any recommendations by the patient's referring physician. The intensity of medical supervision is also guided by the types of patients enrolled in the exercise program, that is, whether patients are early in their post-hospitalization recovery (1-2 weeks postevent) or are more stable, such as those who are participating in the maintenance program and thus are likely to be at lower risk for events. Medical supervision is the most important day-to-day safety factor in CR.

Figure 5.2 suggests various program policies that should help the program staff reduce the risk of events on a daily basis. More intense patient supervision is required during exercise at times of change in health status, symptoms, or other evidence of disease progression and at times when the intensity of the exercise regimen increases, regardless of whether the patient is undergoing continuous ECG monitoring. The monitoring of clinical parameters before, during, and following exercise, provides further safeguards (see guideline 5.4). As a part of clinical supervision, staff members must provide thorough

---

Program policies

- Ensure that all patients have been physician referred and have undergone appropriate assessment before entry into the program and at periodic follow-up intervals.
- Maintain an emergency plan for adverse events and provide for frequent mock emergency practice and critique sessions for all staff members.
- Maintain physicians' standing orders for potential emergent and nonemergent medical events.
- Ensure onsite availability of medical supervision; monitoring and resuscitation equipment, including a defibrillator (as well as maintenance of such equipment); and appropriate medications.
- Emphasize duration of activity over intensity of effort, particularly in higher-risk patients.

Patient education

- Emphasize to patients that they must be alert for warning signs of changes in their condition, both at home and within the program, including chest discomfort or other angina-like symptoms, light-headedness or dizziness, irregular pulse, weight gain, shortness of breath, and so on.
- Educate patients as to the appropriate responses to such changes in their condition.
- Stress the importance of adhering to the exercise prescription (i.e., target heart rate or perceived exertion, exercise workloads, duration of effort, and choices of exercise equipment).
- Emphasize the importance of warming up and cooling down.
- Remind patients to adjust exercise levels according to various environmental conditions such as heat, humidity, cold, and elevation.

During the exercise session

- Evaluate each patient before he or she begins exercise for recent changes in condition, body weight, BP, medication adherence, and ECG (if utilized).
- Use continuous or intermittent ECG monitoring as appropriate.
- If necessary, adjust the intensity and duration of the daily exercise routine based on the patient's condition before exercise and responses to activity.
- Maintain supervision during and following exercise, including periodic checks of any showering or locker-room facilities, until the patient has left the facility.
- Modify recreational activities as appropriate and minimize competition.

Figure 5.2 Reducing CV complications during exercise within CR/secondary prevention programs.

Reprinted from *Cardiology Clinics,* Vol. 19, M.A. Williams, "Exercise testing in cardiac rehabilitation: Exercise prescription and beyond," p. 415-431, Copyright 2001, with permission from Elsevier.

Guideline 5.4 Recommended Methods and Tools for Daily Assessment of Risk for Exercise

The pre-exercise assessment should include the program staff asking the patient about recent signs and symptoms, his or her adherence to the medication schedule, and his or her subjective feelings of well-being. Risk should also be assessed with the following clinical measures:

- Continuous or intermittent ECG monitoring
  - Telemetry or hardwire monitoring
  - "Quick-look" using the defibrillator paddles
  - Periodic rhythm strips
- BP
- HR (by palpation)
- Symptoms and evidence of effort intolerance
- RPE

patient education regarding patient self-assessment and reporting to CR staff changes in symptoms, appearance, well-being, and response to exercise. By communicating with patients and maintaining continuous assessment, not only for well-being but also for compliance with the exercise prescription, the staff will help ensure the safety and efficacy of the exercise program.

Early Outpatient Exercise Program

The early outpatient exercise program is generally defined as beginning within 1 to 2 weeks of discharge from the hospital and lasting up to 12 weeks or longer in some instances, based on medical necessity. Sessions frequently are scheduled 3 d/week, although numbers of sessions per week may vary from one to five per week. The intensity of clinical supervision is usually at its highest level during this phase and may include ECG monitoring. Figure 5.3 outlines the physician's role in the provision of medical supervision. Professionally qualified staff members such as registered nurses or clinical exercise physiologists can provide physicians with documented evidence of unusual or abnormal responses, but in each instance, this documentation should receive the attention of a physician, with additional documentation of such review and plan of action.

ECG Monitoring

The number of ECG-monitored sessions is not a measure of the clinical value of exercise or secondary prevention services or of the duration of an exercise program. ECG monitoring is one of several techniques that program staff may employ for clinical supervision of patients. Nonetheless, reimbursement is frequently tied to a specific number of ECG-monitored exercise sessions and thus, program staff members should make sure they are familiar with the various limitations imposed by each patient's third-party insurance carrier(s). Ideally, length of clinical supervision or the number of ECG-monitored sessions should be determined on an individual basis. Further recommendations for the utilization of ECG monitoring based on risk of exercise events are described in figure 5.4.

ECG monitoring tends to be linked inversely with risk, but no firm predictors exist to help identify patients for whom it may not be necessary.[586] Continuous ECG monitoring is intended to

- detect dangerous dysrhythmias or other significant ECG changes that are amenable to treatment before complications arise;
- monitor compliance with the exercise prescription, especially with respect to heart rate;[7] and
- increase patient self-confidence for independent activity.

Given the variable occurrence of dysrhythmias, however, and that the safety of exercise regimens has been determined only by means of aggregate data, the use of continuous or intermittent monitoring for a specific patient remains a matter of clinical judgment. The type and frequency of ECG monitoring depends on the overall status of the patient and his

- CR services are prescribed and supervised by a physician pursuant to an individualized, written plan of treatment established, reviewed, and signed by a physician every 30 d (in consultation with appropriate staff participating in the program). The plan sets forth the diagnoses; the type, amount, frequency, and duration of the items and services provided under the plan; and the goals under the plan.

- The physician who provides supervision of CR services shall be licensed to practice medicine in the state in which the program is offered, with expertise in the management of patients with cardiac pathophysiology; shall be responsible for the program; and shall provide substantial involvement in directing the progress of individual patients in the program in consultation with appropriate staff.

- The services under the physician's supervision are as follows:
  - Medical evaluation
  - Prescribed exercise
  - Cardiac risk-factor modification
  - Review of patient-specific risk factors, education, counseling, and behavioral interventions
  - Psychosocial assessment and treatment, if needed
  - Outcomes assessment
  - Such items and services that are reasonable and necessary for the diagnosis or active treatment of the individual's condition; are reasonably expected to improve or maintain the individual's condition and functional level; and are furnished pursuant to guidelines relating to the frequency and duration of services, taking into account accepted norms of medical practice and reasonable expectation of patient improvement

- The program is one that is furnished by a hospital, physician's office, or a physician-directed clinic.

A physician shall be immediately available and accessible for medical consultation and for medical emergencies at all times the CR program is conducted. A CR program must ensure that a physician is available to be physically present within 3 min of an identified emergency that occurs while an individual is in the exercise area.

Figure 5.3 Physician supervision of CR and secondary prevention programs.

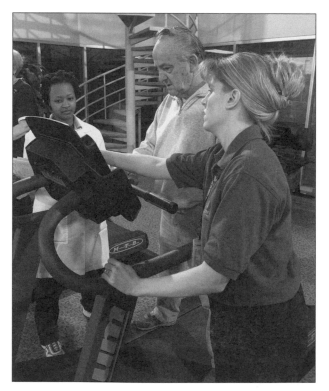

or her response to the exercise session. Intermittent ECG monitoring enables observation when indicated, such as at the time of a suspected change in CV status as assessed by clinical observation, measurement, or symptomatology. The optimal approach balances patient benefit with safety.[58,320,586]

Implementation of Secondary Prevention

The implementation of secondary prevention as described herein can be difficult. Attempting to reduce the cost of health care has become both the trend and the necessity in the current economic environment. Programs are challenged to offer multidisciplinary programming necessary to address the multitude of issues facing patients with CHD but often face limited financial resources; thus, creativity is essential. Identifying available programs offered outside the CR program is often one solution. In the hospital setting and in many communities, resources offer a variety of programs that address general lifestyle

Patients at lowest risk for exercise participation

- Direct staff supervision of exercise should occur for a minimum of 6-18 exercise sessions or 30 d postevent or postprocedure, beginning with continuous ECG monitoring and decreasing to intermittent ECG monitoring as appropriate (e.g., at 6-12 sessions).
- For a patient to remain at lowest risk, his or her ECG and hemodynamic findings should remain normal, there should be no development of abnormal signs and symptoms either within or away from the exercise program, and progression of the exercise regimen should be appropriate.

Patients at moderate risk for exercise participation

- Direct staff supervision of exercise should occur for a minimum of 12-24 exercise sessions or 60 d postevent or postprocedure, beginning with continuous ECG monitoring and decreasing to intermittent ECG monitoring as appropriate (e.g., at 12-18 sessions).
- For a patient to move to the lowest-risk category, ECG and hemodynamic findings during exercise should be normal, there should be no development of abnormal signs and symptoms either within or away from the exercise program, and progression of the exercise regimen should be appropriate.
- Abnormal ECG or hemodynamic findings during exercise, the development of abnormal signs and symptoms either within or away from the exercise program, or the need to severely decrease exercise levels may result in the patient remaining in the moderate-risk category or even moving to the high-risk category.

Patients at highest risk for exercise participation

- Direct staff supervision of exercise should occur for a minimum of 18-36 exercise sessions or 90 d postevent or postprocedure, beginning with continuous ECG monitoring and decreasing to intermittent ECG monitoring as appropriate (e.g., at 18, 24, or 30 sessions).
- For a patient to move to the moderate-risk category, ECG and hemodynamic findings during exercise should be normal, there should be no development of abnormal signs and symptoms either within or away from the exercise program, and progression of the exercise regimen should be appropriate.
- Abnormal ECG or hemodynamic findings during exercise, the development of abnormal signs and symptoms either within or away from the exercise program, or significant limitations in the patient's ability to participate in the exercise regimen may result in discontinuation of the exercise program until appropriate evaluation, and intervention where necessary, can take place.

Figure 5.4 Recommendations for intensity of supervision and monitoring related to risk of exercise participation.

Reprinted from *Cardiology Clinics,* Vol. 19, M.A. Williams, "Exercise testing in cardiac rehabilitation: Exercise prescription and beyond," p. 415-431, Copyright 2001, with permission from Elsevier.

issues such as managing stress, dietary change, and smoking cessation. Program staff may establish links with other in-house programs or outside agencies to offer patients access to these programs, potential discounts, ongoing support, and even periodic assessment. In this way, programs with limited resources may extend services.

Following patients' progress through periodic assessment of the risk factors and a planned follow-up program will help ensure that outcomes are optimized, and thus accurate and detailed record keeping and continued patient contact are critical to long-term success. The process is one of attention to detail, orderly record keeping, and ensuring that established flags alert staff to timely follow-up. Computer software specific to this task, that is, tracking outcomes, is helpful but not an absolute necessity.

Summary

Implementation of multifaceted secondary prevention programs is both prudent and necessary. Assessing patients entering secondary prevention programs for both safety and disease progression helps program staff establish priorities for therapeutic modalities, helps patients understand the health behaviors that require change, and may identify the most efficacious therapy. CR must be more than just an exercise program, and the treatment of risk for disease progression is a multifactorial effort that includes outcome assessment. Clinical supervision, which may include ECG telemetry–monitored exercise, is necessary; the intensity of clinical supervision required depends on individual patient status.

6

Medical Evaluation and Exercise Testing

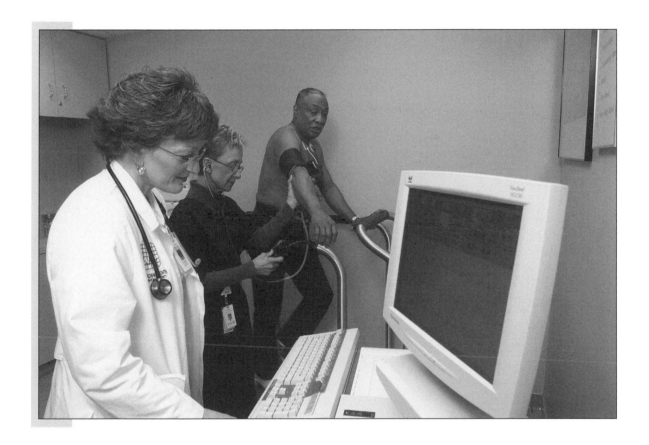

Data gathered from the initial medical evaluation of patients prior to entry into cardiac rehabilitation are used to design and implement an effective program in which specific outcomes are defined and targeted. The AHA guidelines for comprehensive secondary prevention provide a useful framework for evaluation and management (see table 5.1 on page 56).[517] This information is most useful in stratifying the patient in two major ways:

■ It establishes the patient's risk for progression of atherosclerosis and the likelihood of future cardiac events.

■ It establishes the patient's risk for adverse cardiac events during prescribed exercise training, as well as whether exercise is contraindicated, and if not, the level of supervision and monitoring recommended during the initial training period. (Stratification of these factors is discussed separately in chapter 5; see pages 63 and 67.)

OBJECTIVES

This chapter describes

- the components of the physical examination,
- the methods and protocols to be used in exercise testing,
- interpretation of results,
- additional imaging modalities, and
- alternative methods for evaluating physical activity status.

Information from the medical evaluation and exercise testing data may be provided by the patient's primary care physician, cardiologist, and surgeon or through direct evaluation by the medical director of the CR program (guideline 6.1). A medical history, with particular attention to CV status, as well as a detailed review of risk factors and their management are essential components of the initial assessment and will serve to target and customize the program (see figure 6.1). The CR specialist should determine whether patients are experiencing symptoms of angina, dyspnea, palpitations, or syncope and should question patients about previous occurrence of MI, percutaneous coronary intervention, or bypass surgery. Ideally, measurements of left ventricular systolic function and coronary anatomy should be available and noted. A complete list of medications, dosing intervals, and compliance with the drug regimen should be reviewed, because these may affect the response to exercise. Comorbid conditions such as pulmonary, endocrine, and neurological illnesses and behavioral and musculoskeletal conditions should also be evaluated.

Detailed social and occupational histories yield valuable information and allow the tailoring of pro-

gram training and goals to meet individual needs. When developing the patient-assessment protocol for all patients, CR staff should seek consultation from staff from both social services and vocational rehabilitation who are familiar with the array of medical, psychological, economic, and legal factors that influence return-to-work issues. Family and community resources that can assist patients with family concerns and returning to work should also be considered.

Physical Examination

The initial physical examination should be performed by a physician or other appropriately trained and qualified health care provider under the direction of a physician who is actively involved in the routine care of patients with CV disease (guideline 6.2, figure 6.2). A current resting standard 12-lead ECG is useful in assessing HR, rhythm, conduction abnormalities, and evidence of prior MI. The resting ECG serves as an important reference for future comparison, particularly if the patient develops new signs or symptoms suggestive of ischemia or arrhythmias.

Guideline 6.1 Medical Evaluation and Exercise Testing

- To establish a safe and effective program of comprehensive CV risk reduction and rehabilitation, each patient should undergo a careful medical evaluation and exercise test before participating in an outpatient CR program.
- The specific components of the medical evaluation should include a medical history, physical examination, and resting ECG.
- The exercise test should be repeated any time that symptoms or clinical changes warrant as well as in the follow-up assessment of exercise training outcome.

1. **Medical diagnoses**—a variety of diagnoses should be reviewed, including, but not limited to, CV disease, including existing CAD; previous MI, angioplasty, cardiac surgery, angina, and hypertension; pulmonary disease, including asthma, emphysema, and bronchitis; cerebral vascular disease, including stroke; diabetes; peripheral arterial disease; anemia, phlebitis or emboli; cancer; pregnancy; musculoskeletal deficiencies and neuromuscular and joint disease; osteoporosis; emotional disorders and eating disorders

2. **Symptoms**—angina; discomfort (pressure, tingling, pain, heaviness, burning, numbness) in the chest, jaw, neck, or arms; atypical angina, such as lightheadedness, dizziness, or fainting; shortness of breath; rapid heartbeats or palpitations, especially if associated with physical activity, eating a large meal, emotional upset, or exposure to cold

3. **Risk factors for atherosclerotic disease progression**—hypertension; diabetes; obesity; dyslipidemia; smoking; stress; and physical inactivity

4. **Recent illness, hospitalization, or surgical procedure**

5. **Medication dose and schedule, drug allergies**

6. **Other habits**—including alcohol or illicit drug use

7. **Exercise history**—information on habitual level of activity, such as type of exercise, frequency, duration, and intensity

8. **Work history**—with an emphasis on current or expected physical/mental demands, noting upper- and lower-extremity requirements; estimated time to return to work

9. **Psychosocial history**—including living conditions; marital and family status; transportation needs; family needs; domestic and emotional problems; depression, anxiety, or other psychological disorders

Figure 6.1 Components of the medical history.

From Fletcher GF, Balady G, Froelicher VF, et al. Exercise standards, a statement for health professionals from the American Heart Association. AHA medical/scientific statement. *Circulation* 1995;91:580-615.

Guideline 6.2 Physical Examination

The physical examination should focus minimally on the resting HR; BP; and pulmonary, cardiac, vascular, and musculoskeletal areas (see figure 6.2).

1. Body weight, height, BMI, waist-to-hip ratio, waist circumference at the level of the umbilicus

2. Pulse rate and regularity

3. Resting BP

4. Auscultation of the lungs, with specific attention to uniformity of breath sounds in all areas (absence of rales, wheezes, and other abnormal breath sounds)

5. Auscultation of the heart, with specific attention to murmurs, gallops, clicks, and rubs

6. Palpation and auscultation of carotid, abdominal, and femoral arteries

7. Palpation and inspection of lower extremities for edema and presence of arterial pulses and skin integrity (particularly in those with diabetes)

8. Absence or presence of xanthoma and xanthelasma

9. Examination related to orthopedic, neurologic, or other medical conditions that might limit exercise testing or training

10. Examination of the chest and leg wounds and vascular access areas in patients after coronary bypass surgery or percutaneous coronary revascularization

Figure 6.2 Components of the physical examination.

From Fletcher GF, Balady G, Froelicher VF, et al. Exercise standards, a statement for health professionals from the American Heart Association. AHA medical/scientific statement. *Circulation* 1995;91:580-615.

Musculoskeletal complaints and injury are relatively common complications, especially when a patient is initiating an exercise program. Therefore, musculoskeletal function should be assessed before exercise training begins.[330] Assessment of lower-extremity strength and flexibility, especially posterior thigh (hamstrings) and posterior lower leg (gastrocnemius/soleus complex) flexibility, may help prevent injuries related to weight-bearing exercise. CR staff should also determine whether the patient has a history of musculoskeletal injury and assess posture and alignment.

Risk Stratification and Identification of Contraindications for Exercise Training

Recommendations for risk stratifying patients as they enter outpatient CR are described in chapter 5 (see page 61). The classifications are presented as a means of beginning exercise with the lowest possible risk. They do not consider accompanying morbidities (for example, insulin-dependent diabetes mellitus, morbid obesity, severe pulmonary disease, complicated pregnancy, or debilitating neurological or orthopedic conditions) that may constitute a contraindication to exercise or necessitate closer supervision during exercise training sessions. In addition, patients with the following conditions should be excluded from exercise training:

- Unstable ischemia
- Heart failure that is not compensated
- Uncontrolled arrhythmias
- Severe and symptomatic aortic stenosis
- Hypertrophic obstructive cardiomyopathy
- Severe pulmonary hypertension
- Other conditions that could be aggravated by exercise (for example, resting systolic BP ≥200 mmHg or resting diastolic BP ≥110 mmHg, active or suspected myocarditis or pericarditis, suspected or known dissecting aneurysm, thrombophlebitis, or recent systemic or pulmonary embolus)

Exercise Testing

An exercise test is a key component of the initial assessment made before a patient begins an exercise program. Graded exercise tests are used to assess the patient's ability to tolerate increased physical activity, while ECG, hemodynamic, and symptomatic responses are monitored for manifestations of myocardial ischemia, electrical instability, or other exertion-related abnormalities. The exercise test may be used for diagnostic, prognostic, and therapeutic applications, although some limitations do exist with the procedure.[204a] The test may also be a motivational tool for patients as well as verification to the family of the patient's improving condition. Various other published position statements present additional in-depth information regarding applications of exercise testing, methods of conducting exercise tests, and guidelines for managing exercise-testing laboratories.[188,195,223,440]

CR health professionals commonly use exercise tests as a functional rather than diagnostic tool. The test is quite useful in assessing cardiorespiratory status and developing an exercise prescription. It is also used to measure functional changes over time to assess training program outcomes. Exercise tests and simulated work tests also help determine an individual's ability to return to work.[193,612] Not all patients referred for CR services are necessarily candidates for exercise testing or exercise participation, and patients should not be denied participation simply on the basis of their not undergoing pre-entry exercise testing. Information regarding exercise prescription for patients without exercise testing has been published and is described in chapter 8 (see page 117).[370] Figure 6.3 outlines the contraindications to exercise testing.

Safety and Personnel

Exercise is associated with an increased risk of a CV event. For patients with CAD, the risk of an adverse event during exercise testing is 60-100 times greater than during usual activity, and risk is higher in those who are post-MI or with malignant arrhythmias.[223,561] However, the safety of exercise testing is well documented and the overall risk of adverse events is quite low; both MI and death can be expected to occur at a rate of up to 1 per 2,500 tests.[223,561] Patients with recent MI, reduced left ventricular systolic function, exertion-induced myocardial ischemia, and serious ventricular arrhythmias are at highest risk.[189]

Central to the prevention of exercise-induced complications are appropriate screening and risk stratification of patients before they begin exercise. Though the risk of an event is greater in patients with CAD, clinical characteristics are associated with those patients at highest risk, as noted previously in figure 5.1 (see page 63). Matching the patient's medical history and clinical status to established contraindica-

Absolute

- Acute MI (within 2 d)
- High-risk unstable angina
- Uncontrolled cardiac arrhythmias causing symptoms or hemodynamic compromise
- Active endocarditis
- Symptomatic severe aortic stenosis
- Decompensated symptomatic heart failure
- Acute pulmonary embolus or pulmonary infarction
- Acute noncardiac disorder that may affect exercise performance or be aggravated by exercise (e.g., infection, renal failure, thyrotoxicosis)
- Relative acute myocarditis or pericarditis
- Physical disability that would preclude safe and adequate test performance
- Inability to obtain consent

Relative

- Left main coronary stenosis or its equivalent
- Moderate stenotic valvular heart disease
- Electrolyte abnormalities
- Tachyarrhythmias or bradyarrhythmias
- Atrial fibrillation with uncontrolled ventricular rate
- Hypertrophic cardiomyopathy
- Mental impairment leading to inability to cooperate
- High-degree atrioventricular block
- Severe arterial hypertension (systolic BP >200 mmHg and diastolic BP >110 mmHg)

Contraindications can be superseded if benefits outweigh risks of exercise.

Figure 6.3 Absolute and relative contraindications to exercise testing.

tions to exercise and the use of the physical activity readiness questionnaire (PAR-Q) (see figure 6.4), or a modified version of it, should be incorporated into the assessment protocol before the patient gives informed consent and prepares for testing.[189,559] The PAR-Q was designed for use as a general screening tool for patients without CVD, but the seven screening questions are relevant and useful for evaluating cardiac patients. Because many CR programs include primary prevention fitness components within the range of services, the PAR-Q is provided in its entirety.

Before preparing for the exercise test, the patient must give informed consent. An example of a consent form is found in appendix C. The patient should have ample time to read the form prior to testing, and a staff person should ask if the patient has any questions about the consent form or the test procedures and provide satisfactory explanations before proceeding.

Finally, although available research suggests a relatively low risk of patient complications during

exercise testing (and training), maintenance of appropriate emergency equipment, establishment of a workable emergency plan, and regular practice of the plan (with critiques) are fundamental to any contemporary program. Chapter 11 describes the important considerations in managing emergency situations.

The AHA has delineated the degree of exercise-testing supervision required.[440] The level of supervision depends primarily on the type of patients being tested. For patients who are at higher risk (e.g., those with recent MI, heart failure, arrhythmia), a physician must directly monitor the test. In other cases, properly trained exercise physiologists, nurses, physical therapists, and physician assistants can conduct the test and directly monitor patient status throughout testing and recovery, provided there is evidence of training and appropriate credentials. The supervising physician must be available to respond immediately, however. The ACC and the AHA have outlined competencies for supervision of stress tests.[477] For nonphysicians, certification in

PAR-Q & YOU

(A Questionnaire for People Aged 15 to 69)

Regular physical activity is fun and healthy, and increasingly more people are starting to become more active every day. Being more active is very safe for most people. However, some people should check with their doctor before they start becoming much more physically active.

If you are planning to become much more physically active than you are now, start by answering the seven questions in the box below. If you are between the ages of 15 and 69, the PAR-Q will tell you if you should check with your doctor before you start. If you are over 69 years of age, and you are not used to being very active, check with your doctor.

Common sense is your best guide when you answer these questions. Please read the questions carefully and answer each one honestly: check YES or NO.

YES	NO	
❑	❑	1. Has your doctor ever said that you have a heart condition <u>and</u> that you should only do physical activity recommended by a doctor?
❑	❑	2. Do you feel pain in your chest when you do physical activity?
❑	❑	3. In the past month, have you had chest pain when you were not doing physical activity?
❑	❑	4. Do you lose your balance because of dizziness or do you ever lose consciousness?
❑	❑	5. Do you have a bone or joint problem (for example, back, knee or hip) that could be made worse by a change in your physical activity?
❑	❑	6. Is your doctor currently prescribing drugs (for example, water pills) for your blood pressure or heart condition?
❑	❑	7. Do you know of <u>any other reason</u> why you should not do physical activity?

If

you

answered

YES to one or more questions

Talk with your doctor by phone or in person BEFORE you start becoming much more physically active or BEFORE you have a fitness appraisal. Tell your doctor about the PAR-Q and which questions you answered YES.

- You may be able to do any activity you want — as long as you start slowly and build up gradually. Or, you may need to restrict your activities to those which are safe for you. Talk with your doctor about the kinds of activities you wish to participate in and follow his/her advice.
- Find out which community programs are safe and helpful for you.

NO to all questions

If you answered NO honestly to <u>all</u> PAR-Q questions, you can be reasonably sure that you can:

- start becoming much more physically active – begin slowly and build up gradually. This is the safest and easiest way to go.
- take part in a fitness appraisal – this is an excellent way to determine your basic fitness so that you can plan the best way for you to live actively. It is also highly recommended that you have your blood pressure evaluated. If your reading is over 144/94, talk with your doctor before you start becoming much more physically active.

DELAY BECOMING MUCH MORE ACTIVE:

- if you are not feeling well because of a temporary illness such as a cold or a fever – wait until you feel better; or
- if you are or may be pregnant – talk to your doctor before you start becoming more active.

PLEASE NOTE: If your health changes so that you then answer YES to any of the above questions, tell your fitness or health professional. Ask whether you should change your physical activity plan.

<u>Informed Use of the PAR-Q:</u> The Canadian Society for Exercise Physiology, Health Canada, and their agents assume no liability for persons who undertake physical activity, and if in doubt after completing this questionnaire, consult your doctor prior to physical activity.

No changes permitted. You are encouraged to photocopy the PAR-Q but only if you use the entire form.

NOTE: If the PAR-Q is being given to a person before he or she participates in a physical activity program or a fitness appraisal, this section may be used for legal or administrative purposes.

"I have read, understood and completed this questionnaire. Any questions I had were answered to my full satisfaction."

NAME _____

SIGNATURE _____ DATE _____

SIGNATURE OF PARENT _____ WITNESS _____
or GUARDIAN (for participants under the age of majority)

Note: This physical activity clearance is valid for a maximum of 12 months from the date it is completed and becomes invalid if your condition changes so that you would answer YES to any of the seven questions.

© Canadian Society for Exercise Physiology

Supported by: ■✦■ Health   Santé
Canada   Canada

Figure 6.4 PAR-Q physical activity readiness questionnaire.

Source: Physical Activity Readiness Questionnaire (PAR-Q) © 2002. Reprinted with permission from the Canadian Society for Exercise Physiology. http://www.csep.ca/forms.asp.

the clinical track by the American College of Sports Medicine (ACSM) provides evidence of competencies to supervise exercise testing.[195] In addition, the credentialing body for CV technology provides a cardiographic technician certification that encompasses not only exercise testing but also Holter monitoring and pacemaker evaluation.[110a] Successful completion of an advanced cardiac life support (ACLS) course is also recommended. The program's medical director must be responsible for ensuring the availability of the proper equipment and the staffing of the exercise laboratory, including establishing laboratory policies. The physician is further responsible for data interpretation and delivery of emergency care (including ACLS) according to established standards for clinical competence.[189,440,477]

Exercise-Test Protocols

Consideration of the specific outcomes desired should precede the exercise test, with appropriate adjustments made in the exercise-test protocol. Exercise tests may be submaximal or maximal relative to the patient's effort. In addition to common indications for stopping the exercise test (see figure 6.5), submaximal exercise testing has a predetermined endpoint often defined as a peak HR such as 120 bpm or 70% predicted maximum HR, or an arbitrary MET level,

such as 5 METs. Submaximal tests may be used prior to hospital discharge at 4 to 6 d after acute MI. This low-level test provides sufficient data for evaluating the patient's ability to engage in ADL and serves as a baseline for early ambulatory exercise therapy. Test endpoints differ from those of symptom-limited exercise studies and are listed in figure 6.6. Conversely, symptom-limited tests are designed to continue until the patient demonstrates signs and symptoms that necessitate the termination of exercise.[223] Symptom-limited tests are usually selected when testing is performed more than 14 d after acute MI. Minimum required physiological and perceptual measurements to be collected before, during, and following exercise testing are described in figure 6.7. Even after acute MI, it may be desirable to perform a symptom-limited predischarge exercise test with selected subgroups of patients, such as younger, single-vessel-disease patients who have had an uneventful recovery, will be physically active, and need to return to work as soon as possible.

Although several exercise testing protocols are available for both treadmill and stationary-cycle ergometers, it is most important that the protocol be selected according to the individual patient's estimated functional capacity based on age, estimated physical fitness, and underlying disease.[189,195,223,400,421] Patients at risk or clearly deconditioned should

---

Absolute indications

- ST elevation (>1.0 mm) in leads without Q waves (other than V1 or aV$_R$)
- Drop in systolic BP of >10 mmHg (persistently below baseline) despite an increase in workload, when accompanied by any other evidence of ischemia
- Moderate to severe angina (grade 3-4). Figure 6.10 details descriptions and grades for angina scale
- Central nervous system symptoms (e.g., ataxia, dizziness, or near syncope)
- Signs of poor perfusion (cyanosis or pallor)
- Sustained ventricular tachycardia
- Technical difficulties monitoring the ECG or systolic BP
- Patient's request to stop
- Development of bundle branch block that cannot be distinguished from ventricular tachycardia

Relative indications

- ST or QRS changes such as excessive ST displacement (horizontal or downsloping of >2mm), or marked axis shift
- Drop in systolic BP of >10 mmHg (persistently below baseline) despite an increase in workload, in the absence of other evidence of ischemia
- Increasing chest pain
- Fatigue, shortness of breath, wheezing, leg cramps, or claudication
- Arrhythmias other than sustained ventricular tachycardia, including multifocal ectopic, ventricular pairs, supraventricular tachycardia, heart block, or bradyarrhythmias

Figure 6.5 Indications for terminating exercise testing.

- Any of the endpoints noted in figure 6.5
- Exercise HR in excess of peak HR observed in previous graded exercise test. If previous test was a hospital predischarge test, the HR should not exceed 130 bpm.
- Exercise workload in excess of peak workload observed in previous graded exercise test. If previous test was a hospital predischarge test, the exercise workload should not exceed 7 METs.
- RPE >15 (Borg 6-20 grade scale)

Figure 6.6 Submaximal exercise testing endpoints.

From Fletcher GF, Balady G, Froelicher VF, et al. Exercise standards, a statement for health professionals from the American Heart Association. AHA Medical/Scientific Statement. *Circulation* 1995;91:580-615.

Pretest measures
- Minimum of five minutes of rest before initial measures are taken
- Information consent
- Demonstration of equipment (as indicated)
- Definition of maximal effort or desired endpoint(s)
- Explanation of rating scales (use standardized instructions where available)
- 12-lead ECG in supine and in position of exercise
- Blood pressure in supine and in position of exercise
- Assessment of medications, when last taken, and current symptom status

Exercise measures
- 12-lead ECG during last minute of each stage
- Blood pressure and perceived exertion during last minute of each stage
- Other rating scales as appropriate

Post-test measures
- Minimum of six minutes in sitting or supine position, or until near baseline measures are reached. A period of active cool-down may be included in the six-minute recovery period; for functional (nondiagnostic) exercise tests a one-to-three-minute cool-down is recommended, depending on the level of exertion (additional time for heavier exertion) to minimize postexercise effects of venous pooling in the lower extremities.
- 12-lead ECG every minute
- Blood pressure immediately after exercise, then every one or two minutes until normotensive or near-baseline measures are reached.
- Symptomatic ratings each minute as long as they persist after exercise. Patients should be observed until all symptoms have subsided and the ECG is within acceptable limits, as determined by the supervising clinician.

Figure 6.7 Minimum requirements for measures assessed during exercise testing.

engage in a less-aggressive exercise protocol. Most exercise protocols are incremental in nature and are designed to permit the patient to achieve a physiological (HR, BP) steady state so that the relative CV responses (symptoms, ECG) at systematic workloads can be evaluated.

Medications

Although diagnostic exercise tests typically are performed with medications withheld to better assess any underlying ischemic response, functional testing generally should occur with the patient taking medications on the usual schedule. If at all possible, each patient should undergo the functional exercise test at a consistent time following medication ingestion at about the same time of day, preferably when he or she normally exercises.

Modality for Exercise Testing

Treadmill and cycle ergometer testing protocols are summarized in figure 6.8 and table 6.1. Treadmill and cycle ergometers may employ stepped or continu-

Figure 6.8 — Frequently used exercise test protocols.

Functional class	Clinical status	O₂ cost $mL \times kg^{-1} \times min^{-1}$	METs	Bicycle ergometer (1 Watt = 6 KPM/min; For 70 KG body weight KPM/min)	Bruce 3 min stages MPH / %GR	Kattus MPH / %GR	Balke-Ware %Grade at 3.3 MPH, 1 min stages	Ellestad MPH / %GR	USAFSAM MPH / %GR	"Slow" USAFSAM MPH / %GR	McHenry MPH / %GR	Stanford % Grade at 3 MPH	Stanford % Grade at 2 MPH	METs
Normal and I (Healthy, dependent on age, activity)		56.0	16		5.5 / 20		26	6 / 15						16
		52.5	15		5.0 / 18		25		3.3 / 25					15
		49.0	14	1500		4 / 22	24 / 23 / 22 / 21	5 / 15						14
		45.5	13		4.2 / 16		20		3.3 / 20		3.3 / 21			13
		42.0	12	1350		4 / 18	19 / 18	5 / 10			3.3 / 18	22.5		12
		38.5	11	1200		4 / 14	17 / 16		3.3 / 15		3.3 / 15	20.0		11
	(Sedentary healthy)	35.0	10	1050	3.4 / 14	4 / 10	15 / 14			2 / 25		17.5		10
		31.5	9	900			13 / 12	4 / 10	3.3 / 10			15.0		9
		28.0	8	750			11	3 / 10		2 / 20	3.3 / 12	12.5		8
	(Limited)	24.5	7		2.5 / 12	3 / 10	10 / 9	1.7 / 10	3.3 / 5	2 / 15	3.3 / 9	10.0	17.5	7
		21.0	6	600		2 / 10	8			2 / 10	3.3 / 6	7.5	14	6
II		17.5	5	450	1.7 / 10		7 / 6		3.3 / 0	2 / 5		5.0	10.5	5
III	(Symptomatic)	14.0	4	300	1.7 / 5		5 / 4					2.5	7	4
		10.5	3		1.7 / 0		3		2.0 / 0	2 / 0	2.0 / 3	0.0	3.5	3
IV		7.0	2	150			2 / 1		2.0 / 0					2
		3.5	1											1

Reprinted, by permission, from American College of Sports Medicine, 2000, ACSM's guidelines for graded exercise testing and prescription, 6th ed. (Phildelphia: Lippincott, Williams & Wilkins), 98.

Table 6.1 Approximate MET Loads During Cycle Ergometer Assessments

Body weight		Exercise rate (kg · m · min⁻¹ and watts)						
kg	lb	Kpms 300 Watts 50	450 75	600 100	750 125	900 150	1050 175	1200 200
50	110	5.1	6.9	8.6	10.3	12.0	13.7	15.4
60	132	4.3	5.7	7.1	8.6	10.0	11.4	12.9
70	154	3.7	4.9	6.1	7.3	8.6	9.8	11.0
80	176	3.2	4.3	5.4	6.4	7.5	8.6	9.6
90	198	2.9	3.8	4.8	5.7	6.7	7.6	8.6
100	220	2.6	3.4	4.3	5.1	6.0	6.9	7.7

Oxygen uptake ($\dot{V}O_2$) for zero load pedaling is approximately 550 mL × min⁻¹ for subjects weighing 70-80 kg (155-177 lb).

Kpm = kilopond-meter.

Reprinted, by permission, from American College of Sports Medicine, 1991, *ACSM's guidelines for exercise testing and prescription,* 4th ed. (Philadelphia: Lippincott, Williams & Wilkins), 91.

ous ramp protocols. Work-rate increments during stepped protocols can vary from 1 to 2.5 METs (1 MET = 3.5 ml O_2 × kg⁻¹ × min⁻¹ oxygen uptake), whereas those of ramped protocols are less abrupt. Treadmill testing provides a more common form of physiological stress (i.e., walking) in which subjects are more likely to attain a higher oxygen uptake and peak HR. Cycling may be preferable when orthopedic or other specific patient characteristics limit treadmill testing, although it may not necessarily result in significantly greater work rates compared to treadmill testing because of the patient's level of deconditioning. The most frequently used treadmill protocols are the Bruce, the modified Bruce, and the Naughton.[195,223] Ramp protocols are designed to increase gradually until the patient reaches exhaustion. The ramp treadmill or cycle ergometer protocols offer the advantage of steady increases in work rate, which may enhance patient comfort and offer a better estimation of functional capacity.[53,400] Although no standardized ramp protocol is yet widely used, table 6.2 provides a ramp protocol that can be used for patients with functional capacities of less than 12 METs.

The cycle ergometer is smaller, quieter, and less expensive than a treadmill. Because the cycle ergometer requires less movement of the arms and thorax, quality ECG recordings and BP measurements are easier to obtain. Stationary cycling may be unfamiliar to many patients, however, and its success as a testing tool is highly dependent on patient motivation. Thus, the test may end before the patient reaches a true cardiopulmonary endpoint. However, unlike treadmill testing, in which the patient walks unsup-

ported, cycle testing protocols are independent of weight because the seat supports the body weight. Thus, heavier patients may attain higher workloads with leg exercise when not having to support their body weight. The following suggestions are offered to assist in cycling protocol selection:

- Select a protocol appropriate to the patient's weight and fitness level.

- When using a mechanically braked ergometer, keep pedal rpm constant, such as a pedaling rate of 60 rpm.

- After a no-load warm-up of 1 to 2 min, use 25-watt or less (150-kilopond-meter [kpm]) increments for patients who are deconditioned or weigh less than 150 lb. Use 50-watt (300-kpm) increments for more fit or heavier patients.

- Set stages at a minimum of 2 min in duration, increasing the load by 25 watts or less as clinical judgment indicates.

Once the appropriate test equipment and protocol are selected, the exercise component of a symptom-limited exercise test should last approximately 8-12 min.[440] Low-level ramps or protocols that increase metabolic demand by 1 MET per stage are appropriate for high-risk patients with functional capacities of less than 7 METs; metabolic demands of greater than or equal to 2 METs per stage may be appropriate for low- to intermediate-risk patients with functional capacities equal to or greater than 7 METs. Similar considerations must be made when adjusting ramp

Table 6.2 Sample Ramping Protocol

Stage	Duration (sec)	Speed (mph)	Grade %	METs
Rest	Recovery	0.0	0.0	
1	30	1.5	1.5	2.4
2	30	1.6	2.0	2.6
3	30	1.7	2.5	2.9
4	30	1.8	3.0	3.1
5	30	1.9	3.5	3.3
6	30	2.0	4.0	3.6
7	30	2.1	4.5	3.9
8	30	2.2	5.0	4.2
9	30	2.3	5.5	4.5
10	30	2.4	6.0	4.8
11	30	2.5	6.5	5.1
12	30	2.6	7.0	5.5
13	30	2.7	7.5	5.8
14	30	2.8	8.0	6.2
15	30	2.9	8.5	6.5
16	30	3.0	9.0	7.0
17	30	3.1	9.5	7.4
18	30	3.2	10.0	7.8
19	30	3.3	10.5	8.2
20	30	3.4	11.0	8.7
21	30	3.5	11.5	9.2
22	30	3.6	12.0	9.6
23	30	3.7	12.5	10.1
24	30	3.8	13.0	10.6
25	30	3.9	13.5	11.1
26	30	4.0	14.0	11.5
27	30	4.1	14.5	12.0
28	30	4.2	15.0	12.4
29	30	4.3	15.5	12.8

rates. Smaller increments in MET requirements for each stage permit closer delineation of the ischemic or anginal threshold and result in a more accurate estimation of oxygen uptake at the corresponding work rate. The widely used Bruce treadmill protocol (2 to 3 METs per stage) is less effective in this regard.

During treadmill exercise, encourage patients to walk freely, using the handrails for balance only when necessary because excessive gripping alters the blood pressure response and decreases the oxygen requirement (METs) per given workload, resulting in an overestimation of exercise capacity and inaccurate HR- and BP-to-workload equivalents. Most patients will adapt quickly when instructed to lightly rest a finger or two from one hand on the handrail. Exercise capacity can be reasonably estimated for functional purposes from both treadmill or cycle workloads provided the equipment is calibrated regularly. When precise determination of oxygen consumption is necessary, such as in assessing patients for heart transplant, evaluation by expired gas analysis is preferred over estimation. Metabolic assessment is also useful for measuring baseline oxygen consumption and determining the ventilatory threshold for research or advanced clinical use.

Symptom Rating Scales

Before exercising, patients should be completely familiar with the various rating scales that may be used during testing. In addition to perceived exertion (figure 6.9), scales for angina, dyspnea, and claudication are noted in figures 6.10 and 6.11.

Exercise Testing With Ventilatory Gas Analysis

Ventilatory gas exchange analysis during exercise testing is a useful adjunctive tool in the assessment of patients with CVD.[223] Measures of gas exchange primarily include oxygen uptake ($\dot{V}O_2$), carbon dioxide output ($\dot{V}CO_2$), minute ventilation, and ventilatory anaerobic threshold. Oxygen uptake at peak exercise is considered to be the standard index of aerobic capacity and cardiorespiratory function. Such testing is appropriate to achieve the following results:

- Evaluation of functional capacity in selected patients with heart failure to assist in the estimation of prognosis and assess the need for cardiac transplantation

15-grade scale		Patient instructions:
6	No exertion at all	This is a scale for rating perceived exertion. Perceived exertion is the overall effort or distress of your body during exercise.
7	Extremely light	
8		The number 6 represents no perceived exertion or leg discomfort and 20 represents the greatest amount of exertion that you have ever experienced.
9	Very light	
10		At various times during the exercise test you will be asked to select a number that indicates your rating of perceived exertion at the time.
11	Light	
12		Do you have any questions?
13	Somewhat hard	
14		
15	Hard (heavy)	
16		
17	Very hard	
18		
19	Extremely hard	
20	Maximal exertion	

Borg RPE scale
©Gunnar Borg, 1970, 1985, 1994, 1998

Figure 6.9 Borg scales for rating perceived exertion.

Reprinted, by permission, from G. Borg, 1998, *Borg's perceived exertion and pain scales* (Champaign, IL: Human Kinetics), 47.

5-grade angina scale

0	No angina
1	Light, barely noticeable
2	Moderate, bothersome
3	Severe, very uncomfortable
4	Most pain ever experienced

5-grade dyspnea scale

0	No dyspnea
1	Mild, noticeable
2	Mild, some difficulty
3	Moderate difficulty, but can continue
4	Severe difficulty, cannot continue

10-grade angina/dyspnea scale

0	Nothing
0.5	Very, very slight
1	Very slight
2	Slight
3	Moderate
4	Somewhat severe
5	Severe
6	
7	Very severe
8	
9	
10	Very, very severe
	Maximal

Figure 6.10 Frequently used angina and dyspnea rating scales.

- Assistance in the differentiation of cardiac versus pulmonary limitations as a cause of exercise-induced dyspnea or impaired exercise capacity, when the etiology is uncertain

- Evaluation of the patient's response to specific therapeutic interventions in which the improvement of exercise tolerance is an important goal or endpoint

- A more precise determination of the intensity of exercise training through identification of the anaerobic threshold

Normal values for maximal oxygen uptake among healthy adults at different ages are available and may serve as a useful reference in the evaluation of an individual's exercise capacity.[189] Determination of exercise-training intensity to maintain or improve health

0	No claudication pain
1	Initial, minimal pain
2	Moderate, bothersome pain
3	Intense pain
4	Maximal pain, cannot continue

Figure 6.11 Intermittent claudication rating scale.

Adapted, by permission, from Association of Cardiovascular and Pulmonary Rehabilitation, 1995, *AACVPR guidelines for cardiac rehabilitation programs*, 2nd ed. (Champaign, IL: Human Kinetics), 32.

and fitness among individuals with or without heart disease can be derived from direct measurements of peak oxygen consumption (see page 116 in chapter 8). This may be most useful when the HR response to exercise is not a reliable indicator of exercise intensity (e.g., in patients with atrial fibrillation).

The technique of ventilatory gas measurement has a number of potential limitations that hinder its broad applicability. Gas exchange–measurement systems are costly and require meticulous maintenance and calibration for optimal use.[440] Personnel involved with test administration and interpretation must be trained and proficient in this technique. Finally, the test requires additional time as well as patient cooperation.

Diagnostic Utility

Exercise tests are important in the detection of ischemia for diagnostic and management purposes. Abnormalities in exercise capacity, HR, BP, and exercise ECG are important findings. Cardiac events are more likely to occur in patients with lower exercise capacities and those unable to achieve 85% of predicted maximal HR and those who exhibit exercise-induced hypotension.[341a] A poorer prognosis is also seen in patients who exhibit chronotropic incompetence and ventricular ectopy associated with exercise testing as well as abnormal heart rate recovery following exercise testing.[205a,217a,397a] The most common and useful ECG definition of a positive test is a horizontal or downsloping ST depression that is greater than or equal to 1 mm for at least 60 to 80 milliseconds after the end of the QRS complex.[223] The ECG findings must be interpreted in the context of clinical information regarding the patient's cardiac history and current symptoms. Clearly, exercise testing in people with documented CHD (prior MI or coronary angiogram demonstrating significant coronary stenosis) is not used for diagnosis, but rather for the detection of provocable ischemia, disease management, and estimation of prognosis. With patients for whom the diagnosis is in question, the description of symptoms can be most helpful. Typical angina can be defined as substernal chest discomfort (it may also begin in, or radiate into, the arms or jaw) that is provoked by exertion or emotional stress and is relieved by rest and nitroglycerin. Typical or definite angina, particularly in men older than 40 yr and women older than 60 yr, makes the pretest probability of disease so high that the test result does not dramatically change the probability.[223] Atypical angina is defined as chest discomfort that lacks one of the earlier-mentioned characteristics.[223] Unfortunately, it may also include discomfort other than in the chest, arms, or jaw and may include other symptoms such as shortness of breath, all of which serve to complicate the diagnosis. Symptoms of atypical angina generally indicate an intermediate pretest likelihood of coronary disease, particularly in men older than 30 yr and women older than 50 yr.[223]

Sensitivity is the percentage of patients with a disease (i.e., ≥70% lesion of at least one major coronary artery) who will have an abnormal test. *Specificity* is the percentage of patients free of disease who will have a normal test. The sensitivity and specificity of exercise ECG are each approximately 70%. However, those levels will be affected based on the subgroup of patients being evaluated.[152a] *Positive predictive value* of an abnormal test result is the percentage of persons with an abnormal test who have the disease, whereas the *negative predictive value* of a normal test result is the percentage of persons with a normal test who do not have the disease. It is important to understand that the positive and negative predictive values of the test are dependent on the prevalence of disease within the population being tested. Thus, evaluation of the pretest likelihood of disease allows for the most appropriate interpretation of the test results.[223] For example, an abnormal test result is more likely to be a true positive (high positive predictive value) in a 60-yr-old man with typical angina, and more likely to be a false positive (low positive predictive value) in a 25-yr-old woman with atypical symptoms.

Several other factors influence test interpretation. Failure to achieve 85% maximum predicted HR limits the estimation of post-test probability if no abnormalities are detected, because the patient has not reached a diagnostic level of stress from which sensitivity estimates have been derived. The presence of left bundle branch block, left ventricular hypertrophy with repolarization abnormalities, and resting ST segment depression (≥1 mm) and the use of digoxin therapy confound the interpretation of the exercise ECG. In such patients, exercise testing with either nuclear or echocardiographic imaging offers the advantage of greater sensitivity and specificity for the detection of CAD. In severely debilitated patients who are unable to perform an exercise test, pharmacologic testing has been used to evaluate ischemia. Unfortunately, the data from pharmacologic tests are not particularly useful in exercise prescription because hemodynamic and ischemic responses are not directly related to exercise effort. These tests are discussed later in this section.

Exercise Testing With Imaging Modalities

Cardiac imaging modalities are indicated when potential ECG changes are likely to be nondiagnostic, when it is important to determine the extent and distribution of ischemic myocardium, or to exclude or confirm a positive or negative exercise ECG. In addition, patients undergoing prognostic evaluation who have had prior revascularization also will benefit from exercise testing utilizing ECG or nuclear imaging.[24] Cardiac imaging with echocardiography before and after exercise can diagnose and localize the extent of myocardial ischemia. Radioactive agents are used to obtain cardiac perfusion scans at rest and with exercise.

Exercise Echocardiography

Echocardiography can be combined with exercise ECG in an attempt to increase the sensitivity and specificity of stress testing, as well as to determine the extent of myocardium at risk for ischemia. Echocardiographic images at rest are compared with those obtained while the patient bicycles or immediately after treadmill exercise. Images must be obtained within 1 to 2 min after exercise, because abnormal wall motion begins to normalize after this point.

Myocardial contractility normally increases with exercise, whereas ischemia causes hypokinesis, akinesis, or dyskinesis of the affected segments. Therefore, a test is considered positive when wall-motion abnormalities develop in previously normal areas with exercise or worsen in an already abnormal segment.[48] The overall sensitivity and specificity of exercise echocardiography range from 74% to 97% and 64% to 94%, respectively, with higher sensitivities in patients with multivessel disease.[120] Dependent on the patient subgroup studied, levels of specificity and sensitivity may vary greatly.[476a] Patients with a normal exercise echocardiogram have a low risk of future cardiac events, including revascularization procedures, MI, or cardiac death. Exercise echocardiography has been shown to be highly accurate in diagnosing CAD in patients in whom there may be an increased incidence of false-positive exercise ECG (e.g., women).[48,117] Stress echocardiography provides an accurate assessment of CAD and yields important diagnostic and prognostic information in the majority of patients.

Exercise Nuclear Imaging

Exercise tests with nuclear imaging are also performed with ECG monitoring. Thallium or sestamibi is injected 1 min before the end of exercise, and images are obtained. Rest images, taken before or after exercise depending on the nuclear agent used, are compared to exercise images to determine the areas of myocardial ischemia. Perfusion defects that are present during exercise but not seen at rest suggest ischemia. Perfusion defects that are present during exercise and persist at rest suggest previous MI or scar. In this manner, the extent and distribution of ischemic myocardium can be identified. The overall sensitivity and specificity of exercise nuclear imaging range from 83% to 89% and 70% to 88%, respectively.[356] Again, subgroup analyses will impact these levels of sensitivity and specificity.[391a]

Pharmacologic Stress Testing

Patients unable to undergo exercise stress testing for reasons such as deconditioning, peripheral arterial disease, orthopedic disability, neurological disease, or concomitant illness can often benefit from pharmacologic stress testing. Two of the most common tests are dobutamine stress echocardiography (DSE) and nuclear scintigraphy with dipyridamole or adenosine. Indications for these tests include establishing a diagnosis of CAD, determining myocardial viability prior to revascularization, assessing prognosis after MI or in chronic angina, and evaluating cardiac risk preoperatively.[444] Little information can be gained for the specifics of exercise prescription such as heart response or ischemic threshold in relationship to exercise. Pharmacologic studies can, however, provide information regarding ventricular function and the extent of myocardium that may become ischemic; thus they are useful in determining the level of risk stratification, particularly as it relates to the exercise program.

Dobutamine is a synthetic catecholamine and acts predominantly as a beta-1 agonist but also has some beta-2 and alpha-1 stimulatory effects. At lower doses, it increases cardiac output by causing an increase in contractility and HR. At higher doses, its principal effect is to bring about an increase in HR. Patients who have inadequate HR response to dobutamine may also receive an additional infusion of atropine to further stimulate HR response. As a result of the increased cardiac work, myocardial oxygen demand increases. If significant coronary artery stenoses are present, an oxygen supply-and-demand mismatch may occur, resulting in ischemia and abnormal wall motion.[638]

Dipyridamole and adenosine cause maximal coronary vasodilation in normal epicardial arteries, but not in stenotic segments. It has been suggested that as a result, a coronary steal phenomenon occurs, with a relatively increased flow to normal arteries and a relatively decreased flow to stenotic arteries. However, increased myocardial oxygen demand resulting from hypotension and reflex tachycardia, which unmasks a reduced endocardial myocardial blood flow, also has been indicated as a primary mechanism of vasodilator-induced regional dysfunction in CAD.[80a] Nuclear perfusion imaging under resting conditions is then compared with imaging obtained after coronary vasodilation.[584]

Alternative Opportunities for Evaluating Physical Activity Status

Several opportunities exist for the evaluation of physical activity status in addition to symptom-limited exercise testing. These include the submaximal exercise evaluation, a 6- or 12-min walk assessment, estimation of exercise tolerance from the clinician-patient interview and questionnaires, and controlled job simulation.

Submaximal Exercise Evaluations

Obtaining consistent data for comparison and for optimization of the exercise prescription is fundamental. The submaximal evaluation is a useful alternative to maximal exercise testing when assessing HR and BP responses to graded exercise, as, for example, when medications have been changed that are known to alter such responses (guideline 6.3). In patients who are clinically stable and have been participating regularly in a supervised program, submaximal assessments may be done with telemetry monitoring at the time of a regular exercise session using modest increases in treadmill or cycle ergometer intensity (e.g., increases at 3 min using 1-MET workload increases). In the event of previous abnormalities during exercise testing or training, the submaximal evaluation should be terminated below the point at which the abnormalities were observed. Additional recommendations for evaluation termination are presented in figures 6.5 and 6.6. Such testing should not be used to evaluate new symptoms or

Guideline 6.3 | Submaximal Assessment of Exercise Response

In the absence of routine clinical exercise testing, submaximal assessment of exercise response should be used to assess functional outcome and provide a mechanism for revision of the exercise prescription.

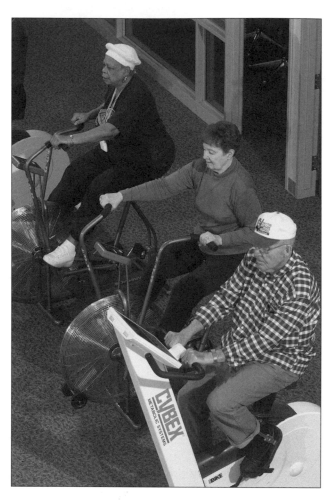

suspicious findings for a patient's current medical history. Patients must be actively enrolled in the supervised program, and such submaximal evaluations may be supervised only by staff designated by the medical director.

Six-Minute Walk Assessment

The 6- or 12-min walk assessment has been used with increased frequency in recent years, primarily as an objective measure of exercise tolerance in patients with lung disease, but also in low-functioning cardiac patients such as those with heart failure and in cardiac patients with a COPD comorbidity.[359a] In addition to collecting data during the assessment, a number of clinicians use this functional test to determine whether the patient is likely to tolerate a more-sophisticated exercise assessment. Given the increased frequency of use, standardization of the assessment is important. The 6-min walk assessment protocol is found in appendix D.[535]

Clinician-Patient Interview and Questionnaires

Although they are not a substitute for exercise testing, clinicians may obtain rough estimations of exercise tolerance by using MET activity tables and questioning patients about those activities that induce fatigue or symptoms.[10,401] In addition, a number of physical-activity surveys have been used to quantify activity.[334] The Duke Activity Status Index, the Functional Status Questionnaire, the Human Activity Profile, and the Specific Activity Scale are specific examples of such scales.[186,229,275,295]

Controlled Job Simulation

Data from an exercise test can be compared to readily available MET tables to assist in making recommendations for safe vocational and avocational activities.[10] However, mechanical efficiency, specific job-task requirements, and environmental and psychological stressors can substantially alter the responses measured in the laboratory.[189,198] Controlled laboratory simulation of physical tasks can aid physicians and employers in determining whether a patient can safely return to work.[612]

Summary

A careful evaluation of the patient's medical status and exercise testing results prior to participation in an outpatient CR and secondary prevention program is essential to identifying limitations to exercise participation, describing a patient's CVD progression risk-factor profile, and facilitating the development of patient and staff goals as they relate to expected outcomes. Recognizing the appropriate methodologies for accomplishing these objectives and understanding potential alternatives to the evaluation of physical activity status are keys to the success of the secondary prevention intervention program.

Education and Behavior Modification for Risk-Factor Management

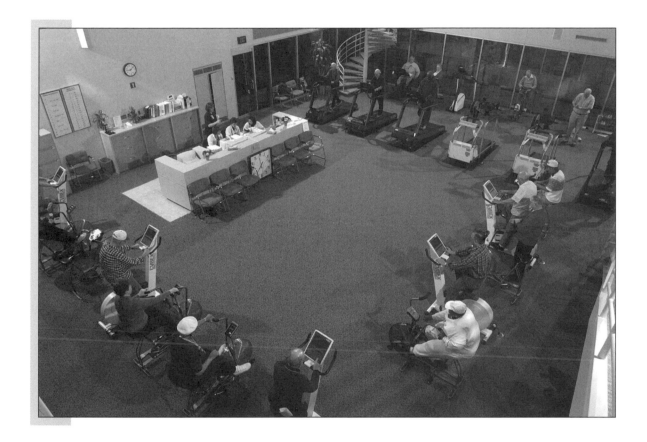

Research has clearly demonstrated that comprehensive risk-factor management can benefit cardiac patients. Risk-factor management benefits these patients in the following ways:

- It delays the progression of atherosclerosis (in some cases, leading to regression).
- It promotes plaque stabilization and prevents plaque rupture.
- It reduces the risk of reinfarction.
- It decreases the need for interventional procedures, such as CABGS and percutaneous transluminal coronary angioplasty (PTCA).

- It reduces hospitalizations for coronary disease.
- It improves quality of life.
- It reduces the risk of death.[141,495,511,600]

Despite these potential benefits, however, only one-third of coronary disease patients implement lifestyle changes that would enable them to reap these rewards. Many are never exposed to a truly comprehensive secondary prevention program either by choice, absence of referral, lack of access due to location or cost, or insufficient insurance reimbursement, or because the program they have

7

Education and Behavior Modification for Risk-Factor Management

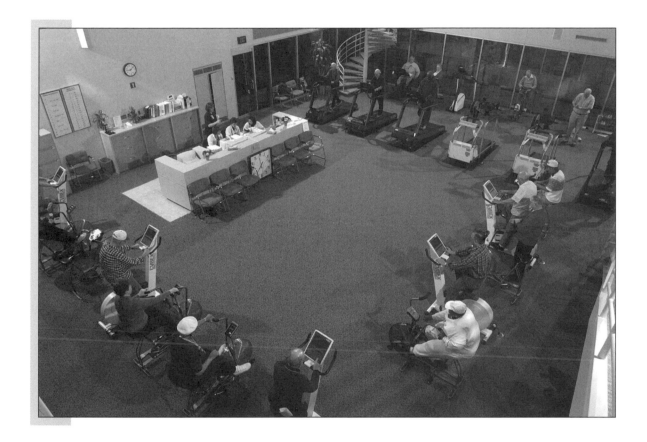

Research has clearly demonstrated that comprehensive risk-factor management can benefit cardiac patients. Risk-factor management benefits these patients in the following ways:

- It delays the progression of atherosclerosis (in some cases, leading to regression).
- It promotes plaque stabilization and prevents plaque rupture.
- It reduces the risk of reinfarction.
- It decreases the need for interventional procedures, such as CABGS and percutaneous transluminal coronary angioplasty (PTCA).

- It reduces hospitalizations for coronary disease.
- It improves quality of life.
- It reduces the risk of death.[141,495,511,600]

Despite these potential benefits, however, only one-third of coronary disease patients implement lifestyle changes that would enable them to reap these rewards. Many are never exposed to a truly comprehensive secondary prevention program either by choice, absence of referral, lack of access due to location or cost, or insufficient insurance reimbursement, or because the program they have selected is not comprehensive.[107] Among those patients who do participate in risk-factor modification programs, more than half discontinue changes within 1 yr.[518] Thus, it is vital that program professionals include assessments and interventions aimed at education and behavior modification for all cardiac risk factors and that they individualize treatment to accommodate the needs and preferences of the patient and his or her family (see guideline 7.1).

OBJECTIVES

This chapter reviews

- basic counseling skills,
- strategies for promoting patient independence,
- principles of adult learning and behavior modification,
- theories of social learning and readiness for change,
- inpatient and outpatient settings, and
- selection of educational materials.

Chapters 8 and 9 provide content to be included in individual risk-factor education and behavior-modification components.

Guideline 7.1   Education and Behavior Modification

To achieve an optimal program of education and behavior modification, program professionals should address the following points:

- Resources should be allocated to education and behavior modification for *all* modifiable risk factors.
- Plans for risk-factor modification using current clinical practice methodologies should be developed.
- Staff should be trained in health-counseling skills.
- A variety of strategies and materials should be employed to take into account the patient's and family's individual needs and preferences, culture, and spiritual beliefs.
- The program should foster patient independence.
- Resources should be allocated to facilitate transition to full independence postdischarge.
- The patient's potential for social isolation should be evaluated before discharge from the hospital.
- The program should include written teaching plans and documentation of progress toward goals.
- Smoking cessation should be addressed immediately on an inpatient basis.
- All risk factors, disease processes, management of cardiac emergencies, maintenance of psychosocial health, and adaptation to limitations should be addressed on an outpatient basis.

A plan for returning to work and the need for job retraining should be addressed, where appropriate, on an outpatient basis.

Basic Counseling Skills

Counseling skills are at the heart of any behavioral intervention because it is through interpersonal communication that professionals develop rapport and a sense of empathy with patients, obtain accurate assessments, help manage transient life crises, and ultimately facilitate change. Program professionals must therefore become aware of, develop, and incorporate the counseling skills discussed in this chapter into their practices.[127]

Nonverbal Communication

Nonverbal communication includes body movements, eye contact, voice inflections, changes in voice volume, facial expressions, body position, interpersonal distance, touch, and room and seating arrangements. Staff should be aware of any discrepancies that exist between nonverbal communication and verbal communication. For example, a patient who answers that he feels fine but expresses himself in a sad, low-energy tone is providing a mixed message. This is a clue to the skilled practitioner to investigate further. By the same token, patients sense practitioners' nonverbal communication clues and will respond to energy levels, voice inflections, and gestures. Eye contact is particularly important to convey a sense of interest in the patient. The way the room is arranged can be a subtle force as well. For example, individual counseling sessions might be better suited to a small space where patient and staff member sit diagonal to each another with only a corner of a table or desk between them. Conversely, group sessions are probably more effective when participants and staff are arranged in a circle so that everyone can see everyone else and discussion can flow freely. In either case, privacy and quiet are important contributors to the success of the interaction.

Active Listening

Staff can convey empathy and a desire to understand patients through *active listening*. Active listening refers to a variety of responses, including paraphrasing, reflection, clarification and probing, summary, and confrontation. All of these responses tell patients, "I hear you," and demonstrate a desire to comprehend. A brief description and example of each response follow.

■ **Paraphrase.** Paraphrasing means saying the same thing a patient has said but in a slightly different way. Example: "So people brought around food you really liked and you found it difficult to say 'no'," in response to a patient's statement, "I tried really hard to stay on the diet, but every morning someone came in with doughnuts or something, and I haven't lost a single pound."

■ **Reflection.** Staff can reflect a feeling or emotion that the patient's words convey. Example: "You sound pretty disappointed with your weight," in response to the patient's earlier statement.

■ **Clarification and probe.** The staff's response can clarify a patient's statement or probe for additional information. Example: "So, are you saying you haven't lost any weight at all?" in response to the patient's statement.

■ **Summary.** Summarize several statements or ideas and bring the patient back on track. Example: Staff might respond to a patient's somewhat rambling account of an episode of angina with this summary statement: "So you were having terrible chest pain and you took your nitro just like you were supposed to, but it didn't stop. So then you went to the hospital."

■ **Confrontation.** Staff can use gentle confrontation to help patients see discrepancies in their beliefs, thoughts, and actions. This technique should be used with caution and usually after a relationship has been established. Example: "You have told me how important it is for you to be alive and healthy so that you can watch your grandchildren grow up, but you are continuing to put yourself at risk by not taking your medication. I'm wondering what thoughts run through your head when you decide not to take your medication."

Encouraging Independence

Comprehensive secondary prevention programs typically provide staff-directed classes or support groups as the core of risk-factor interventions. These are often supplemented by individual counseling sessions and informal counseling and education during exercise sessions. Program staff must take care, however, not to inadvertently foster patients' dependence on staff to solve day-to-day challenges in lifestyle modification. To effect lifelong behavior change, programs must include techniques to promote patients' confidence in their own problem-solving abilities.

Foster independence by teaching and encouraging patients to develop strategies for self-learning, self-motivation, and social support external to the program and staff. A wide variety of strategies should be employed so that patients can choose those that meet their particular needs and preferences. Strategies might include providing supplemental audio-tapes, books, health magazines, computer programs,

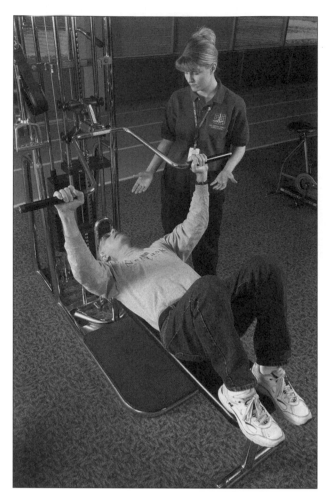

the benefits of the program. Staff should use e-mail with caution, however, in that typically it is not a secure mode of communication and therefore is not appropriate for relaying sensitive or confidential information.

Principles of Adult Learning

Adults bring a great deal of experience and knowledge with them to the rehabilitation program, and they are generally accustomed to having control over their environment. Thus, it serves rehabilitation staff well to incorporate the following principles of adult learning into the design and implementation of educational interventions.

- Readiness to learn is achieved when the learner is physically stable, has adequate energy, is emotionally stable, and is aware of the problem or need to learn.
- Adults learn only if and when they are ready to learn.
- Adults prefer to be self-directed, to participate in making decisions relative to their health and treatment, and to be actively involved in the learning process.
- Adults use their cumulative experience as a learning resource.
- Adults learn by problem solving and learn best in the immediate timeframe.[121,135]

Principles of Behavior Modification

Principles of behavior modification are derived from research on factors affecting behavior change. Because behavior change is necessary to modify cardiac risk, these principles should be incorporated into cardiac rehabilitation interventions. The following is a general summary of these principles.

Goal Setting

Staff should work with patients to set specific, realistic, measurable goals for both the long and short term. A long-term goal might be, "I will eventually walk five days a week for 30 minutes," whereas a short-term goal might be, "This month I will walk three days a week for 10 minutes." It is important that the short-term goals be achievable so that the patient can experience success and avoid undue discomfort. By setting achievable short-term goals

and Web sites and inviting guest teachers (who offer classes in the community) to give demonstrations or presentations as part of the rehabilitation program or support group. Though it may not be possible to include onsite all the strategies mentioned, many can be recommended for patients to try offsite. In any case, from the beginning, the program should incorporate strategies that foster independence, and these should continue for the duration of patients' participation.

In addition to encouraging independence during the time the patient is actively participating in the program, staff should allocate resources to facilitate full independence from the program after discharge. One way to accomplish this transition is for staff to e-mail or make telephone calls to discharged patients at regular intervals (for example, every week for 1 month, every month for 3 months, and once at 12 months postdischarge) to offer additional support and encouragement and to ensure that patients are staying on track. Telephone calls or e-mail may also facilitate collection of outcome data, which can provide payers with important information about

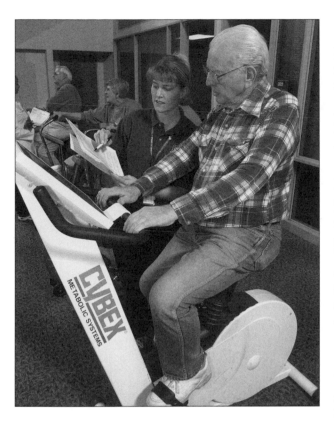

in small, gradually increasing steps, the patient can eventually attain his or her long-term goal. If the patient does not reach the short-term goals, patient and staff should reconsider and possibly reset them. One way of testing whether a particular goal is realistic is to ask the patient to rate on a scale of 0 to 100 how confident he or she is of achieving the goal. If a patient is more than 70% confident, then the goal is probably realistic. If the patient is less than 70% confident, the patient and staff may wish to consider a more achievable goal.[552]

If despite achieving behavioral goals a patient continues to be unable to reach clinical outcomes (for example, LDL <100 mg/dL, BP <140/90 mmHg, fasting blood sugar [FBS] <126 mg/dL), staff should discuss the situation with other members of the team. The patient's rehabilitation case manager and referring physician may need to discuss initiating, adjusting, or changing an intervention in such instances.

Contracts and Agreements

A written contract between the patient and a staff member, family member, or friend, with goals clearly stated, can increase the patient's commitment to the behavior-change process. Similarly, agreements between staff and patient outlining what each will contribute to the process can also be helpful.

Feedback

Patients need feedback on progress to maintain the motivation they need to continue the behavior. Thus, it is important to schedule regular measurements (such as lipids, BP, weight, dietary intake, etc.) and provide clear and timely feedback. Graphs are particularly helpful in providing patients with information regarding their progress over time.

Self-Monitoring

Patients should be taught how to monitor their behaviors with written records, logs, or diaries. The record serves not only as a prompt to perform the desired behavior but also as a way of measuring compliance as well as a means for providing feedback on performance. Records, logs, or diaries should be simple and easy to use and, whenever possible, easy to carry in a pocket or wallet.

Prompts

When a patient is unaccustomed to a new behavior, prompts can be particularly helpful reminders. Prompts can be as simple as a log on the refrigerator or a note on a calendar, or they can take the form of telephone calls or e-mails from staff, friends, or family.

Rewards

When patients have achieved their short- or long-term goals, they should be rewarded. Rewards need not be expensive or fancy, and they certainly should not be unhealthy. Appropriate rewards include praise, seeing a movie, or getting a favorite book, and inappropriate rewards include having an ice cream sundae, a beer, or a cigar. When the behavior itself can be reinforcing (for example, when the exercise is swimming and the patient enjoys swimming very much regardless of the health benefits), it is more likely that the patient will maintain the behavior. For this reason, it is important to attempt to find behavior types, times, and situations that patients find appealing.

Social Support

Social support from staff, family, and friends is a critical component in any behavior-change process. Staff can encourage social support by allowing spouses or friends to participate actively in the program, by instituting a buddy system for patients, or by providing patients with each other's phone numbers or e-mail addresses (with their

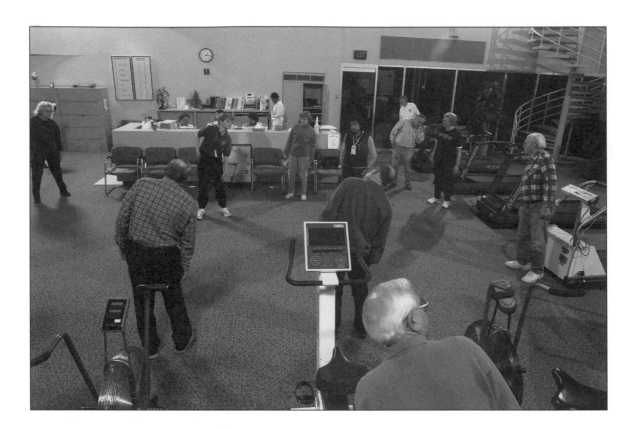

permission, of course). Two national organizations, Mended Hearts (www.mendedhearts.org) and the National Coalition for Women with Heart Disease (www.womenheart.org), also can provide a strong social-support network.

Social Learning Theory

Social learning theory postulates that human behavior develops through the interaction of behavioral, cognitive, and environmental systems and that behavior change results when the patient believes that he or she can perform that behavior.[59,60,123,225] This belief, known as self-efficacy, can be estimated in a fashion similar to that used with goal setting by asking patients to rate on a scale of 1 to 100 how confident they are that they can make a specific behavior change. It has been observed that if confidence levels are greater than 70%, the behavior-change process often goes smoothly, but that problems can be expected at lower confidence levels.[390] This type of ballpark assessment can be useful in determining how to allocate resources and how much support from the family the patient might need. Self-efficacy can be influenced by persuasion from an authority figure, observation and modeling, successful performance, and physiological feedback.[61] The following are descriptions and

examples of how rehabilitation staff can incorporate these factors into their interventions.

Persuasion by Authority

Patients respond to consistent and repeated verbal instructions and explanations of the need for specific behavior changes from multiple sources, particularly from health care professionals. Messages should be simple and firm. For example, "You need to work on lowering your LDL to less than 100" will probably be more persuasive than "You might want to think about lowering your cholesterol." Program professionals should make sure that all members of the team, including the primary care physician, are providing similar messages to the patient and delivering them consistently and repeatedly. Also, some patients learn well by reading newsletters or viewing Web sites authored by reputable health care sources. Providing those who desire more information with resources can support the educational efforts.

Observation and Role Models

Patients learn from watching what others do, particularly those in similar situations, and model those they most admire. Thus, it is extremely important for program staff to model heart-healthy behavior themselves. Role models can also be provided through videotapes, guest speakers, or other patients who have been successful in making changes.

Successful Performance

Experiencing success in performing a particular behavior makes that behavior much easier to perform the next time. Conversely, failures, including those in the near or distant past, can be barriers to the behavior-change process. For this reason, it is crucial that rehabilitation professionals inquire about previous experiences with specific behavior changes and address the issues that led to past failures so that they can be avoided. Additionally, to ensure successful performance, encourage the patient to set realistic goals and to make changes in small, achievable steps toward lifestyle changes. For example, the program professional might help a patient set a short-term goal of taking three deep abdominal breaths per day after lunch rather than asking the patient immediately to perform full-body progressive muscle relaxation on a daily basis.

Physiological Feedback

The patient's perception of the physical or psychological effects of a particular behavior change can enable or disable the change process. For example, muscle soreness and discomfort can deter a patient from continuing to exercise, whereas feeling more flexible and energetic is more likely to motivate a patient to continue exercising. Similar perceptions may occur with other interventions such as heart rate response to exertion or the physical or emotional responses to smoking cessation. Staff members who serve as health educators must suggest methods to aid patients in their ability to understand the immediate and long-term physical or psychological effects of specific interventions or changes in behavior. Education to alert patients of these potential effects is critical to the success of behavior modification.

Readiness-for-Change Theory

Stages of patients' readiness for change have been identified as the following:

- Precontemplation stage—the patient is not seriously considering making a change

- Contemplation stage—the patient has begun to consider the idea of making a change

- Preparation and action stage—the patient has taken the first steps toward making a change

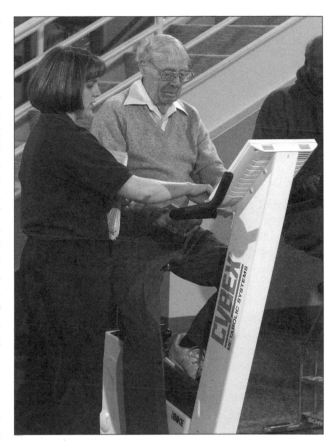

- Maintenance stage—the patient has maintained a change for 6 months or more[449]

It is critical that the program staff assess where the patient falls within this scheme, because educational and behavioral strategies should vary accordingly. The answers to a few straightforward questions, such as the following, will usually provide a reasonable estimate:

- Is the patient already performing the desired behavior regularly? If so, for how long has he or she been performing it?

- Has the patient made any steps toward changing?

- Is the patient considering making the behavior change?

If the answer is "yes" to the first question and the patient has been performing the desired behavior for 6 months or more, the patient is already in the maintenance stage. A patient who has been performing the behavior for less than 6 months and has made steps toward changing would fall into the preparation and action stage. A patient who is seriously considering making the change would fall into the contemplation stage. A patient answering "no" to all three of the questions would fall into the precontemplation stage.

Once determined, the stage can guide the professional in choosing appropriate strategies. However, program staff should be aware that patients can move quickly and unexpectedly forward or backward on this continuum due to influences within and outside the rehabilitation program.

Precontemplation

At the precontemplation stage, when patients may have little or no interest in changing, repeated, gentle confrontation from multiple sources may be helpful. One way to accomplish this is to ask the patient's physician to discuss at every office visit the importance of a certain behavior change. It is important to keep in mind that confrontation is most effective when the topic is personally relevant. For example, a patient is more likely to respond positively to a statement such as "Lowering your LDL can help you avoid having a second heart attack and to be able to spend more time with your grandchildren" than "It is important for you to lower your LDL." Some other sources that might help patients move to the next stage include bulletin boards, brochures, books, newsletters, videotapes, personal experiences, newspaper articles, television shows, guest speakers, and other positive role models.

Contemplation

In the contemplation stage, interventions should be aimed at providing information in the form of written materials, videotapes, role models, and so on. Discussions with the patient regarding the particular behavior should include an appeal to whatever seems to be a motivating force for that person. Common examples include a desire to be slim, to be able to engage in a favorite recreational activity (e.g., golf, hunting), or to perform a valued service (e.g., cutting grass, bringing in groceries). In addition, at this stage a cost-benefit analysis is often quite useful. Accomplish this by helping the patient write down all the "costs" (negative consequences) and "benefits" (positive consequences) of making a particular change (for example, having to give up french fries to follow a low-fat diet on the cost side, and feeling less bloated on the benefit side). Program staff should be aware that most patients will need help listing immediate benefits. However, this is probably staff time well spent in that unless the patient is able to see that the short- and long-term benefits truly outweigh the costs, he or she is unlikely to conclude that the behavior is worth changing. Once this cost-benefit list

is developed, it is useful to have the patient keep this list for future reference during difficult times.

Preparation and Action

Most interventions are designed for the preparation and action stage. This is the skills-building stage when staff and patients begin setting goals, implementing plans of action, tracking systems, giving rewards, and practicing actual behaviors. Building in social support for the behavior is an important consideration at this stage as well.

Maintenance

The maintenance stage is, of course, the stage that is the longest, the most important, and the most difficult to sustain. Patients and staff should emphasize problem-solving skills in this stage to ensure that the patient can handle novel or difficult situations, for example, how to maintain a low-fat diet in an Italian restaurant. The concept of lapse versus relapse should also be discussed. The patient should understand that a lapse (temporary discontinuation of a behavior) does not necessarily lead to a relapse (long-term

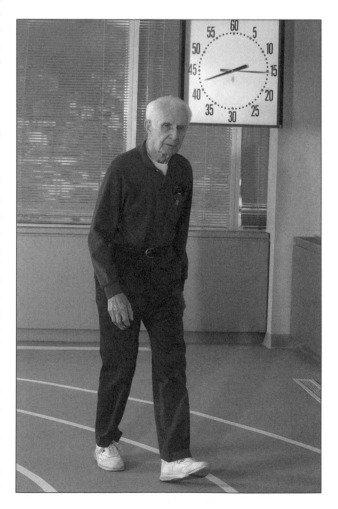

discontinuation of the behavior). Program staff and patients should discuss situations in which the patient is most at risk for lapse and develop a coping strategy or plan of action for those particular situations to prevent relapse (for example, a telephone number to call or a card to take out and read that prompts the patient not to let the lapse become a relapse). In addition, because stress is a common reason for lapse and relapse, it is important to include relaxation training and stress management at this stage. Finally, the patient should be encouraged to take ownership of and responsibility for his or her actions so that the behavior change can be maintained after discharge from the program and sustained indefinitely. Family and friends should be enlisted to provide social support outside the program for this reason as well.

Inpatient Interventions

The highest priority in the inpatient setting is meeting the immediate needs of the patient and his or her family.[489] With the exception of smoking, risk-factor education is generally not the highest priority. Smoking is an exception in part because of its critical impact on CVD and in part because research has demonstrated that efforts at smoking cessation initiated in the hospital setting are more successful than those initiated postdischarge (see page 98 in chapter 8).[555]

Outpatient Interventions

Educational interventions should be aimed at

- improving cardiac risk (through a low-fat diet, BP management, lipid management, smoking cessation, diabetes management, and stress management);
- managing cardiac emergencies (such as angina, possible heart attack, or pain or discomfort during exercise);
- understanding the disease process (atherosclerosis, high BP, diabetes);
- maintaining psychosocial health (addressing sexual function, social relationships, depression, anger, hostility); and
- adapting to limitations imposed by the disease process (changing roles in the family, jobs at work, hobbies and recreational activities).

Education and behavior-modification content can be delivered individually, in group settings, or

through in-home programs with telephone or Internet-based monitoring and follow-up, depending on the needs and preferences of the patient and his or her family. Controlled studies have shown that home-based programs using books, audiotapes, videotapes, computers, CD-ROMs, and interactive computer programs can be effective options for improving patient access to information. Telephone monitoring and immediate feedback, with clinic visits once every 1 to 2 months for evaluation and follow-up, have demonstrated excellent success.[553] Regardless of the type of delivery, all programs should have written plans for providing education and behavior-modification services and a method for documenting implementation and patient progress.

Selecting and Developing Educational Materials

Patient and family instructive materials should be

- consistent with national guidelines,
- developed by health care professionals,

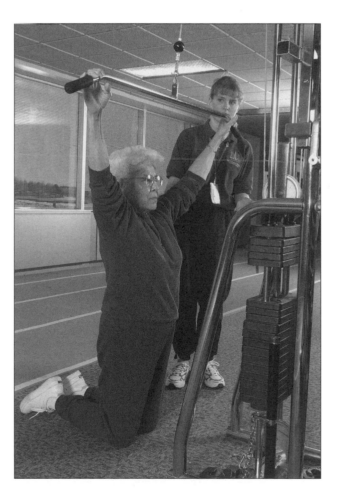

- developed from behavior and education programs with documented success,
- reviewed and commented on by patients and families, and
- approved by the appropriate institutional administrative structure.

In all cases, local, regional, and national consensus information should provide the foundation for recommended behaviors. Additionally, staff should tailor materials to the individual needs and preferences of the patient and his or her family. Thus, in selecting and developing materials, staff should take the following factors into consideration.

Reading Level of the Patient and Family

Program staff should keep in mind that the average reading level in the United States is grade seven, and that one in seven adults reads below a fourth-grade level, with some being illiterate.[423] Research has shown that many cardiac patient-education materials are written at or above the college reading level. If these materials are used, technical words should be reviewed separately with patients to reduce their anxiety and improve comprehension. Elderly patients generally find materials with large print on nonglossy paper more readable.

Language and Culture

Some patients do not speak English, or English is a second language for them. For this reason, it is helpful to have some materials in other languages, appropriate to the community. Many publishers and pharmaceutical companies can readily supply these types of materials. The AHA and other producers of educational materials have translated their products into the Spanish and Chinese languages. Much more attention needs to be directed to these efforts.

Computer-Aided Instruction

Secondary prevention programs may also benefit from using computer-assisted instruction (CAI) to supplement printed educational materials and group-based instruction. CAI in the form of multimedia CD-ROMs has been shown to be as effective as, if not more effective than, traditional educational materials and classes in areas such as hypertension, asthma, and diabetes.[125,353] In addition to their effectiveness, these innovative teaching materials and techniques also save valuable staff time. Similarly, the Internet offers a wide variety of health-education sites. However, staff should caution and instruct patients regarding the selection of Web sites that provide accurate information. As patient acceptance of these new learning modalities increases, programs should incorporate them both onsite, using computers at the program, and offsite, by recommending CD-ROMs and Internet sites for use at home.

Summary

The process of modifying risk of future events of morbidity and mortality in patients with CHD is complex and not without individual successes and challenges. In most instances, it is the modification of behavior, through education and psychosocial-focused interventions, that can create an environment for risk reduction. All rehabilitation staff attempting to modify behavior in both inpatient and outpatient settings should consider employing the principles of basic counseling skills and adult and social learning theories. Program staff should individualize interventions through careful selection of education materials and counseling approaches, being mindful of the variety of patient learning, cultures and languages, and social skills.

Modifiable Cardiovascular Disease Risk Factors

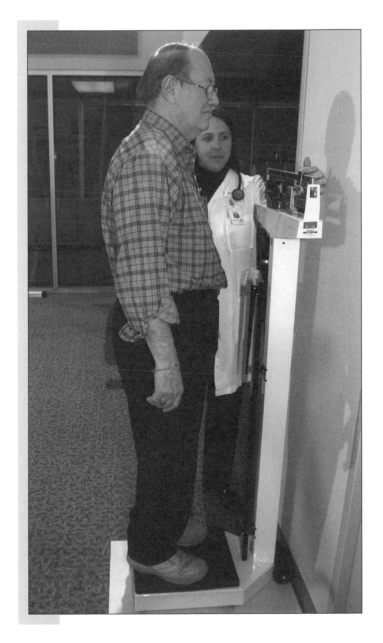

A comprehensive approach to CVD risk-factor management is essential to the secondary prevention efforts applied through CR programming.

This chapter describes the basis for assessment and intervention strategies related to modifiable CVD risk factors.

OBJECTIVES

This chapter describes the basic assessment and intervention strategies for the following modifiable CVD risk factors:

- smoking,
- abnormal lipids levels,
- hypertension,
- physical inactivity,
- psychosocial concerns, and
- weight management.

Smoking

One in five deaths from CVD is attributable to smoking. Moreover, the global mortality from tobacco use is expected to climb from 3 million deaths in 1990 to 10 million in 2025.[31] Smoking is associated with an increased risk of CVD events in patients with established disease including recurrent MI, sudden death, and restenosis after coronary angioplasty.[214] As a result of the high rates of relapse upon cessation even weeks, months, and years after quitting, the U.S. Public Health Service Clinical Practice Guideline on Treating Tobacco Use and Dependence suggests that tobacco dependence must now be considered a chronic condition that requires repeated intervention (guideline 8.1).[185]

Guideline 8.1 — Evaluation of Tobacco Use

To reduce the risk associated with tobacco use, all health care professionals must take every opportunity to

- identify smokers in all practice settings, and
- provide an environment that facilitates repeated interventions.

Smoking causes numerous problems within the CV system. Nicotine, the most important by-product of smoking, promotes catecholamine release, increasing HR and BP and thus increasing myocardial oxygen demand. In addition, nicotine constricts peripheral arteries, interfering with blood flow to tissues; lowers the threshold for ventricular fibrillation; and increases platelet activation. Finally, nicotine causes adverse effects on the lipoprotein panel, decreasing HDL and increasing the oxygenation of LDL, promoting atherogenesis. Carbon monoxide, another by-product of smoking, injures vascular endothelium and interferes with the ability of red blood cells to carry oxygen, thus reducing the amount of oxygen delivered to the heart muscle.

The improved outcome associated with smoking cessation in those with CVD is apparent soon after quitting and in people of all age groups, including the elderly. For example, cessation is associated with a 25-50% reduction in overall mortality in those suffering an MI, with a 50% decline observed in the first year of quitting. Smoking cessation improves morbidity and mortality in those over the age of 70 who have undergone coronary surgery.

Assessment of Tobacco Use

The clinical practice guideline suggests that health care professionals take every opportunity to identify smokers in all practice settings.[185] Because numerous patients are identified for rehabilitation programs at the time of hospitalization, this setting serves as an important entryway for smoking-cessation intervention. Moreover, at the time of hospitalization, patients are focused on their health, experience the worst of withdrawal in the first 48-72 h of quitting, and are forced to follow hospital smoking bans. Thus, a mechanism for identifying all smokers at the time of hospitalization such as including smoking status as a vital sign or using chart or computer prompts is critically important for patient outcomes. In outpatient rehabilitation programs, health care professionals can identify smokers through the use of health-risk appraisals, intake forms that collect information about risk factors, or through interviews that are often part of taking a medical history. Due to the enforcement of hospital smoking bans, many smokers view themselves as having stopped smoking once they have entered the hospital. Therefore, it is critical that interviewers ask the appropriate question to identify smokers. The question "Have you smoked any tobacco products in the past 30 days?" is more specific than "Do you smoke tobacco products?"

Once patients have been screened, the next step in intervening is determining an individual's willingness to quit smoking. Staff members may simply ask, "Are you willing to quit smoking now?" or "Are you willing to make an attempt to quit smoking now?" The clinical practice guideline indicates that those patients who are willing to quit tobacco should be provided appropriate treatments (see *Intervention* section on page 98).[185] In addition, those who are unwilling to make an attempt to quit smoking should be offered a brief intervention designed to enhance their motivation. Enhancing motivation is accomplished by

- encouraging patients to indicate why quitting smoking is personally relevant to them,
- helping patients to identify the acute, long-term, and environmental risks associated with continued smoking,

- helping patients determine potential benefits of quitting by selecting personal rewards,
- identifying barriers or roadblocks to quitting, and
- repeating the intervention (motivational interview) as often as possible at every patient encounter (figure 8.1).

A key to remembering the structure of such an intervention is to focus on the five Rs:

- relevance,
- risks,
- rewards,
- roadblocks, and
- repetition.

For patients who are ready to make an attempt to quit smoking, additional information about their smoking status is helpful and allows individualized counseling. However, the clinical practice guideline also notes that smoking-cessation interventions should not depend solely on formal assessments referring to questionnaires, the clinical interview, or physiological measures such as carbon monoxide or pulmonary function measures to guide them.[185] These assessments do not consistently produce higher long-term quit rates than nontailored interventions of equal intensity. Thus, time allotted to undertake these assessments must be weighed against the time available for counseling and intervention.

A smoking history (see appendix E) may provide additional information useful for individualizing counseling about smoking. Documenting whether other household members smoke may help determine the patient's level of support and whether family members may also benefit from counseling. Determining a patient's past experience with

Relevance	Personalize why quitting is relevant (i.e., wishes of family members, health)
Risks	Ask patient to identify negative consequences of tobacco use
	• Acute risks: Shortness of breath, chest discomfort
	• Long-term risks: MI, stroke, chronic obstructive pulmonary disease (COPD)
	• Environmental: Respiratory infections in children, heart disease in spouses
Rewards	Ask patient to identify benefits of stopping smoking (e.g., improved symptoms, saving money, setting a good example for children)
Roadblocks	Ask patient to identify barriers to quitting (e.g., weight gain, depression, withdrawal symptoms)
Repetition	Repeat this intervention at every clinic visit or within any other setting

Figure 8.1 Motivational interview.

serious attempts to quit and length of cessation, success with previous smoking interventions, and previous use of pharmacological therapies can be helpful in planning an appropriate intervention. People with a history of depression have more difficulty quitting than those without such a history. Therefore, using standardized tools to measure depression as part of an evaluation of the patient's psychosocial status, or incorporating single-item measures such as the scale depicted in figure 8.2 that has been shown to correlate with other clinical measures of depression, can be useful in counseling.[556] Moreover, patients who are depressed are appropriate candidates for the use of buproprion SR to help them quit smoking.

Alcohol use is another important question to address when individualizing counseling for people attempting to quit smoking. Smokers who consume large amounts of alcohol or abuse alcohol find it difficult to quit. Success with quitting is extremely low, and little research has been conducted showing the efficacy of smoking interventions in this population. Confronting patients about inappropriate alcohol use may be necessary when intervening with them. Determining the frequency of use and weekly consumption, as well as screening for alcohol abuse, provides important insights useful for counseling. The CAGE questionnaire (see appendix F) is the most common screening tool for potential alcohol abuse.[174] A "yes" response to any of the questions may indicate potential alcohol abuse, and two or more positive responses increases the probability of past or present abuse. Questions found in the smoking history (appendix E) related to alcohol consumption are also useful in this regard. The frequent underreporting of alcohol use, and the cardiotoxic effects of high consumption in patients with CVD, require health care professionals to assess and openly discuss this issue.[324] Referral to an alcoholism-treatment program may be warranted.

Intervention

The clinical practice guideline highlights evidence from randomized controlled trials suggesting several key findings that are important when intervening with smokers:

- The more intense the treatment, the greater the rate of cessation.

- Treatment can be maximized by increasing the length of individual sessions to greater than 10 min and the number of treatment sessions to greater than or equal to 4 sessions ($\geq$30 min contact time).

- Use of multiple types of providers (physicians, nurses, pharmacists, etc.) enhances cessation rates.

- Proactive telephone calls and individual and group counseling are effective cessation formats.

- Practical counseling (problem solving and skills training) and use of social support significantly improves cessation outcomes.

- Pharmacological therapies increase cessation rates and should be encouraged for all quitters except where contraindications exist.

- Treatments are effective for diverse populations varied by age, gender, and ethnicity.[185]

Many of the preceding recommendations have been applied in helping cardiac patients to quit smoking.[413,473,555] In general, exercise training alone as part of rehabilitation has not been shown to improve smoking-cessation rates in this population. Although some of the highest rates of cessation have been noted in patients who suffer from CVD, specifically post-MI patients, smoking relapse rates continue to be as high as 50-65% following hospital discharge.[516,554] In addition, patients who suffer from CVD but do not sustain an event have lower rates of cessation.[388,555] Finally, because most smokers do not attend formal cessation programs, which often provide individuals with behavioral skills training over 10-12 weeks, offering education and reinforcement for quitting is important on an ongoing basis.

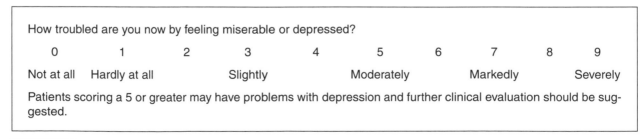

How troubled are you now by feeling miserable or depressed?

0	1	2	3	4	5	6	7	8	9
Not at all	Hardly at all		Slightly		Moderately		Markedly		Severely

Patients scoring a 5 or greater may have problems with depression and further clinical evaluation should be suggested.

Figure 8.2 Example of a single-item measure of psychological status.

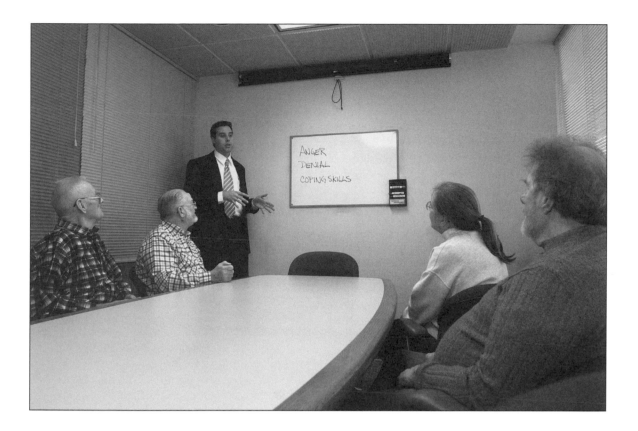

Because smokers move along a continuum from contemplation to preparation to action to quitting, numerous health care providers strongly reinforcing the message about the need to quit may help a patient to take action.[448] Physicians' advice to quit is extremely powerful, and rehabilitation specialists should not only encourage patients to quit but also cue physicians when available to provide the same strong message. Personalizing the message to include information about the smoking hazards related to the disease offers patients a greater understanding of the risks associated with continuing to smoke.

At a minimum all health care professionals involved in secondary prevention can help people to quit smoking by

- identifying them at every encounter;
- asking if they are willing to make an attempt to quit smoking (see *Assessment of Tobacco Use*);
- aiding the smoker in using interventions, including providing strong advice about the need to quit and self-help materials such as videotapes and pamphlets for those willing to quit and community resources for those unwilling to quit; and
- arranging for follow-up, either in person or via telephone.

In addition, rehabilitation specialists should provide behavioral counseling and monitor the effects of pharmacological therapies for those patients interested in quitting. An algorithm for patients who are smoking at the time of an encounter with a secondary prevention program is highlighted in appendix G. Due to the high risk of recurrent events, all patients who choose not to quit should also be offered follow-up. Contracting with them to limit the number of cigarettes they smoke each day, aggressively modifying other CVD risk factors, and ensuring that patients are well protected with other interventions known to affect prognosis, such as angiotensin-converting enzyme (ACE) inhibitors, antiplatelet agents, beta-blockers, statins, and antihypertensive medications, may improve overall survival and in time alter their perspective on quitting smoking.

A person who has not quit smoking but is interested in doing so will need help with cessation. Patients should set a quit date within 1 to 2 weeks of the encounter so that their commitment to cessation does not wane. They must also decide whether to quit "cold turkey" or use other methods, such as switching brands or decreasing the number of cigarettes smoked in the days before they quit. People may benefit from the use of pharmacological therapies such as buproprion SR in the weeks before they quit and during the initial period of abstinence (see

Pharmacological Therapy). Health care professionals can use this opportunity to review the smoking history, highlighting the most relevant items, such as success with previous attempts, availability of social support, use of alcohol, and problems that may have hindered past success. In addition, rehabilitation specialists should prepare individuals for their "quit day" by asking them to remove all ashtrays and tobacco products, informing family members of their intent to quit, and obtaining pharmacological therapies if they have not done so already.

For patients who have quit smoking during hospitalization, relapse-prevention counseling and other behavioral interventions, such as contracting, aid them. Relapse-prevention training has been used with great success for those with addictive behaviors such as excessive gambling, obesity, alcoholism, and smoking. Slips or lapses into the old behavior are common when a person gives up smoking, and they often relate to emotional states such as frustration, boredom, or depression; interpersonal conflict with family members, friends, or colleagues; or social pressure. Relapse-prevention interventions to help people cope involve

- helping individuals identify those high-risk situations likely to cause relapse;
- determining both behavioral and cognitive coping skills and practicing them through role rehearsal;
- using lifestyle changes such as relaxation, imagery, and exercise to support the quitting effort; and
- knowing what to do if a slip occurs.

In addition to the preceding, as noted in the algorithm, people also need counseling about

- potential weight gain,
- common withdrawal symptoms that may pose an important need for pharmacological therapy,
- the difficulty in quitting associated with alcohol use,
- integrating social support networks such as family members and friends to aid in quitting,
- the psychological craving associated with quitting that occurs through urges, and
- the psychological sense of loss associated with giving up cigarettes.[389]

Exercise through CR also helps individuals as they quit smoking by improving psychological well-being and minimizing weight gain and withdrawal symptoms. Thus, program professionals should encourage active participation in exercise rehabilitation. Self-help materials such as pamphlets, videotapes, and audiotapes developed by the AHA, American Lung Association, and the American Cancer Society should also be used to supplement counseling and to reinforce information provided by program specialists. An abundance of reputable Internet sites offer resources to help smokers through the early stages of quitting, to complement in-person counseling.

Pharmacological Therapy

The clinical practice guideline indicates that all patients should be encouraged to use pharmacological therapies for smoking cessation except in special circumstances.[185] Numerous studies now indicate a lack of association between the use of nicotine products and acute cardiovascular events.[76,305,359] Precautions with the use of nicotine-replacement products continue to exist for patients who are within 2 weeks of an MI, those with serious arrhythmias, and those with serious or worsening angina. However, with some patients, one must also weigh the risks associated with continued smoking, noting that the amount of nicotine is far greater in cigarettes than in nicotine-replacement products.

Presently, five first-line medications are indicated to help smokers in their attempts to quit. These include buproprion SR, nicotine gum, nicotine inhaler, nicotine nasal spray, and the nicotine patch. Personal preference and previous use can often guide the choice of which agent to use, because further research is needed to determine which agents are most efficacious in helping individuals to quit smoking. One should consider some important facts about the use of these agents, including the following: (1) 4 mg nicotine gum is more useful for highly dependent smokers than 2 mg gum; (2) buproprion SR has been especially helpful for those with a history of depression; and (3) pharmacological therapies (nicotine patch or gum and buproprion) have not been shown to prevent weight gain—it is simply delayed. Most patients benefit from the use of an agent for 8-12 weeks, with a small proportion needing therapy for 24 weeks. Rehabilitation specialists should offer appropriate education and counseling regarding the administration of these agents. Education can be reinforced through written instructions developed to support these pharmacological aids.

Follow-up carried out through visits, telephone contacts, and e-mail increase the success of smoking-cessation interventions. Studies suggest an increase in cessation rates when four or more contacts are used to follow up with CHD patients.[388,555] Telephone contacts may provide a convenient, effective method to provide positive reinforcement, to problem solve difficulties the patient encounters in quitting, and to help patients set another quit date if relapse has occurred. These telephone contacts are especially helpful in the early stages of quitting.

Abnormal Lipids

Approximately 50% of American adults have blood cholesterol levels of 200 mg/dL or higher. The prevalence of elevated serum cholesterol is similar for black and white men and women. However, black and white women over age 55 have demonstrated a higher prevalence of elevated cholesterol compared with men over 55.[31] Strong evidence supports the benefits of lowering serum cholesterol levels in patients with CHD, particularly among those who have suffered MI. Reductions in cardiovascular mortality, recurrent cardiac events, hospitalizations, and angiographic progression of atherosclerotic disease with cholesterol lowering have been demonstrated.[236,511,604] Benefits have also been shown in women and the elderly.[487] Unfortunately, however, evidence suggests that despite the measurable benefit associated with lowering cholesterol levels, many patients who have been identified as having CHD continue to exhibit elevated cholesterol levels.[16,108,342] The results of these studies justify aggressive cholesterol evaluation and management as early as possible in patients with known CHD (guideline 8.2).

Cholesterol is a fatlike substance (lipid) that is present in cell membranes and is a precursor of bile acids and steroid hormones. Cholesterol travels in the blood in distinct particles containing both lipid and proteins. These particles are called lipoproteins. The cholesterol level in the blood is determined partly by inheritance and partly by acquired factors such as diet, calorie balance, and level of physical activity.

Three major classes of lipoproteins are found in the blood: LDL, HDL, and very low density lipoprotein (VLDL). LDL typically contains 60-70% of the total serum cholesterol, and both are directly correlated with risk for CAD. HDL normally contains 20-30% of the total cholesterol, and HDL levels are inversely correlated with CHD risk. VLDL contains 10-15% of the total serum cholesterol along with most of the triglyceride in fasting serum. VLDL is a precursor of LDL and some forms of VLDL, particularly VLDL remnants, appear to be atherogenic.[403]

LDL cholesterol is estimated from measurements of total cholesterol, total fasting triglycerides, and HDL cholesterol. If the triglyceride value is below 400 mg/dL, then its value can be divided by 5 to estimate the VLDL-C level. Because the level of total cholesterol is the sum of LDL-C, HDL-C, and VLDL-C, LDL-C can be calculated as follows (all quantities are in mg/dL):

$$LDL\text{-}C = \text{total cholesterol} - HDL\text{-}C - (\text{triglycerides}/5)$$

To convert cholesterol values in mg/dL to millimoles per liter, divide by 38.7. To convert triglyceride values in mg/dL to millimoles per liter, divide by 88.6. Because the LDL-C value is estimated from measurements that include triglycerides, blood samples should be collected from patients who have fasted for 9-12 h, having taken nothing by mouth except water and medications. For patients with triglyceride values over 400 mg/dL, estimation of LDL-C as described previously is not accurate. In such cases, direct measurement of LDL by ultracentrifugation in a specialized laboratory is recommended if available. It is recommended that measurement of cholesterol occur within the first 24 h following the event or that it wait until 4-6 weeks after the event or procedure to establish a true baseline on which therapeutic decisions can be made.[215,403,497,517] This is not to suggest, however, that therapeutic management and education should not begin immediately, especially in those patients whose lipids were previously found to be abnormal.[191] In all adults over the age of 20 a fasting lipoprotein profile should be obtained every 5 yr.[403]

Clinical evaluation in patients with abnormal lipids should include a detailed history to determine potential contributors to elevated lipid levels such as various disease states, inappropriate diet, or in some instances, medications. Some secondary causes of abnormal lipids include

Guideline 8.2	Evaluation of Lipids

All patients with established CHD should have a lipoprotein analysis for LDL-C determination after an overnight fast on two occasions 1-8 weeks apart, initiated at 4-6 weeks postevent or postprocedure.[403,517]

- diabetes mellitus;
- hypothyroidism;
- nephrotic syndrome;
- obstructive liver disease; and
- drugs that may raise LDL-C levels or lower HDL-C, particularly progestins, anabolic steroids, corticosteroids, and certain antihypertensive agents. Thiazide diuretics and loop diuretics can cause an elevation of total cholesterol, LDL, and triglycerides.

Although limited in their impact, beta-adrenergic blocking agents without intrinsic sympathomimetic activity (ISA) or alpha-blocking properties increase serum triglycerides and lower HDL. However, it should be noted that these drugs are not contraindicated in the presence of abnormal lipids. Their use must be considered in the context of their benefit in treating other disorders versus their potential adverse effect on the lipid profile.

Because abnormal lipids often are caused by familial genetic disorders, a careful family history can help to determine the etiology and management of LDL-C elevations in affected patients as well as potentially identifying family members who need therapy for high cholesterol levels. Increasing evidence shows that additional factors such as homocysteine, lipoprotein (a), fibrinogen levels, and immune responses interact with lipids in ways that can also increase coronary risk (see *Emerging Risk Factors* on page 133).

Specific areas of the physical examination (see page 70 in chapter 6) relevant to abnormal lipids include a careful examination of the eyes to document corneal arcus, a funduscopic examination to detect retinal changes due to abnormal lipids, and an examination of the skin to detect xanthoma and xanthelasma. Specific laboratory assessment in the hyperlipidemic patient should include thyroid-stimulating hormone, fasting blood glucose, serum creatinine, and alkaline phosphatase and liver function tests. Each patient's lipids should be measured regularly to make sure that the patient is achieving and maintaining goals and has no medication-related side effects.

LDL-C, Traditional Risk Factors, and CHD Risk

The NCEP was developed after evidence from epidemiological studies revealed a significant relationship between elevated cholesterol and CHD. Studies were then undertaken to determine whether cholesterol lowering would result in a decrease in CHD. The NCEP Expert Panel on Detection, Evaluation, and Treatment of High Blood Cholesterol in Adults (Adult Treatment Panel III, ATP III) provides clinical guidelines for cholesterol testing and management. ATP III focuses on lowering LDL while also emphasizing primary prevention in persons with multiple risk factors. The most recent classifications are described in figures 8.3 and 8.4.

In addition to using risk factors in the determination of overall treatment goals and intervention strategies, ATP III emphasizes the need to assess 10-yr CHD risk (MI or coronary death) as a part of this process. Risk of development of CHD over a 10-yr period using Framingham risk scoring for men and women is grouped into three categories (figure 8.5).

Risk factors used in the estimation of 10-yr risk for a cardiac event include age, total cholesterol (an average of two readings), systolic BP on the day of assessment, HDL, and smoking (yes/no, any amount or type) (figure 8.6). Each risk factor is given points depending on the age group. Points are totaled to determine 10-yr risk in a percentage.[403] The risk can be recalculated as the patient makes lifestyle changes to demonstrate reductions in CHD risk.

LDL Cholesterol Goals, Therapeutic Lifestyle Changes, and Drug Therapy

It is important to recognize that the recommendations for target LDL-C levels as well as levels for the initiation of non-pharmacological (therapeutic lifestyle

Total cholesterol (mg/dL)	
<200	Desirable
200-239	Borderline high
≥240	High
LDL-C (mg/dL)	
<100	Optimal
100-129	Near optimal/above optimal
130-159	Borderline high
160-189	High
≥190	Very high
HDL-C (mg/dL)	
<40	Low
≥60	Desirable

Figure 8.3 APT III classification of cholesterol, HDL, and LDL.

From National Cholesterol Education Program (NCEP). Executive summary of the third report of the Expert Panel on Detection, Evaluation and Treatment of High Blood Cholesterol in Adults (Adult Treatment Panel III). *JAMA* 2001;285:2486-2497.

Positive risk factors*

- Age: Men ≥45 yr; women ≥55 yr
- Family history of premature CHD
  - CHD in male first-degree relative <55
  - CHD in female first-degree relative <65 years
- Cigarette smoking
- Hypertension ≥140/90 mmHg or on antihypertensive medication
- Low HDL-C <40 mg/dL

Negative risk factor

- High HDL-C ≥60 mg/dL (presence of this negative risk factor removes one positive risk factor from the total number of risk factors)

Figure 8.4 Traditional CVD risk factors.*Diabetes is regarded as a CHD risk equivalent.

From National Cholesterol Education Program (NCEP). Executive summary of the third report of the Expert Panel on Detection, Evaluation and Treatment of High Blood Cholesterol in Adults (Adult Treatment Panel III). *JAMA* 2001;285:2486-2497.

High risk

Individuals in this category have a >20% risk for a new or recurring cardiac event (MI or coronary death) in a 10-yr period and should be treated the most aggressively:

- Those with documented CHD
- Those at high CHD risk equivalent, including patients with symptomatic carotid artery disease, peripheral arterial disease, abdominal aortic aneurysm, or diabetes

Moderate risk

Individuals in this category have a 10-20% risk for a cardiac event (MI or coronary death) in a 10-yr period:

- Those with 2 or more traditional risk factors for CHD

Lowest risk

Individuals in this category have a <10% risk for a cardiac event (MI or coronary death) in a 10-yr period:

- Those with 0-1 other traditional risk factors

Figure 8.5 Risk categories for development of CHD in 10 yr.

From National Cholesterol Education Program (NCEP). Executive summary of the third report of the Expert Panel on Detection, Evaluation and Treatment of High Blood Cholesterol in Adults (Adult Treatment Panel III). *JAMA* 2001;285:2486-2497.

---

changes [TLC]) and pharmacological therapies are based on stratification of 10-yr risk. Table 8.1 identifies the three risk categories and associated goals.

Therapeutic Lifestyle Changes

Treatment of dyslipidemia must include therapeutic lifestyle changes, including dietary intervention, physical activity, and weight loss, as a part of any risk-reduction program. The most recent guidelines have condensed previous recommendations of the AHA step 1 and step 2 diets, which gradually lowered cholesterol and saturated fat intake, to one diet that represents most of what was a part of the step 2 diet (figure 8.7). These dietary guidelines provide a range of 25-35% of total calories to be derived from total fat intake (which is especially helpful for people who have diabetes or are insulin resistant) but still recommend that intake of calories from saturated fat intake be kept below 7% of total calories.[331] If the patient does not reach the LDL goals, other options include increasing or adding plant stanols/sterols and viscous fiber.

Dietary evaluation and counseling should serve as the foundation of treatment for patients with abnormal lipids. A registered dietitian or other appropriately trained individual specializing in dietary lipid management should perform a careful assessment of current eating habits and dietary composition. This assessment should include an estimation of total daily caloric requirements to achieve and maintain

Estimate of 10-yr Risk for Men (Framingham Point Scores)

Age (yr)	Points
20-34	−9
35-39	−4
40-44	0
45-49	3
50-54	6
55-59	8
60-64	10
65-69	11
70-74	12
75-79	13

Total cholesterol, mg/dL	Points				
	Age 20-39	Age 40-49	Age 50-59	Age 60-69	Age 70-79
<160	0	0	0	0	0
160-199	4	3	2	1	0
200-239	7	5	3	1	0
240-279	9	6	4	2	1
≥280	11	8	5	3	1

	Points				
	Age 20-39	Age 40-49	Age 50-59	Age 60-69	Age 70-79
Nonsmoker	0	0	0	0	0
Smoker	8	5	3	1	1

HDL, mg/dL	Points
≥60	−1
50-59	0
40-49	1
<40	2

Systolic BP, mmHg	If untreated	If treated
<120	0	0
120-129	0	1
130-139	1	2
140-159	1	2
≥160	2	3

Point total	10-yr Risk, %
<0	<1
0	1
1	1
2	1
3	1
4	1
5	2
6	2
7	3
8	4
9	5
10	6
11	8
12	10
13	12
14	16
15	20
16	25
≥17	≥30

Estimate of 10-yr Risk for Women (Framingham Point Scores)

Age (yr)	Points
20-34	−7
35-39	−3
40-44	0
45-49	3
50-54	6
55-59	8
60-64	10
65-69	12
70-74	14
75-79	16

Total cholesterol, mg/dL	Points				
	Age 20-39	Age 40-49	Age 50-59	Age 60-69	Age 70-79
<160	0	0	0	0	0
160-199	4	3	2	1	1
200-239	8	6	4	2	1
240-279	11	8	5	3	2
≥280	13	10	7	4	2

	Points				
	Age 20-39	Age 40-49	Age 50-59	Age 60-69	Age 70-79
Nonsmoker	0	0	0	0	0
Smoker	9	7	4	2	1

HDL, mg/dL	Points
≥60	−1
50-59	0
40-49	1
<40	2

Systolic BP, mmHg	If untreated	If treated
<120	0	0
120-129	1	3
130-139	2	4
140-159	3	5
≥160	4	6

Point total	10-yr Risk, %
<9	<1
9	1
10	1
11	1
12	1
13	2
14	2
15	3
16	4
17	5
18	6
19	8
20	11
21	14
22	17
23	22
24	27
≥25	≥30

Figure 8.6 Estimate of 10-yr risk for men and women.

From National Cholesterol Education Program (NCEP). Executive summary of the third report of the Expert Panel on Detection, Evaluation and Treatment of High Blood Cholesterol in Adults (Adult Treatment Panel III). *JAMA* 2001;285:2486-2497.

Table 8.1 Target LDL Goals and Recommendations for Therapeutic Lifestyle Changes and Pharmacologic Therapy Stratified by Risk Category

Risk category	LDL goal	LDL level to initiate therapeutic lifestyle changes	LDL level to consider drug therapy
CHD or CHD risk equivalent* (10-yr risk >20%)	<100 mg/dL	≥100 mg/dL	≥130 mg/dL 100-129 mg/dL drug optional
2+ risk factors 10-yr risk 20%	<130 mg/dL	≥130 mg/dL	≥130 mg/dL for patients at 10-20% risk ≥160 mg/dL for patients at <10% risk
0-1 risk factor	<160 mg/dL	≥160 mg/dL	≥190 mg/dL 160-189 mg/dL drug optional

*Clinical CHD, symptomatic carotid artery disease, peripheral arterial disease, abdominal aortic aneurysm, diabetes.

Data from National Cholesterol Education Program (NCEP). Executive summary of the third report of the Expert Panel on Detection, Evaluation and Treatment of High Blood Cholesterol in Adults (Adult Treatment Panel III). *JAMA* 2001;285:2486-2497.

Diet

- Saturated fat <7% of total calories; cholesterol <200 mg/day
- Consider increased viscous (soluble) fiber (10-25 g/d and plant stanols/sterols (2g/d) as therapeutic options to enhance LDL lowering

Weight management

Increased physical activity

Figure 8.7 Therapeutic lifestyle changes.

From National Cholesterol Education Program (NCEP). Executive summary of the third report of the Expert Panel on Detection, Evaluation and Treatment of High Blood Cholesterol in Adults (Adult Treatment Panel III). *JAMA* 2001;285:2486-2497.

desirable body weight (see *Obesity* section beginning on page 129 of this chapter); total caloric intake; and dietary composition, including, at least, an estimate of the percentage of total calories from fat, percentage of total calories from saturated fat, and daily cholesterol intake. Dietary intervention should not preclude the immediate use of pharmacological therapy to appropriately lower lipid levels to the desirable range as outlined by ATP III.[403]

Insulin Resistance and the Metabolic Syndrome

Substantial evidence now exists to suggest a correlation between insulin resistance and coronary heart disease.[453,459,462,637] Although the LDL goal is still the primary target of therapy, other lipid and nonlipid goals will also be targeted. The first-line therapy for people who are insulin resistant includes weight loss and exercise, both of which can have a great impact on

insulin resistance and reduce CHD risk. Both weight loss and physical activity will reduce insulin resistance, lower triglycerides (and VLDL-C), increase HDL, and possibly decrease blood pressure.[369,536] In helping to identify patients at risk for insulin resistance, ATP III recommends evaluating the characteristics listed in table 8.2, which are associated with insulin resistance. If three of the five characteristics are present, a patient is considered at risk for the metabolic syndrome. Insulin resistance is related to both genetic and environmental factors.[459,460] Increasing weight and lack of physical activity can contribute to this syndrome. Upon recognition of those characteristics in table 8.2, initiation of a treatment plan as described in figure 8.8 is appropriate.

Elevated Triglycerides

People who are insulin resistant often have elevated triglycerides, with or without elevated cholesterol

Table 8.2 Clinical Identification of the Metabolic Syndrome*

Risk factor	Defining level

Abdominal obesity**
   Men***
   Women
	Waist circumference**
	   >102 cm (>40 in.)
	   >88 cm (>35 in.)

Triglycerides	≥150 mg/dL

HDL-C
   Men
   Women
	
	 <40 mg/dL
	 <50 mg/dL

BP	≥130/≥85 mmHg
Fasting glucose	≥110 mg/dL

* The presence of three or more of these characteristics identifies the metabolic syndrome.

** Both obesity and overweight are associated with insulin resistance and the metabolic syndrome. The presence of abdominal obesity, however, is more highly correlated with the metabolic risk factors than is an elevated BMI. Therefore, the simple measure of waist circumference is recommended to identify the body weight component of the metabolic syndrome.

*** Some male patients can develop multiple metabolic risk factors when the waist circumference is only marginally increased (e.g., 94-102 cm [37-39 in.]). Such patients may have a strong genetic contribution to insulin resistance. The benefit they gain from changes in lifestyle habits is similar to that of men with categorical increases in waist circumference.

Data from National Cholesterol Education Program (NCEP). Executive summary of the third report of the Expert Panel on Detection, Evaluation and Treatment of High Blood Cholesterol in Adults (Adult Treatment Panel III). *JAMA* 2001;285:2486-2497.

levels, and are at further increased risk for CHD.[50,215,533] In these cases, other goals may be necessary after the LDL goal is obtained. Non-HDL-C is total cholesterol minus HDL-C.[206] Using non-HDL cholesterol (total cholesterol minus HDL-cholesterol) as a goal when elevated triglyceride levels are present is a new addition to the guidelines. Specific guidelines for levels of elevated triglycerides are listed in figure 8.9.

Treatment goals and intervention recommendations for elevated triglycerides and low HDL are

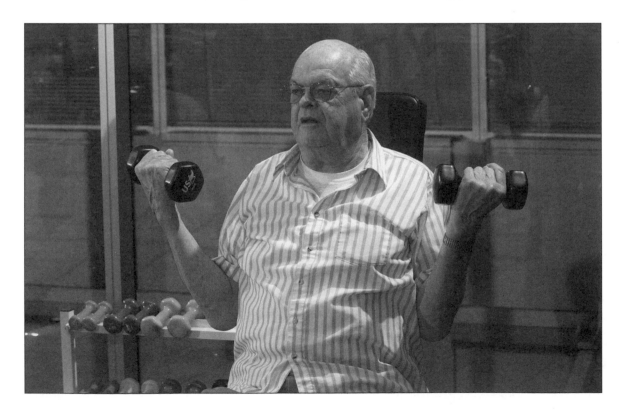

First-line therapies:

- Increasing physical activity
- Intensifying weight loss

Treat lipid and nonlipid risk factors if they persist despite these lifestyle therapies.

- Treat hypertension

Use aspirin for CHD patients to reduce prothrombotic state.

Figure 8.8 Treatment of insulin resistance–metabolic syndrome.

From National Cholesterol Education Program (NCEP). Executive summary of the third report of the Expert Panel on Detection, Evaluation and Treatment of High Blood Cholesterol in Adults (Adult Treatment Panel III). *JAMA* 2001;285:2486-2497.

<150	Normal
150-199	Borderline high
200-499	High
≥500	Very high

Figure 8.9 ATP III classification of serum triglycerides (mg/dL).

From National Cholesterol Education Program (NCEP). Executive summary of the third report of the Expert Panel on Detection, Evaluation and Treatment of High Blood Cholesterol in Adults (Adult Treatment Panel III). *JAMA* 2001;285:2486-2497.

described in table 8.3 and figures 8.10 and 8.11. As mentioned, intensifying weight management and increasing physical activity are always part of the treatment regime.[403]

General Treatment Guidelines for the CHD Patient

The optimal LDL goal for patients with CHD or CHD risk equivalent is <100 mg/dL.[403] Recommendations in figure 8.12 should be incorporated at the same time as pharmacological therapy (figure 8.13). If baseline LDL is ≥130 mg/dL, begin therapeutic lifestyle changes and an LDL-lowering drug to attain the goal. If LDL level is 100-129 mg/dL, either at baseline or with LDL-lowering therapy, consider the following treatment options:

■ Begin or intensify lifestyle and drug therapies to lower LDL.

■ Initiate or intensify weight reduction and increased physical activity in persons with insulin resistance.

■ Institute treatment of other lipid or nonlipid risk factors. If the patient has elevated triglycerides or low HDL, consider the use of nicotinic acid or fibric acid.

■ If baseline LDL cholesterol is less than 100 mg/dL, emphasize controlling other lipid or nonlipid risk factors and treating insulin resistance if present.[403]

Pharmacological Therapy

Details regarding pharmacological therapy are beyond the scope of these guidelines and are covered comprehensively by the NCEP.[403] Pharmacological therapy includes the use of one or more of the following drugs targeted to reduce LDL and triglycerides.

■ **HMG Co-A reductase inhibitors (statins).** This class of drugs inhibits HMG Co-A reductase, the rate-limiting enzyme in cholesterol biosynthesis, causing up-regulation of LDL receptors, decreasing LDL and VLDL, and increasing HDL. Aside from their effects on lipids, clinical investigations have revealed that statins can exert a number of cardioprotective and anti-inflammatory actions through up-regulations of endothelial function.[116a,266a,346a,450a,470a,480a] These drugs are generally well tolerated but rarely can cause liver enzyme elevation and creatine phosphokinase (CPK) elevation with myositis. They may also occasionally cause skin rash, stomach upset, and headaches. Additionally, statins should be used cautiously in persons with significant comorbidities who are on multiple medications. This class of drugs is considered first-line therapy in CAD patients with LDL greater than 130 mg/dL.[245,517]

■ **Cholestyramine and colestipol.** Cholestyramine and colestipol are ion exchange resins that bind bile acids; increase conversion of liver cholesterol to bile acids; and up-regulate LDL receptors in the liver, thus decreasing plasma LDL by about 20%. Furthermore, because the resins are nonsystemic, this class of medications may be very useful in younger patients with CAD or at very high risk of developing CAD who face a lifetime of lipid-lowering therapies. Side effects include bloating and constipation, elevation

- Helping the patient identify ways to remember doses
- Anticipating common side effects and teaching the patient to identify and manage them
- Providing updates on the effects of treatment
- Ensuring mechanisms for patients to contact the health care professionals who are overseeing their lipid management

According to the NCEP, follow-up of lipid measurements should include

- remeasuring at 4-6 weeks and again at 3 months if the patient has not reached the goal;
- following up at 8- to 12-week intervals through week 52 once the patient has reached the goal; and
- following up with the patient at 4- to 6-month intervals after the goal has been maintained for 1 yr (LDL should be measured once a year; at other times total cholesterol measures will suffice).

Hypertension

One in four adult Americans has hypertension. It is more common in men than in women until age 55, when the prevalence in men is about equal to that in women. Hypertension is more common among elderly black Americans and black and white adults who live in the southeastern United States.[31] Not surprisingly, hypertension is highly prevalent among people with CHD; it is noted in 30-38% of patients with MI enrolled in large clinical trials.[251,481] Importantly, hypertension has been reported to be present in 47-65% of patients enrolled in CR programs (guideline 8.3).[109,342]

The etiology of hypertension in 90-95% of cases is not known. Nonetheless, secondary prevention

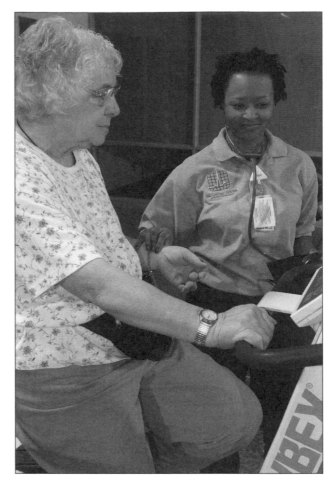

staff can effectively work with the patient's primary care physician to evaluate and manage this important modifiable risk factor. Table 8.4 lists the Joint National Committee—VII (JNC-VII) classification of BP for adults.

Pertinent medical histories should include many items recommended for the initial evaluation of patients entering the secondary prevention program (see figure 6.1, page 71), with a particular focus on dietary sodium intake, excessive alcohol consumption, excessive consumption of calories, and low

Guideline 8.3 Assessment of Hypertension

- Hypertension should not be diagnosed on the basis of a single measurement.
- Initial elevated readings should be confirmed on at least two subsequent visits over a period of one to several weeks (unless systolic BP is >180 mmHg or diastolic BP is >110 mmHg), with average levels of systolic BP of 140 mmHg or higher or diastolic BP of 90 mmHg or higher required for diagnosis.[304]

Table 8.4 Classification and Management of Blood Pressure for Adults Aged 18 Years or Older

BP classificaiton	SBP mmHg*		DBP mmHg*	Lifestyle modication	Management — Initial drug therapy: Without compelling indication	Management — Initial drug therapy: With compelling indications
Normal	<120	and	<80	Encourage		
Prehypertension	120-139	or	80-89	Yes	No antihypertensive drug indicated.	Drug(s) for the compelling indications.†
Stage 1 hypertension	140-159	or	90-99	Yes	Thiazide-type diuretics for most; may consider ACE inhibitor, ARB, BB, CCB, or combination	Drug(s) for the compelling indications. Other antihypertensive drugs (diuretics, ACE inhibitor, ARB, BB, CCB) as needed.
Stage 2 hypertension	≥160	or	≥100	Yes	Two-drug combination for most (usually thiazide-type diuretic and ACEI or ARB or BB or CCB).‡	Drug(s) for the compelling indications. Other antihypertensive drugs (diuretics, ACE inhibitor, ARB, BB, CCB) as needed.

SBP = systolic blood pressure; DBP = diastolic blood pressure. ACE = angiotensin-converting enzyme inhibitor; ARB = angiotensin-receptor blocker; BB − beta-blocker; CCB − calcium channel blocker.

*Treatment determined by highest BP category.

†Treat patients with chronic kidney disease or diabetes to BP goal of <130/80 mmHg.

‡Initial combined therapy should be used cautiously in those at risk for orthostatic hypotension.

Reprinted from National Cholesterol Education Program (NCEP), 2003, "Executive Summary of the third report of the Expert Panel on Detection, Evaluation and Treatment of High Blood Cholesterol in Adults (Adult Treatment Panel III). *JAMA* 289(19):2560-2572.

levels of physical activity. The initial physical examination should include two or more BP measurements taken 2 min apart after 5 min of rest with the patient seated and legs uncrossed, followed by verification in the contralateral arm (if values are different, the higher value should be used). Other important aspects of the physical examination related to the evaluation of hypertension that an appropriately trained health care professional should perform and document include

- examination of the neck for carotid bruits, distended veins, or an enlarged thyroid gland;
- examination of the heart for increased rate, increased size, precordial heave, clicks, mur-

Guideline 8.4 Hypertension Intervention

- Secondary prevention professionals should start all patients with BP of 140 mmHg systolic or higher or 90 mmHg diastolic or higher on a documented program of weight control, physical activity, alcohol moderation, and moderate sodium restriction.

- BP medication, individualized to other patient requirements and characteristics (i.e., age, risk factors, comorbidities, race, need for drugs with specific benefits), should be added if BP is not less than 140 mmHg systolic or 90 mmHg diastolic in 3 months or if initial BP is 180 mmHg systolic or higher or 110 mmHg diastolic or higher.[304,517,604]

Table 8.5 Lifestyle Modifications to Manage Hypertension*

Modification	Recommendation	Approximate SBP reduction, range
Weight reduction	Maintain normal body weight (BMI = 18.5-24.9).	5-20 mmHg/10-kg weight loss
Adopt DASH eating plan	Consume a diet rich in fruits, vegetables, and low-fat dairy products with a reduced content of saturated and total fat.	8-14 mmHg
Dietary sodium reduction	Reduce dietary sodium intake to no more than 100 mEq/L (2.4 g sodium or 8 g sodium chloride).	2-8 mmHg
Physical activity	Engage in regular aerobic physical activity such as brisk walking (at least 30 minutes per day, most days of the week).	4-9 mmHg
Moderation of alcohol consumption	Limit consumption to no more than 2 drinks per day (1 oz or 30 mL ethanol; e.g., 24 oz beer, 10 oz wine, or 3 oz 80-proof whiskey) in most men and no more than 1 drink per day in women and light-weight persons.	2-4 mmHg

* For overall cardiovascular risk reduction, stop smoking. The effects of implementing these modifications are dose and time dependent and could be higher for some individuals. SBP = systolic blood pressure; BMI = body mass index calculated as weight in kilograms divided by the square of height in meters; DASH = Dietary Approaches to Stop Hypertension.

Reprinted from National Cholesterol Education Program (NCEP), 2003, "Executive Summary of the third report of the Expert Panel on Detection, Evaluation and Treatment of High Blood Cholesterol in Adults (Adult Treatment Panel III). *JAMA* 289(19):2560-2572.

murs, arrhythmias, and third (S_3) and fourth (S_4) heart sounds;

■ examination of the abdomen for bruits, enlarged kidneys, masses, and abnormal aortic pulsation;

■ examination of the extremities for diminished or absent peripheral arterial pulsations or the presence of bruits or edema; and

■ a neurologic assessment.

A few laboratory tests should be performed routinely before hypertension therapy begins. These include urinalysis; a complete blood count; and a blood glucose (fasting, if possible), potassium, calcium, creatinine, uric acid, and lipid profile. A 12-lead ECG should be used to identify the presence of left ventricular hypertrophy. Based on this evaluation, appropriate and tailored therapy can be initiated (guideline 8.4).

Expert opinion supports exercise and education as important components of a multifactorial intervention that should also include counseling, behavioral intervention, and pharmacological approaches to the management of hypertension.[604] Secondary prevention programs can greatly assist the primary care physician in the treatment and close monitoring of patients with hypertension. Lifestyle modifications are the foundation for treatment of hypertension (see table 8.5). Moreover, lifestyle modifications complement pharmacological therapy when the patient neither achieves nor is expected to achieve treatment goals by lifestyle changes alone, or when more urgent control of BP is needed.

The JNC-VII underscores the importance of lifestyle modifications, which include weight reduction (if the patient is overweight), increased physical activity, and moderation of diet, that can be used as definitive or adjunctive therapy for hypertension. Dietary modifications should include several components: (1) individualizing diet to achieve and maintain a healthy body weight (see *Obesity* section beginning on page 129); (2) limiting alcohol intake to less than 1 oz of ethanol/d; (3) limiting sodium intake to 2.4 g/d; (4) emphasizing intake of fruits, vegetables, and low-fat dairy products; and (5) reducing fat in general.[45,331,547] The DASH diet has been shown to reduce BP in both hypertensive and nonhypertensive people, and particularly in African Americans.[331,547] The DASH diet emphasizes five to nine servings of fruits and vegetables a day and two to four servings of low-fat dairy products a day. The diet includes whole grains, fish, poultry, and nuts and is low in fat, red meat, sweets, and sugar-containing beverages. This diet is also rich in potassium, magnesium, and calcium. Increased intake of these minerals, particularly potassium, has been associated with lower BP. In addition to these recommendations, stress, which is associated with increased adrenaline/norepinephrine levels, must

that these are separated into safety factors, which help to set the clinical oversight of the program, and those characteristics (associated factors) that may influence the parameters of the exercise prescription as well as the balance between endurance and resistive exercise components. Setting the safe upper limit for exercise intensity should be a foremost consideration when exercise induces abnormal signs and symptoms. Figure 8.15 provides guidelines in this regard, although specific policies should be adopted based on the consensus of the staff and medical director.

Exercise-Intensity Parameters

Several approaches may be taken to prescribe exercise intensity (see table 8.6). The methods may be used independently or in an associative fashion (i.e., using RPE at the HR or MET level observed during evaluation), but in any case they should result in exercise training parameters that are beneath the criteria noted in figure 8.15. The frequency, intensity, and duration of exercise training may be manipulated to achieve specific fitness or health-related outcomes (such as weight loss), as previously described. The intensity of

Guideline 8.5 Exercise Prescription

The following key variables must be considered in preparation for the exercise prescription:

Safety Factors

1. Clinical history
2. Risk stratification, exercise risk
3. Degree of left ventricular impairment
4. Ischemic and anginal threshold
5. Any cognitive or psychological impairment that might result in nonadherence to exercise limits

Associated Factors

1. Vocational and avocational requirements
2. Orthopedic limitations
3. Premorbid and current activities
4. Personal health and fitness goals

Other noncardiac diagnostic considerations

- Onset of angina or other symptoms of cardiovascular insufficiency
- Plateau or decrease in systolic blood pressure, systolic blood pressure of >240 mmHg, or diastolic blood pressure >110 mmHg
- >1mm ST-segment depression, horizontal or down sloping
- Radionuclide evidence of reversible myocardial or echocardiographic evidence of moderate-to-severe wall motion abnormalities during exertion
- Increased frequency of ventricular arrhythmias
- Other significant ECG disturbances (e.g., 2nd or 3rd degree A-V block, atrial fibrillation, supraventricular tachycardia, complex ventricular ectopy)
- Other signs or symptoms of exertional intolerance

Figure 8.15 Signs and symptoms below which an upper limit for exercise intensity should be set.

The peak exercise HR should generally be at least 10 bpm below the HR associated with any of these criteria. Other variables (e.g., corresponding systolic BP response and perceived exertion), however, should also be considered when establishing the exercise intensity.

exercise necessary for functional improvement might be as low as 50% of exercise capacity in patients with low initial levels of cardiovascular fitness. As fitness level increases, the exercise intensity threshold necessary for further improvement in cardiovascular fitness likewise increases. Thus, for lower-fitness patients, the exercise intensity might be set at 50% of the patient's exercise capacity, and this could be as high as 80% in higher-fitness patients. The exercise intensity that results in measured improvement is physiologically associated with the anaerobic, or ventilatory, threshold. The anaerobic threshold can be identified by objective criteria including measured oxygen uptake and lactate measurements, and more indirectly by plotting ventilation against workload, although these measurements require sophisticated technology and trained personnel.

More practically, estimations of peak oxygen uptake and associated submaximal percentages, as well as assessment of RPE, can help identify an appropriate threshold. It has been fairly well established that RPE ratings of 12-16 are consistent with improvements in exercise tolerance (see figure 6.9 on page 80).[189,195] Given the conservative nature of most clinicians and in view of literature citing the benefits of moderate exercise, an RPE range of 11-15 is frequently used. Thus, in addition to traditional HR techniques to prescribe exercise intensity, an appropriate alternative is using the exercise HR associated with appropriate RPE ratings, provided the patient can reliably utilize the RPE rating scale. Importantly, patients should be able to maintain the prescribed exercise intensity for the duration needed to yield the desired energy (caloric) expenditure. If not, in most cases patients will best meet long-term exercise goals by lowering the exercise intensity to permit an adequate volume of exercise.

Once the initial exercise prescription is set, patients should progress gradually toward the goals determined after the evaluation. There is no set format with respect to progression because many factors, including fitness level, motivation, and orthopedic limitations, influence the speed at which a patient might advance. In general, it is prudent to change one variable and provide some time (a minimum of one exercise session) to assess the patient's adaptation to the new load before progressing further. When time permits, increases in duration should precede increases in intensity. Modest increases in intensity, when appropriate, are likely to be tolerated and should be based on the observations of the staff and subjective responses of the patient, provided the changes remain within the limits set through the most recent evaluation.

In recent years, the issue of lower-intensity leisure-time physical activity of a habitual nature has been promoted as an alternative to moderate or higher-intensity exercise programs. Evidence suggests that habitual activity, rather than fitness per se, provides the basis for significant health-related benefits.[83,426]

Table 8.6 Exercise Prescription Methodologies

Exercise intensity method	Description
% of peak heart rate (PHR)	Prescribes a target HR as a percentage of the PHR obtained during the exercise test. Underestimates equivalent oxygen consumption value by about 15% (i.e., 70% PHR = 55% peak METs).
Heart rate reserve (HRR)	Defines an HRR based on peak HR and resting HR, calculating the target HR based on the reserve and adjusting for resting HR. Example: PHR 150 – rest 70 = 80 reserve. If the target is 60%, 80 × .6 = 48. The resting HR of 70 is added to 48 to provide a target HR of 118. This method usually is close to equivalent oxygen consumption values (i.e., 70% HRR = 70% of peak METs).
METs	Prescribes the exercise intensity by workloads or activities associated with desired MET values. Best when used in an environmentally controlled area and ergometers or treadmills are used as exercise modalities (to reduce variability in estimating METs).
RPE	For patients who can reliably use the RPE scale, this can be an excellent adjunct to HR guidelines, and it is especially useful when medication changes affect HR or when the patient cannot assess HR accurately. It is important to use standardized RPE instructions and to verify the RPE ratings during an exercise session, because they may differ slightly from those obtained during the exercise test.

Though some view this as contradictory to traditional exercise approaches, clinicians should view the prescription of exercise in the context of desired health outcomes. Certainly, the lowest appropriate common denominator should be an overall increase in leisure-time activities. For greater improvements in cardiovascular fitness and functional performance, a more aggressive program (one of moderate intensity) should be incorporated.

A guiding principle, then, should be progression of the exercise program in such a way that the patient eventually achieves desired caloric volume thresholds. In general, this threshold might range from 500 calories per week to upward of 1,500 calories per week for improvements in fitness and weight loss, respectively. In this regard, patients exercising at a lower exercise intensity, such as those with left ventricular dysfunction or a low ischemic threshold, should benefit from compensatory increases in the frequency (which might include multiple sessions per day as well as additional days) and duration of exercise. If the MET requirement of the chosen exercise mode can be estimated, either by metabolic equation, by plotting from the exercise test at the prescribed HR, or from published MET tables, the clinician can reasonably estimate the caloric expense of exercise and adjust the prescription accordingly.

Exercise Prescriptions for Patients Without Recent Exercise Tests

For patients entering a secondary prevention program without an entry exercise test, staff should implement exercise programs conservatively with close patient surveillance. The medical director and referring clinician should advise the upper safe HR limit for exercise. Initial exercise intensities can be determined according to the length of time from cardiac event and discharge from the hospital and from the information obtained during the patient's entry interview (e.g., ADL and home walking program, walking distances during hospital admission, etc.).

At a minimum, monitoring should include ECG, signs and symptoms, BP, RPE, and signs of overexertion. A submaximal exercise evaluation with conservative endpoints can be helpful to determine exercise-session parameters. Initial exercise intensities usually range from 2 to 3 metabolic equivalents (METs) or 1 to 3 mph, 0% grade on the treadmill, or 25 to 50 watts on a cycle ergometer with gradual increments of 0.5 to 1.0 MET as tolerated. Advancement can be based on the patient's signs and symptoms, monitored response, and RPE. If the patient remains asymptomatic, exercise intensity may be gradually increased up to a perceived exertion of 12-13 (moderately hard on the 6 to 20 Borg scale), or to the upper safe limit as documented by the medical director or referring clinician. The HR at that intensity may be used as the patient's new training threshold. Exercise duration and type of exercise can be similar to those used for patients in general.

Exercise Format and Modalities

Patients can benefit from both continuous exercise as well as alternating short (i.e., 5-min) bouts of exercise with rest periods (1-2 min or longer, if needed) when limited by fatigue or symptoms. Optimal gains in fitness likely occur between 20 and 60 min of continuous exercise, depending on the prescribed intensity.[189,195,447] With intermittent exercise, clinicians should attempt to maintain the prescribed volume of exercise, necessitating a longer overall exercise session. Walking, jogging, cycling, and swimming have been complemented in recent years by a variety of large-muscle-group activities like climbing and using skiing machines and elliptical trainers. Provided that exercise goals are achieved and orthopedic risk is minimized, patients should be encouraged to choose a variety of modalities to maximize peripheral adaptation, keeping in mind the principle of exercise specificity; that is, the choice of exercise mode(s) and muscle groups employed should be consistent with the patient's vocational and leisure-time requirements. In summary, many options are available to improve fitness; the patient and clinician should arrive at a program that meets the patient's needs while enhancing health.

Physical Activity in Weight Management

Data demonstrating the positive effect of exercise training as a singular modality to achieve normal body composition in cardiac patients are few. This scarcity underscores the need to reevaluate current exercise, dietary, and behavioral strategies in regards to overweight patients. Volume of exercise prescribed for most cardiac patients may be the limiting factor. Typically, secondary prevention programs consist of low- to moderate-intensity endurance exercise for 20-60 min in a 3-d/week program.[447] As an example, a typical exercise prescription for an outpatient with a 7-MET functional capacity might be 30 min at a HR or RPE that would yield an exercise intensity approximating 4 METs. The following formula from the AHA provides a method to estimate caloric costs of exercise:[189]

$$\text{calories per minute} = [\text{METs} \times \text{body weight (kg)} \times 3.5]/200$$

Because activities rated at 4 METs also include the resting component (1 MET), the caloric cost of exercise is 3 METs. Thus, a 100-kg (200-lb) patient exercising 3 d/week would expend approximately 5.3 kcal/min, 160 kcal/session, or only about 480 kcal/week. Though patients clearly improve exercise tolerance following this exercise format, the estimated total caloric cost of exercise falls short of the weekly threshold of 1,000-1,500 exercise calories that ACSM recommends.[195] As an example, 40-min sessions 5 d/week at the same intensity would result in an expenditure of 1,060 kcal/week. Thus, adjustments must be made with regard to frequency and duration of exercise based on the desired outcome(s), with a higher exercise volume required for weight loss. These adjustments must be made, however, with the caveat that although it is prudent to increase exercise volume progressively, staff must carefully consider the risk that a higher-volume program may lead the patient to drop out.[63] Overweight patients must be sensitized to the need to develop and maintain fitness as the core of their exercise programs, with the additional volume of exercise facilitating weight-loss goals.

Initial determination of caloric goals for the purposes of exercise prescription necessitates estimation of body composition or excess weight. Various techniques to accomplish this are described later in this chapter (see the *Obesity* section beginning on page 129). The initial exercise prescription should be based on low to moderate intensity and progressively longer durations of activity. On the basis of each person's response to the initial exercise program, program staff should eventually work toward increasing the intensity to bring the patient into a target HR range suitable for cardiorespiratory conditioning. The higher intensity will allow for a shorter duration per session or fewer sessions per week to achieve the same weekly energy expenditure. In addition, the transition to higher-intensity exercise will increase the number of opportunities for the patient to incorporate activities that naturally require a higher rate of energy expenditure. However, for many patients—for example, older or obese patients—a walking or other low-intensity exercise program may be all they desire, and movement toward a more intense program may not be warranted. For obese patients to achieve long-term weight management, their needs and goals must be individually matched with the proper exercise program.

Resistance Exercise Training

Improving muscle-force production through the inclusion of resistance exercise training has become an accepted component of comprehensive exercise programs. Though the caloric effect of resistance exercise and its influence on risk-factor modification is less than with traditional endurance exercise, increased muscle mass correlates with an increased basal metabolic rate, a major component of 24-h energy utilization. Resistance exercise training also improves skeletal muscle strength and endurance, and evidence exists that exercise tolerance may be improved as well. This is important for the safe return to ADL and vocational and avocational activities and may well prolong independence in frail and elderly patients, through reduced susceptibility to falls. Other chronic conditions for which resistance training has been shown to be beneficial include low-back pain, osteoporosis, obesity and weight control, and diabetes.[445]

The long-standing perception that resistive exercise is harmful to cardiac patients, or at the least is not beneficial, is not supported by the scientific literature. Lower myocardial oxygen demand as compared to dynamic exercise, attenuation of ischemic responses, and increases in subendocardial perfusion have all been observed in studies of resistance exercise training in cardiac patients.

Although ample evidence supports the safety and efficacy of resistance exercise, careful selection of patients is prudent. Figure 8.16 outlines guidelines to assist the clinician in this regard. Once a patient has been cleared for participation, some measure of baseline muscle strength is appropriate. The results may be used to determine a resistance exercise plan as well as to assess subjective and objective responses. Patients should be monitored for HR, BP, and ECG response throughout the evaluation of baseline muscle strength. BP can be measured before and immediately after the lift. Several methods used for baseline assessment of strength include the following:

- One repetition maximum (1RM)—determining the maximal amount of weight that a person can lift once but not twice, maintaining correct technique without straining
- Modified 1RM (90% of repetition maximum)—progressively increasing the weight load at 2-min intervals to find the greatest weight that a person can lift twice but not three times, maintaining correct technique without straining
- Isokinetic testing—determining muscle-force production at varying rates of muscle contraction, using an isokinetic dynamometer

Although a number of established secondary prevention programs safely use both the 1RM and modified 1RM techniques, others simply choose to start patients at very low weight loads and increase as tolerated, following the recommendations outlined in figure 8.17.

Typically, the goals of the resistance program are to improve general muscular fitness to complement the endurance-training component so the patient may better engage in avocational activities and ADL with less fatigue and decreased risk of injury. In other instances, the resistance program may be specifically designed to improve muscular strength for occupational requirements. Thus, a plan that emphasizes the necessary muscle group(s) and the needs of the patient (strength, endurance) must be thoughtfully developed. Guidelines regarding sets, repetitions, loads, and frequencies may differ depending on the source, but the underlying rationale should remain consistent.[180,446]

It is important to recognize that resistance exercise spans a continuum of devices, including elastic

---

- Minimum of 5 weeks after date of MI or cardiac surgery, *including* 4 weeks of consistent participation in a supervised endurance training CR program**
- Minimum of 3 weeks following transcatheter procedure (PTCA, other), *including* 2 weeks of consistent participation in a supervised endurance training CR program**
- No evidence of the following conditions:
  - congestive heart failure
  - uncontrolled arrhythmias
  - severe valvular disease
  - uncontrolled hypertension. Patients with moderate hypertension (systolic BP >160 mmHg or diastolic BP >100) should be referred for appropriate management, although these values are not absolute contraindications for participation in a resistance training program
  - unstable symptoms

Figure 8.16 Patient criteria for a resistance exercise program.*

*In this figure, a resistance exercise program is defined as one in which patients lift weights 50% or greater of 1RM maximum. The use of elastic bands, 1- to 3-lb hand weights, and light free weights may be initiated in a progressive fashion at phase II program entry, provided no other contraindications exist.

**Entry should be a staff decision with approval of the medical director and surgeon as appropriate.

- To prevent soreness and minimize the risk of injury, the initial load should allow 12-15 repetitions comfortably. If a 1RM protect is used, this load would be approximately 30-40% 1RM for the upper body and 50-60% for hips and legs. Low-risk-stratified, well-trained patients may progress to higher relative loads depending on program goals.
- Perform 1 set of 6-8 exercises (major muscle groups) 2-3 d/week. An additional set may be added, but additional gains are not proportionate.
- Some specific considerations are as follows:
  - Exercise large muscle groups before small muscle groups.
  - Increase loads by 5% when the patient can comfortably lift 12-15 repetitions.
  - Raise weights with slow, controlled movements; emphasize complete extension of the limbs when lifting.
  - Avoid straining.
  - Exhale (blow out) during the exertion phase of the lift (e.g., exhale when pushing a weight stack overhead and inhale when lowering it).
  - Avoid sustained, tight gripping, which may evoke an excessive BP response to lifting.
  - Minimize rest periods between exercises as tolerable to maximize muscular endurance.
  - An RPE of 11-13 may be used as a subjective guide to effort.
  - Stop exercise if warning signs or symptoms occur, especially dizziness, arrhythmias, unusual shortness of breath, or anginal discomfort.

Figure 8.17 Resistance training guidelines.

bands, light hand weights, progressively heavier free weights, and various types of weight machines. The amount of force the patient must generate can be quite low, providing a stimulus to skeletal muscle with minimal load on the myocardium. Thus, a distinction should be drawn between lower- and higher-load resistance programs. Figure 8.17, for example, lists criteria for patients enrolled in a program where the loads for leg work are ≥50% or greater of 1RM maximum. A person entering an outpatient program can immediately begin using elastic bands, light (1-3-lb) hand weights, and light free weights in a progressive fashion, provided there are no other general contraindications to exercise. Patients can then easily progress to heavier loads and the use of weight circuits based on their adaptation (see figure 8.18). The recommendations listed in figure 8.17 should be applied to patients engaged at any level of resistance-exercise training.

The guidelines presented in this chapter reflect a combination of scientific evidence and clinical experience, and clinicians are encouraged to develop program guidelines that best fit their programs. A guiding principle should be the development of a resistance program that is progressive in nature, is safe, and does not supersede the physiological limits set for the endurance training component.

Flexibility Exercise

Optimal musculoskeletal function requires that a patient maintain an adequate range of motion in all joints.[195,446,447] It is particularly important to maintain flexibility in the lower back and posterior thigh regions. Lack of flexibility in these areas may be associated with an increased risk for the development of chronic lower-back pain. Therefore, preventive and rehabilitative exercise programs should include activities that promote the maintenance of flexibility. Lack of flexibility is prevalent in the elderly and contributes to a reduced ability to perform ADL. Accordingly, exercise programs for the elderly should emphasize proper stretching, especially for the upper and lower trunk, the neck, and the hip regions.

Properly performed stretching exercises can help a person improve and maintain range of motion in a joint or series of joints. Flexibility exercises should be performed in a slow, controlled manner, with a gradual progression to greater ranges of motion. A wide variety of recommendations exist regarding the parameters for flexibility exercises, but duration of the stretch appears to be important to achieve deformation in connective tissue and neuroinhibitory effects.[450] A general exercise prescription for achieving and maintaining flexibility should adhere to the following recommendations:

- Frequency: 2-3 d/week
- Intensity: Hold to a position of mild discomfort (not pain)
- Duration: Gradually increase to 30 s, then as tolerable to 90 s for each stretch, breathing normally
- Repetitions: Three to five repetitions for each stretch
- Type: Static, with a major emphasis on the lower back and thigh areas

Elastic bands	Inexpensive, available in varying lengths and thickness, provide for progressive resistance through full range of motion.
Cuff and hand weights	Portable, inexpensive, may range from 1 to 5 lb. Wrist cuffs and handheld weights add to the energy cost of activity and provide for increased strength, depending on weight load and range of motion.
Free weights and dumbbells	Relatively inexpensive and generally available in 1- to 5-lb increments. Dumbbells are handheld; free weights are lifted with both hands using a barbell. Dumbbells provide for greater increases in strength through a range of motion, whereas the use of free weights requires skill, proper form, and additional personnel for spotting, as necessary.
Wall pulleys	Require little space and relatively inexpensive. Resistance is easily set; generally have lower weight increments than weight-training machines.
Weight machines	Usually multistation machines in a circuit format. Probably optimal for comprehensive conditioning. Requires substantial space; increases both initial and ongoing maintenance expenses.

Figure 8.18 Progressive resistance options.

Patients Requiring Special Consideration

A variety of common diagnoses for cardiac patients may alter the parameters of the exercise prescription. Some of these diagnoses and associated precautions are described in table 8.7.

Exercising in Various Environmental Conditions

External environmental conditions influence a person's physiological response to exercise. Clinicians must therefore take them into account, particularly for patients with CVD, especially those with ischemic thresholds. The most commonly encountered conditions are heat and cold stress, altitude, and air pollution.

Because approximately 75% of the heat generated with exercise is exchanged with the environment, factors that inhibit heat release such as excessive clothing or an environment that is significantly warmer and more humid than normal indoor conditions will alter HR response to exercise as well as raise the risk of heat-induced symptoms or injury, including heat cramps, syncope, dehydration, exhaustion, and heatstroke. It is difficult to establish clear-cut guidelines for patients because factors such as fitness and degree of acclimatization, along with intrinsic physiological differences, may all alter individual response to heat stress. Nonetheless, guidelines using the wet bulb globe temperature (WBGT), an index that is derived from air temperature and measures of dew point temperature or relative humidity have been established. Of these latter two measures, the most practical measure is the dew point temperature, because it is usually readily available and remains relatively constant throughout the day provided the weather remains stable. Table 8.8 reflects the WBGT or heat index using the dew point temperature. Use of relative humidity and the actual wet bulb temperature may be found elsewhere.[78]

Table 8.7	Common Diagnostic Characteristics Requiring Special Considerations in Exercise Prescription and Supervision
Diagnostic characteristic	**Special considerations**
Angina	Monitor the occurrence of symptom onset, frequency, duration, triggers (e.g., upper-body exercise), and associated exercise intensity or workload
Revascularization (PTCA, stent, atherectomy, CABGS)	Monitor for the occurrence of pretreatment signs and symptoms, especially during the first 6 months postprocedure
Left venticular dysfunction, CHF	Recognize the increased potential for complex arrhythmias, hypotension, sudden weight gain, SOB, lower-extremity edema, and unusual fatigue
Pacemakers/implantable cardioverter defibrillators (ICDs)	Review the type of device and reason for placement and discharge threshold of ICD
Heart transplant	Recognize the potential for altered HR, BP, and symptom response
Leg claudication	Evaluate responses to varying exercise modalities including symptom onset, walking distance, and pain ratings
Diabetes	Recognize the importance of glucose management and specific symptoms related to the exercise
COPD	Monitor for the occurrence of oxygen desaturation and understand the role of supplemental oxygen and dyspnea ratings
Hypertension	Recognize the BP responses to varying activities
Obesity	Recognize the potential for orthopedic stress and understand the behavioral factors associated with the disease
Arthritis	Limit excessive joint stress by altering the exercise format

Table 8.8 Table for Estimation of WBGT From Air Temperature and Dew Point Temperature

Tdp °F	60	65	70	75	80	85	90	95	100	105	110	Tdp °C
95	86	88	90	91	93	95	97	99	101	103	105	35
90	80	83	85	87	89	91	93	95	97	99	101	32
85	76	78	80	83	85	87	89	91	93	96	98	28
80	72	74	77	79	81	83	86	88	90	93	95	27
75	69	71	73	76	78	81	83	85	88	90	92	24
70	66	65	71	73	76	78	80	83	85	88	90	21
65	63	66	68	71	73	76	78	81	83	86	88	18
60	61	64	66	69	71	74	76	79	82	84	87	16
55	60	62	64	67	70	72	75	77	80	83	85	14
50	58	60	62	66	68	71	74	76	79	81	84	13
45	58	59	62	64	67	70	72	75	78	80	83	7
40	56	58	61	63	66	69	71	74	77	80	82	4
35	54	57	60	62	66	68	71	73	76	79	82	2
30	53	56	59	62	64	67	70	73	75	78	81	-1
	16	18	21	24	27	29	32	35	38	41	43	

* For outdoor exercise, WBGT can be estimated from the current air temperature and the dew point temperature that has been recorded in the last few hours. If the exercise occurs in direct sunlight, add 4 °F to the estimated WBGT.

Data from Bernard TE. Environmental considerations: Heat and cold. In *ACSM's resource manual for guidelines for exercise testing and prescription,* 4th ed. JL Roitman, et al. (eds.). Baltimore: Williams & Wilkins, 2001, pp. 209-216.

One method used to guide physical activity programming using the WBGT index is as follows:[78]

■ Adjustments for external factors:

Step 1. Determine environmental WBGT (heat index) using air temperature and dew point temperature.

Step 2. If the patient is not acclimated (no recent heat stress exposure), add 3 ∞F to the index.

Step 3. If the metabolic rate is light (e.g., walking), subtract 2 ∞F from the index. If the metabolic rate is heavy, add 2 ∞F to the index.

Step 4. If the patient is wearing multiple layers of clothing, add 6 ∞F to the index. If clothing is impermeable to water, add 15 ∞F to the index.

■ Level of heat stress: WBGT description (heat index)

< 80 °F — No appreciable heat stress

80-85 °F — Low heat stress: Implement personal protective practices (seek relief from heat stress, adequately hydrate, avoid heat stress during acute illness, decrease intensity of exercise, and so on).

86-88 °F — Moderate heat stress: Increased risk; ensure adequate breaks; avoid strenuous exercise.

>88 °F — High heat stress: Significant risk; consider cancellation of exercise.

Exposure to cold stress increases various indices of cardiac work, including arterial pressure. In patients with CVD, exposure to cold stress, particularly when the wind chill index is 25 °F, should be avoided.[195] Cold temperature may also induce exercise bronchospasm and angina in susceptible patients. Employ common sense in advising patients about exercising in the cold, such as dressing in layers; wearing a simple mask for those with cold-induced angina or bronchospasm; drinking warm, noncaffeinated beverages; seeking relief from prolonged exposure, and particularly using caution with respect to heavy exertion such as shoveling snow.[196] Interestingly, moderate to vigorous exercise in the cold may ultimately present problems associated with the heat, particularly when patients are overdressed and unable to shed layers of clothing. Increased sweating during more prolonged activity may also lead to dehydration. Patients should be reminded about fluid intake.

Exercising at higher altitude (>5,000 feet above sea level) results in increased cardiovascular strain manifested by decreased arterial oxygen saturation and reduced maximal exercise capacity. Increased work of breathing and associated breathlessness is also observed above 5,000 feet.[633] A reduction in cardiovascular strain is associated with 5-10 d of acclimatization, but sea-level responses should not be expected.[195] Counseling patients for whom altitude presents additional cardiovascular stress regarding an appropriate reduction in exercise intensity is especially prudent. Patients should be reminded that HR responses to exertion are usually elevated compared to the same activity at sea level. Target HRs continue

to be useful, although staff should remind patients that they should reduce workloads to maintain appropriate HR responses.

Psychosocial Concerns

Many recovering cardiac patients and their families struggle with the adaptive challenges that come with illness and rehabilitation.[520,521] There is increasing evidence of the detrimental effects of depression, hopelessness, social isolation, and acute mental stress on the recovery process and risk for disease progression.[19,113,173,200,605] Successful psychosocial adjustment has been shown to have a positive effect on such crucial rehabilitative issues as adherence to medical recommendations, vocational adjustment, morbidity, and mortality (see guideline 8.6).[419] Initial clinical

| Guideline 8.6 | Assessment and Outcomes Related to Psychosocial Concerns |

Assessment

- Staff should identify clinically significant levels of psychosocial distress using a combination of clinical interview and psychosocial screening instruments at program entry, exit, and periodic follow-up.

Outcomes

- Clinical: The patient should experience emotional well-being as evidenced by the absence of
  - psychosocial distress indicated by clinically significant levels of depression, social isolation, anxiety, anger, and hostility;
  - drug dependency; and
  - chronic or excessive psychophysiological arousal.
- Behavioral: Program services should enhance the patient's ability to
  - describe the recovery and rehabilitation process;
  - develop realistic health-related expectations;
  - assume responsibility for behavior change;
  - demonstrate problem-solving capabilities;
  - engage in regular physical exercise and incorporate relaxation techniques, such as meditation, into the daily schedule;
  - demonstrate effective use of other cognitive-behavioral stress-management skills;
  - obtain effective social support;
  - comply with psychotropic medications if prescribed;
  - reduce or eliminate alcohol, tobacco, caffeine, or other nonprescription psychoactive drugs; and
  - return to meaningful social, vocational, and avocational roles.

trials designed to reduce psychological distress in post-MI and post-CABGS surgery patients have had promising effects on morbidity and mortality.[103] Unfortunately, the psychosocial needs of recovering cardiac patients are often ignored or undertreated in both inpatient and outpatient settings.

Secondary prevention specialists should approach psychosocial evaluations with the attitude that patients and their families are generally emotionally healthy individuals facing a frightening and unusual situation.[480] The psychosocial component of secondary prevention programs should contain at least four elements: assessment; feedback; brief interventions; and, where needed, referral for specialized intervention. The structure and focus of psychosocial services might differ in inpatient and outpatient settings; however, assessments in both settings should answer the following questions:

- Has a crisis been caused by the illness or by entry into secondary prevention?
- Has the illness disrupted the patient's ability to adapt to daily demands of living?
- Does the patient show affective or cognitive impairment in the ability to cope with the adaptive demands of illness or those of secondary prevention?
- Is the patient receiving adequate psychosocial support to aid in coping with the stressors of medical intervention or secondary prevention?
- Does the patient show any behavioral patterns that warrant aggressive, immediate psychosocial intervention? Behaviors such as smoking, overeating, or substance abuse might be included here.
- What are the major concerns of the patient and family regarding anticipated psychosocial adjustment challenges in the immediate future?

With these questions as a backdrop, the following specific guidelines can help clinicians implement psychosocial assessment in inpatient and outpatient settings (see guideline 8.7).

Inpatient Evaluation

Three specific domains frame the recommendations for structuring psychosocial services in inpatient rehabilitation settings. These include crisis management, ability to relax, and need for special consultation.

Crisis Management

Patients and their families often experience the stressors associated with cardiovascular illness as unrelenting and overwhelming. As such, momentary episodes of psychosocial struggle are normal and to be anticipated during rehabilitation. Guidelines exist, however, for identifying patients at high risk for problems with psychosocial adjustment and adherence to rehabilitation prescriptions.[41,424,480,624] The following populations of patients should be considered at higher risk for adjustment difficulties necessitating additional evaluation and support:

- Patients who live alone
- Patients who are not married and do not have a confidant
- Patients who are recently divorced or widowed
- Patients who are socially isolated
- Patients from multiproblem families
- Patients with low education levels
- Patients with low incomes
- Patients who smoke,
- Patients who are obese
- Patients who have multiple chronic illnesses
- Patients without spiritual or religious comfort
- Patients with a history of mental health difficulties

Guideline 8.7 | Inpatient Evaluation

Staff should

- determine the manner and success with which the patient is coping with the medical crisis;
- assess the patient's ability to relax; and
- determine if referral for specialized consultation is needed due to the presence of depression, smoking, alcohol abuse, significant anxiety, excessive frustration or anger, or spiritual crisis.

- Patients who have cultural or religious values that conflict with a philosophy of self-reliance and optimism
- Patients who have impaired cognitive functioning

Ability to Relax

The importance of preoperative mood on the outcome of medical interventions has long been recognized. Relaxation can facilitate coping with fear, anxiety, and pain. The CR professional should explore for signs and symptoms of stress and investigate how the patient attempts to relax.

Need for Specialized Consultation

Specialized consultation from a mental health professional is suggested for any patient who has protracted adjustment struggles, who does not respond to brief interventions geared toward crisis management, or whose recovery may be impeded by psychosocial problems. When signs and symptoms of distress are clinically significant, the patient should be referred back to the primary care provider or to a mental health specialist. The findings of a formal psychological evaluation can greatly aid the efforts of rehabilitation staff who are not mental health professionals. Such assessments typically incorporate data from extended clinical interviews with patients and spouses and the results of a battery of standardized personality, neuropsychological, and family systems inventories.[480] Furthermore, the rehabilitation specialist can provide significant input into this process by identifying several factors that may contribute to psychosocial concerns. Some of these are described here.

■ **Does the patient smoke or abuse alcohol?** Patients who continue to smoke following a coronary event experience twice the risk of death as their counterparts who quit. Efforts to promote smoking cessation initiated during the inpatient stay appear to be particularly effective.[555] See the section on *Smoking* on page 96 of this chapter. It is estimated that 25% of patients in the hospital abuse alcohol or are alcohol dependent.[17] The increased risk associated with excessive alcohol intake and other substance abuse makes this an important area for assessment. Substance abusers routinely downplay the severity and effect of their use, making it all the more difficult to uncover. One particularly useful set of standardized questions can be used during a clinical interview in both the inpatient and outpatient settings (see appendix F).

■ **Does the patient exhibit signs or symptoms of clinical depression?**[574] Signs or symptoms suggesting clinical depression include the following:

- Ongoing struggle to control mood or to sustain sufficient energy to cope with daily stressors
- Preoccupation with fears, regrets, aches, pains, and thoughts of death
- Loss of the ability to experience pleasure
- Changes in sleep patterns, eating patterns, and sexual drive
- Recurring sense of being overwhelmed by current stressors
- Agitation and frustration
- Self-blame and pessimism
- Irritation with others
- Obsessive insecurities about the future
- Psychomotor retardation
- Disrupted concentration and memory
- Failure of supportive interaction with others to alleviate symptoms of depression.

■ **Does the patient exhibit signs or symptoms of anxiety disorders?** These signs or symptoms include the following:

- Nervousness, agitation
- Weakness
- Numbness
- Stomach churning
- Shortness of breath
- Blurred vision
- Feeling unable to cope
- Dizziness
- Heart palpitations
- Trembling and shaking
- Feelings of paralysis
- Sweating
- Pressure in head or chest
- Feeling that things are not real

■ **Is the patient in need of evaluation for psychotropic medication and psychotherapy?** Between 30% and 50% of recovering cardiac patients suffer clinically significant levels of anxiety or depression. These symptoms dissipate spontaneously within 6 to 9 months in most patients. However, depressed patients remain at a higher level of cardiovascular risk until remission or dissipation of these symptoms. Hence, rehabilitation specialists should very carefully consider medical evaluation of the need for antidepressant or anxiolytic therapy for a patient who has a history of anxiety or depression, who exhibits an elevated score on a questionnaire assessing negative affect (e.g., SCL-90R, Beck Depression Inventory, Profile of Mood States, Center for Epidemiologic Studies Depression Inventory [CES-D], Spielberger State-Trait Anxiety Inventory, etc.), or whose current functioning is significantly compromised by any combination of the signs and symptoms.[69,149,373,457,528,547]

In addition, patients who suffer from anxiety disorders often report a combination of terrifying fears, including panic attacks involving fears of dying, fainting, going crazy, having a heart attack, losing control, causing a scene, or not being able to get back to a safe environment (i.e., home). Many patients become hyperattuned to visceral or body feedback perceived to be consistent with these fears.

■ **Is the patient in need of spiritual counseling?** Many medical patients experience spiritual crises during the course of secondary prevention, manifested as questioning or anger directed toward one's god, urgent appeal to one's higher power for help in coping, or anxiety over being separated from one's spiritual support system. Some patients may believe that anxiety equates with a lack of spiritual strength or trust. This can result in even greater anxiety and stress. Here, as in all aspects of psychosocial intervention, the rehabilitation specialist should provide appropriate responses to the patient's needs but still remain within the provider's personal comfort zone. Minimally, patients should be asked whether they wish consultation from a pastoral counselor or religious leader.

Inpatient Interventions

The patient and family should be encouraged to conceptualize the crisis of illness as an opportunity for physical, mental, and spiritual growth. Viewing the crisis as a challenge leads to more optimistic thoughts and increases the likelihood of successful outcomes. The importance of family participation in needed areas of health care management (such as smoking cessation, exercise, or dietary modification) should be underscored. Families should be encouraged, and where appropriate, coached, to reach a common understanding regarding secondary prevention recommendations. They should also be advised of the importance of mutual participation, supportive interaction, positive reinforcement of healthy lifestyle changes, and avoidance of relationship patterns that involve excessive policing, monitoring, blaming, shaming, or criticizing.[520,521] Programs should develop and offer ongoing support groups for patients, their families, and couples on an outpatient basis.

Where possible, rehabilitation specialists should plan a brief telephone follow-up regarding psychosocial concerns within the first month after hospitalization, particularly for those with elevated levels of psychological distress or depression.[555] If telephone follow-up is not possible, a postcard reminder of key points covered in the discharge plan should be sent.

Inpatient rehabilitation services present an early opportunity to assist patients in transitioning into outpatient services while providing support, education, and counseling related to those areas described in guideline 8.8. CR specialists should include a variety of components as part of inpatient services.

Support, Education, and Guidance

Patients and their families should be assisted in managing the health crisis and prepared to meet the challenge of secondary prevention. Crisis-intervention theory offers useful guidelines for helping patients and their families cope with the stresses of hospitalization. The rehabilitation specialist should provide

---

Guideline 8.8 | **Inpatient Intervention**

CR staff should

- provide individual counseling and small-group education regarding adjustment to illness and smoking cessation;

- provide a supportive rehabilitation environment to enhance the patient's and family's level of social support; and

- refer patients experiencing clinically significant post-traumatic stress, depression, anxiety, or hostility for further mental health evaluation and treatment.

multiple, brief interventions consisting of support, education, and anticipatory guidance. Patients and their families should be assured that their concerns and fears are normal and should receive practical suggestions for the management of novel stressors that come with hospitalization. Reassure patients and their families that the hospital staff is providing excellent care for the whole family. The practitioner should emphasize to family members the importance of providing the patient with support; the rehabilitation specialists, in turn, should provide that support.[157] Long-term behavior change is most successful when the entire family system is viewed as an integral component of the rehabilitation process.

Relaxation Training

A variety of brief interventions geared toward teaching the patient to relax can be incorporated into routine cardiac care. For example, patients can be given instruction in abdominal breathing. Where applicable, they can be encouraged to recall previously learned relaxation strategies, such as the breathing techniques used in Lamaze training. Patients can also be instructed to focus attention on soothing stimuli or visual imagery. Preparatory education regarding prognosis and scheduled interventions seems to have a positive effect on many patients' tension levels. Some patients, however, may actually respond with higher levels of anxiety when presented with more detail related to their conditions. Hence, clinicians need to assess the effect of such education on patients' anxiety levels and adjust the level of detail accordingly.

Specialized Consultation Referral

Signs and symptoms of clinical depression, anxiety, hostility, or substance abuse noted during the clinical interview, or elevated scores on psychometric measures of these conditions, suggest the need for specialized consultation.[548] People with these characteristics may need psychotropic medications, psychotherapy, or spiritual counseling.

In the event that referral for specialized counseling is necessary, the rehabilitation specialist should make every effort to communicate with the counselor. For example, where alcohol abuse counseling is indicated, the rehabilitation specialist should, within the limits of confidentiality, inform the counselor of any observed changes in tolerance, symptoms of withdrawal, or odor of alcohol on the patient's breath.

Smoking Cessation

For any patient with a recent history of nicotine dependence, CR staff should give firm yet compassionate advice regarding the need for continued smoking cessation after hospitalization. Given the complexity of nicotine addiction and the relative safety of nicotine-replacement therapy (NRT), NRT should be encouraged for any patient for whom it is deemed medically safe. Some physicians, however, may prefer to use the medication buproprion SR as a cessation aid, either alone or as an adjunct to NRT. In either case, coaching in behavioral strategies for smoking cessation should always accompany NRT or buproprion SR.[227]

Discharge Planning Session

The discharge-planning session sets the stage for much that is to come for recovering cardiac patients and their families. Given the importance of family systems operations in secondary prevention, discharge-planning sessions should be delivered simultaneously to the patients and their most significant others.[523] They should all be warned of the likelihood of homecoming depression, anxiety, and increased family tensions as they struggle to adjust to this illness and the demands of secondary prevention and the consequences of relapse.[519-521] They should also be told that periods of grieving are normal and likely, for both patients and family members. In addition, the CR specialists should also proactively address concerns regarding the sexual consequences of illness and medications, offering reassurance and practical advice.[519,522,594]

Outpatient Services

Both the patient's perception of health status and the family's attitudes toward secondary prevention can significantly affect overall psychosocial adjustment following illness. A number of useful questionnaires and interviewing guidelines are available for assessing these important variables.[390,480] At minimum, the patient and his or her significant other should be questioned about their attitudes toward secondary prevention (see guideline 8.9). The patient's goals should be solicited upon entry into secondary prevention, and where possible, secondary prevention prescriptions should be framed as aids to accomplishing these goals (see guideline 8.10). This is particularly salient when CR specialists are assisting the patient's return to work. The patient's perceptions of current and anticipated flexibility, strength, and exercise tolerance should be identified and compared to perceptions of work skills and energy requirements. Patients perceiving an inability to meet these requirements may need referral to a vocational-rehabilitation counselor for further evaluation and guidance.

Guideline 8.9 | Outpatient Evaluation

Staff should

- determine if there is evidence of post-traumatic stress syndrome;
- assess for the presence of significant negative affect, particularly depression;
- evaluate for the presence of substance abuse;
- determine the patient's and family's perception of health status;
- identify the patient's goals with regard to sexual adjustment and problem behaviors (e.g., type A behavior, smoking, overeating, hostility, etc.);
- determine the level of social support; and
- assess the effectiveness of the patient's stress-management strategies.

Guideline 8.10 | Outpatient Interventions

Staff should

- provide individual counseling and small-group education regarding stress management to include cognitive and behavioral techniques to address type A behavior, anger or hostility, job strain, smoking, and overeating;
- provide a supportive rehabilitation environment to enhance the patient's and family's level of social support; and
- refer patients experiencing clinically significant post-traumatic stress, depression, substance abuse, anxiety, or hostility for further mental health evaluation and treatment.

Outpatient Evaluation

For patients recently discharged from the hospital, inquiry regarding symptoms of post-traumatic stress syndrome that may occur secondary to the trauma of hospitalization and medical interventions is essential. CR specialists should consider the presence of post-traumatic stress syndrome if the following symptoms persist for more than 1 month after hospitalization:

- Recurrent, distressing dreams or recollections of the trauma
- Obsessive ruminations regarding details of the trauma
- Recurrent tearfulness or anxiety
- Sleep disturbances
- Uncontrollable startle responses
- Avoidance of stimuli associated with the trauma
- Difficulty controlling mood, concentration, or irritability

If negative affect is manifested, the rehabilitation specialist should try to differentiate whether the patient is mourning losses associated with the illness or is suffering from clinical depression.[519] The symptoms of grief and clinical depression overlap in many ways. Grief associated with illness, however, typically dissipates within approximately 2 months of diagnosis or hospitalization and is often relieved by supportive discussion and input from others. The symptoms of clinical depression, on the other hand, tend to persist despite the support and guidance normally offered in secondary prevention.

Sexual dysfunction is common in patients with heart disease. Contributing factors include depression, medication side effects, hormonal changes associated with menopause, and vascular insufficiency. In addition, lack of information regarding the safety of sexual activity in heart disease patients can provoke anxiety in both patient and partner. It is therefore essential to incorporate questions regarding past and present sexual functioning when eliciting the patient's general medical and health history.

Outpatient Interventions

Secondary prevention settings can provide a broad range of potentially helpful psychosocial interventions. Although interventions are often prepackaged, effort should be made to tailor the message as much as possible to the needs of the individual patient. Effective psychoeducational interventions can be provided in either group or individualized formats. Regardless of the format, topics to be covered should include the following:

- Sexual adjustment throughout the life cycle and the effects of cardiopulmonary illness and medications on mood and sexual response (see figure 8.19)[22]

- Strategies for modifying problem behaviors, such as smoking or overeating

- The dangers of unchecked hostility and depression on health

- The importance of ongoing social support in promoting secondary prevention and wellness

- General stress-management strategies

- Training in relaxation techniques

Biological issues
- Variations of sexual-performance problems
- Effects of the aging process
- Sexual effects of organic factors related to the illness
- Safety of sexual activity
- Effects of medication
- Evaluation and treatment options

Behavioral factors
- Setting the appropriate sexual context
- Specific sexual technique

Emotional factors
- Importance of relaxation and comfort
- Sexual effects of antierotic emotions such as anger

Cognitive factors
- Anxiety-provoking beliefs
- Myths versus realities

Personality factors
- Need for education, permission, or therapy

Relationship factors
- Issues that relate to overall intimacy
- Sex versus sexuality in context

Sensory factors
- Sensate focus as an antidote to anxiety
- Advisability of self-stimulation

Figure 8.19 Issues to address in sexual counseling with heart disease patients.

Adapted, by permission, from Sotile W.M., 1996, *Psychosocial interventions for cardiopulmonary patients.* (Champaign, IL: Human Kinetics), 209.

Secondary prevention programs benefit from a relationship with a mental health specialist who is knowledgeable about secondary prevention and is willing to become an active member of the team. Such professionals can serve as inpatient consultants and outpatient therapists and group leaders. In addition, an increasing number of resources are available to guide CR specialists in the development and implementation of psychosocial services.[15,367,522,625] Extended psychotherapy can enhance overall psychosocial adjustment and adherence to medical recommendations. Psychotherapeutic services can be provided in individual, marital/family, or small-group formats either within the context of a secondary prevention program or as an adjunct to the program. All patients and their families should be encouraged to participate in these services as appropriate to their needs. These activities should be a major therapeutic thrust for those with clinically significant levels of emotional or interpersonal distress.

Finally, a crucial and often overlooked aspect of the psychosocial component of secondary prevention is follow-up. To assess and educate patients upon their entry into formal rehabilitation without follow-up makes no more sense within the psychosocial realm than within any other realm. Hence, CR staff should include questions regarding psychosocial adjustment in all follow-up interviews, mailed questionnaires, or telephone contacts performed and communicate findings from this evaluation, particularly if problems persist, to the patient's primary care physician.

Obesity

Obesity has been determined to be an important risk factor for CVD among men and women.[161] Obesity appears to interact with or amplify the effects of other risk factors by mechanisms that as yet remain unknown. Alarming data from the National Health and Nutrition Exam Surveys show that the prevalence of overweight and obesity among Americans has increased over the past 20 yr, such that nearly 55% of adult Americans are deemed to be overweight. Thus, obesity should be viewed as a prevalent; serious; and, to date, refractory public health problem.[104,176,542]

In several large consecutive series of patients enrolled in CR programs, the prevalence of obesity is 50-80%.[52,109,342] Surprisingly, weight management and obesity, despite their strong link to other risk factors, have not been a primary focus in CR. This is evidenced by the paucity of scientific data on this subject in the CR literature. It is very clear, however, that more data are needed and that additional focused interventions must be performed and evaluated. Obesity should be viewed as a heterogeneous problem that stems from genetic, biologic, and behavioral factors. Accordingly, the expert panel of scientists at the Prevention III Conference called for a new generation of integrated basic and clinical research to focus on the following questions:[542]

- Who should lose weight?
- Who can lose weight?
- How much weight can be lost?
- What is the best approach for a person to lose weight?
- How can weight maintenance be enhanced?

Secondary prevention programs need to focus concentrated efforts on the careful evaluation and treatment of overweight patients (guideline 8.11). Program specialists must identify patients in need of weight management in order to provide appropriate further evaluation and focused intervention (see *Dietary Assessment and Intervention* on page 131).

Evaluation of Body Weight, BMI, and Body Mass Determination

Well-defined and reliable indices of weight and body composition should be assessed at baseline, because simple height and weight measures do not adequately assess adiposity. In addition to height and weight, BMI should be determined and waist circumference should be measured. Waist circumference is correlated with abdominal fat content, and the presence of excess fat in the abdomen is an independent predictor of risk factors and morbidity.[161]

Guideline 8.11 | Weight Management

- Weight-management interventions should be targeted to those patients whose weight and body composition place them at increased cardiac risk, and whose weight may adversely affect other risk factors such as diabetes, abnormal lipids, and hypertension.

- Patients generally at risk include those with BMI ≥25 kg/m² and waist >40 inches in men (102 cm) and >35 inches (88 cm) in women.

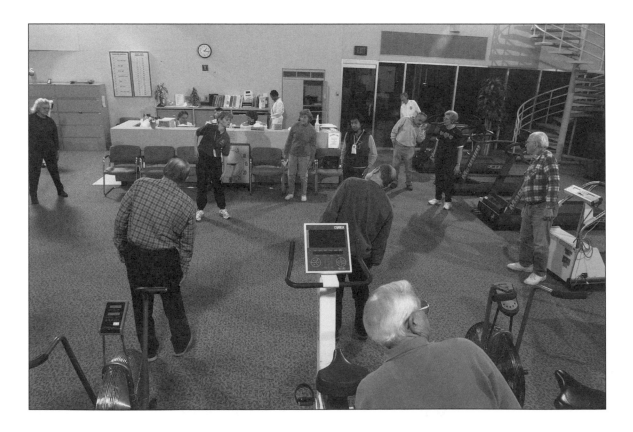

Waist circumference provides a simple, fast, and clinically acceptable measurement of assessing abdominal fat. Using these measures, the levels of overweight and obesity can be determined (table 8.9).

Clinical research tools such as hydrostatic weighing, computerized tomography (CT), magnetic resonance imaging (MRI), and dual-energy X-ray absorptiometry (DEXA) are most accurate but are generally not practical for use in secondary prevention settings.[298,587] Various alternative approaches to estimating body composition have been employed in CR programs, including bioelectrical impedance (BIA), near-infrared interactance (NIR), and skin-fold measures. Of these, the validity of BIA and NIR techniques in overfat or obese adults remains questionable and, at the least, must be measured under strict conditions. Although skinfold measurements are easily obtained estimates of percentage of body fat, inter- and intra-observer variability in measurements and estimation of recommended weights from these measures can be problematic. Used as absolute measures rather than for the determination of percentage of fat, individual skinfold, in addition to BMI, can provide meaningful and comparative feedback to patients throughout their participation in the program.

BMI may be calculated as follows:

$$BMI = weight_{(kg)} / height^2_{(meters)}$$

or

$$BMI = weight_{(lb)} \times 703 / height^2_{(inches)}$$

A complete educational module for BMI, including a chart to calculate BMI, is available at the following Web sites: http://www.shapeup.org and http://www.nhlbisupport.com/bmi. In general, a BMI of <25 is desirable, whereas a BMI ≥25 is associated with increased health risks.

Because patient behavior is integral to the success of any weight-loss program, practitioners should assess the patient's motivation to begin weight-loss therapy, assess the readiness of the patient to implement the plan, and then take appropriate steps to motivate the patient for treatment. All patients should achieve and maintain an appropriate or desirable weight and should begin diet management and physical activity as appropriate.

Dietary Assessment and Intervention

Dietary evaluation is an essential component of a weight-management program. Patients should be assessed for total daily caloric intake, fat and cholesterol intake, and adequate nutrient and fiber content of their diet. Evaluation of eating habits, including time of day they eat, portion sizes, snacking, triggers, and sociocultural influences, is important. Caloric expenditure during domestic, occupational, and leisure tasks as well as during exercise is helpful to estimate caloric balance. The presence of underlying metabolic abnormalities (including hypothyroidism, Cushing's disease, and other endocrine disorders) should be noted. Family history of obesity as well as the patient's weight history should also be assessed to evaluate possible genetic influences. Finally, assessment of the patient's personal perception of weight and appearance can be helpful in setting reasonable short-term and long-term goals.

Interventions to promote weight loss in patients determined to be at an undesirable body weight and composition should focus on the following areas:

- Identifying and treating underlying metabolic disorders when possible
- Adjusting caloric intake via dietary counseling

Table 8.9 Classification of Overweight and Obesity

Weight class	BMI (kg/m²)	Disease risk* associated with waist circumference >40 inches (102 cm) in men and >35 inches (88 cm) in women
Normal	18.5-24.9	Increased
Overweight	25.0-29.9	High
Class 1 obesity	30.0-34.9	Very high
Class 2 obesity	35.0-39.9	Very high
Class 3 obesity	≥40	Extremely high

* Disease risk for diabetes, hypertension, and cardiovascular disease.

Data from Krauss RM, Eckel RH, Howard B, et al. AHA Dietary Guidelines: Revision 2000: A statement for healthcare professionals from the Nutrition Committee of the American Heart Association. *Circulation* 2000;102:2284-2299.

- Increasing caloric expenditure via increased daily physical activity and a regular program of exercise

- Implementing behavioral interventions to promote long-term adherence

- Considering pharmacological therapy in patients whose obesity has been determined to be seriously detrimental to their health, and only as an adjunct to a comprehensive weight-control program.

Secondary prevention programs that combine exercise, dietary education, counseling, and behavioral interventions designed to reduce body weight can help patients lose weight. These multifactorial cardiovascular risk–reduction interventions are recommended as components of secondary prevention. Because of the potential adverse effects of appetite-suppressant medications, these drugs should be considered only for those patients with a BMI of 30 or greater with no concomitant obesity-related risk factors or diseases, or for those patients with a BMI of 27 or greater with concomitant obesity-related risk factors or diseases. Weight-loss drugs should never be used without lifestyle modification. When used, continual assessment of drug therapy for efficacy and safety is essential.[161]

Individualized recommendations for dietary modification should be made with consideration of reasonable goals and likelihood of compliance. Involvement of the patient's spouse or live-in partner in nutritional counseling sessions is important to foster compliance and support, particularly if this person is primarily involved with food shopping and meal preparation. Nutrition instruction should emphasize helping the patient to establish a new eating style that is low in sugar, fat, and cholesterol and high in nutrients, complex carbohydrates, and fiber. In the initial stages of weight loss, both total daily caloric intake and percentage of fat calories should be reduced. A diet that is individually planned to help create a deficit of 500-1,000 kcal/d should be an integral part of any program.

Most women do well on 1,200-1,500 kcal/d and men on 1,500-2,000 kcal/d, depending on their age, height, weight, and activity level. Much of the calorie moderation tends to occur spontaneously as patients focus on higher-nutrient choices. A rate of weight loss of 1-2 lb/week (.5-1 kg/week) or 1% of body weight/week is considered safe.[104] An initial goal of reducing body weight by approximately 10% from baseline should be considered, but the timeframe to accomplish this must be individualized. Randomized controlled diet studies suggest that this can be accomplished within 6 months of therapy. With success, further weight loss can be attempted, if indicated.[176] A multivitamin/mineral supplement is recommended in that it is difficult to ensure nutritional adequacy on diets of less than 1,800 kcal/d.

Patients should be counseled to avoid skipping meals or undertaking periods of nutritional deprivation. Instead, they should adopt a regular eating pattern that begins with breakfast and includes four to six small feedings per day spaced 3-4 h apart. In addition to improving metabolic regulation, this recommended eating pattern eliminates the intense feelings of physical deprivation that may characterize erratic, large-meal eaters and commonly lead to indiscriminate food choices and recurrent binges.[104] The use of very low calorie diets (VLCD) are beyond the scope of typical CR programs. Information regarding VLCD programs can be found elsewhere. [104,176,244]

As with all patients, increased daily physical activity should be recommended for those trying to control weight. Patients can incorporate walking, stair climbing, gardening, and recreational activities (e.g., bowling, golf, tennis) into their daily and weekly schedule to promote general health and caloric expenditure. The exercise program should be designed to promote at least 250-300 kcal of energy expended per session by the point of completing 12 weeks of early outpatient exercise training, with the long-term goal of 1,000-2,000 kcal/week, which would include additional daily physical activity.[195] This may be difficult to attain for cardiac patients who may have a low exercise capacity. Therefore, additional or lengthier exercise sessions may be useful with these patients. The choice of exercise modalities is particularly important for the person aiming to lose weight. Weight-bearing activities appear to provide the greatest caloric expenditure and should be recommended whenever possible after considering any musculoskeletal limitations.[638] Other concerns include body-weight limits for use of treadmills and stair climbers, increased difficulty of obtaining adequate ECGs during telemetry monitoring, and modification of training equipment to optimize efficacy and comfort for the obese individual. Larger seats for stationary and recumbent cycles and a platform step to utilize equipment are suggested. Some patients may have to walk in hallways or on an adjacent track (if available) until they reach a weight appropriate for the treadmill. If the overweight patient cannot use a treadmill or stationary cycle to perform the initial exercise test, a 6-min walk test may be used for exercise prescription and functional capacity assessment.

Behavioral interventions designed to reinforce changes in diet and physical activity, beyond basic educational sessions, are important. Additionally, CR specialists should assess measures of patient compliance, including attendance rates and activities during each session. Periodic structured outcome measures should assess both short-term and long-term results and the factors that may affect them. Referral to specialized validated weight-loss programs should be considered if the patient does not attain weight-loss goals. A weight-maintenance program of diet, physical activity, and behavior therapy is essential to prevent regain of weight.

Emerging Risk Factors

Several additional risk factors for atherosclerotic disease are emerging. In general, these risk factors relate directly or indirectly to thrombus formation and dissolution and to atherosclerotic initiation and progression processes, such as inflammation or endothelial dysfunction. The following factors have received considerable attention.

Homocysteine

Altered homocysteine metabolism can lead to elevations in the plasma concentrations of homocysteine beyond the normal level of 10 mmol/L. A large series of cross-sectional and retrospective case-control studies indicates that levels greater than 15 mmol/L are associated with increased risks of CHD, peripheral artery disease, stroke, and venous thromboembolism.[88,493] Elevated homocysteine levels may be linked to atherosclerosis and thrombosis by several pathophysiologic mechanisms, including endothelial cell injury and impairment of endothelial function, increased proliferation of vascular smooth muscle cells, adverse modification of LDL particles, increased propensity for coagulation, and increased oxidative stress. Although treatment of hyperhomocysteinemia with vitamin supplementation (folic acid, vitamin B6, and vitamin B12) is effective in lowering the plasma levels of homocysteine, appropriate clinical trials are under way to evaluate the proper dose and subsequent effect of these vitamin supplements on atherosclerosis. Until these data become available, population-wide screening for elevated homocysteine levels is not recommended.[361] In selected patients with personal or family history of premature CVD, especially without other known risk factors, evaluation of homocysteine levels may be prudent. In those patients with levels >10 mmol/L, it may be advisable to increase their intake of vitamin-fortified foods (vegetables, fruits, legumes, fortified grains and cereals), and to suggest the use of supplemental vitamins (folate, vitamin B6, and vitamin B12). Such treatment, however, is still considered experimental, pending the results from trials that demonstrate that homocysteine lowering favorably affects atherosclerosis and adverse cardiovascular events.[361]

Lipoprotein(a) and Other Factors Related to Thrombosis

Although Lp(a) is technically a lipid, this molecule plays a regulatory role in atherothrombosis. Unlike other lipid molecules, which participate in the process of atherosclerosis, Lp(a) is thought to compete with plasminogen in binding to fibrin. This results in a potential direct inhibition of endogenous fibrinolysis.[491] Clinical data supporting a role of Lp(a) in CAD remain inconclusive. Even among the positive studies, only a modest association has been found between levels of Lp(a) and subsequent risk. Although the use of niacin has been associated with lower levels of Lp(a), again the question whether this effect reduces coronary risk remains unresolved.[492,504] Elevated fibrinogen levels, and elevated levels of tissue-type plasminogen activator (tPA) have also been shown to be associated with increased cardiovascular risk.[169,469] As methods for detection of these factors improve, future studies may provide additional evidence that either prove or negate the need for continued consideration of these factors as important targets for evaluation and possible treatment.

C-Reactive Protein and Other Markers of Inflammation

Because it is now recognized that atherosclerosis is an inflammatory process, several plasma markers of inflammation have also been evaluated as potential tools to predict the risk of coronary events. Many are now being studied and include high-sensitivity C-reactive protein (hs-CRP), heat shock protein, interleukin-6, and soluble intercellular adhesion molecule type 1 (sICAM-1). Of these, hs-CRP has been the most widely evaluated. Only hs-CRP has an established World Health Organization standard, and high-sensitivity assays for this parameter appear to provide reliable results.[349,469,470] Therefore, hs-CRP has potential for future clinical use as a readily obtainable marker that may guide preventive treatment strategies.

The possibility that infectious agents can cause vascular inflammation and subsequently lead to atherothrombosis is intriguing. New evidence linking microorganisms such as *Chlamydia pneumoniae* to atherosclerosis is indeed provocative, and several studies report that an association does exist, having found the organism in atherosclerotic tissue.[238] However, the finding of an association does not prove causation. To date, there are no definitive findings from secondary prevention antibiotic treatment trials.[240] Currently, two large trials are under way to evaluate whether Chlamydia pneumoniae plays a causative role in atherosclerosis, and whether antibiotic treatment directed against Chlamydia pneumoniae will decrease the complications of atherosclerosis.[158,239]

Summary

The interaction of the various CVD risk factors that have been described in this chapter contribute to the overall potential for events of morbidity and mortality in patients with CHD. Our attempts to identify and assess and subsequently provide appropriate interventions are of paramount importance in the process of reducing risk for such sequelae. Patients, particularly those with multiple risk factors, may find the task of simultaneously reducing the level of each risk factor overwhelming. In such instances, rehabilitation staff members should educate patients as to the significance of each risk factor, perhaps prioritizing, with the patient's input, the structure of the various risk factor interventions. Clearly the elimination of habitual smoking; the control of hypertension, dyslipidemia, and obesity; increasing physical activity; and treatment of anxiety and depression are keys to reducing the risk of subsequent MI and death resulting from heart disease. However, secondary prevention staff members must approach each patient from a case-management perspective, thus providing an organized plan for intervention services.

9

Special Considerations

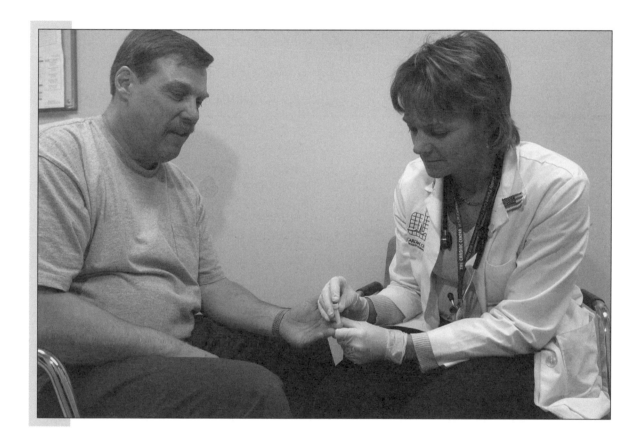

Contemporary secondary prevention programs deliver individualized programs of prescribed exercise and risk-factor modification that focus on the attainment of well-defined, measurable goals. The attainment of these specific goals predicts improved clinical and quality-of-life outcomes. The AHCPR Clinical Practice Guideline *Cardiac Rehabilitation*, published in 1995, provided the model for CR practice and secondary prevention.[604] This model identified the need to

- emphasize the roles of education and behavior-modification aspects of CR as equal to that of exercise, and

- individualize available rehabilitation services rather than package them into a rigid, repetitive program structure.

OBJECTIVES

This chapter describes the basis for assessment and intervention strategies related to specific groups of patients within the overall secondary prevention model, providing individualized program considerations for

■ older and younger patients;

■ women;

■ patients of racial and cultural diversity;

■ patients who have undergone revascularization or valve surgery;

■ patients with a history of complex arrhythmias or placement of a pacemaker or implantable cardioverter defibrillator (ICD);

■ patients with heart failure;

■ patients who have undergone cardiac transplantation; and

■ patients with diabetes, pulmonary disease, or peripheral arterial disease.

The resulting services for both exercise and behavioral change individualize CR to the different collection of problems and needs each cardiac patient brings to the rehabilitation setting. This personalized approach works well in a case-management environment in which an increasing number of subgroups of cardiac patients are in CR (see guideline 9.1).

Guideline 9.1   Implementation of Cardiac Rehabilitation in Special Populations

CR specialists should

■ prepare a list of special population groups likely to participate in their facility, for example, older and younger adults; women; those of ethnic diversity; patients who have undergone revascularization or valve replacement; and patients with a history of dysrhythmias, heart failure, heart transplant, diabetes, COPD and heart disease, and peripheral arterial disease;

■ identify major safety concerns and outline strategies to minimize safety problems and respond to safety incidents should they occur for each group;

■ prepare a plan of care outlining how secondary prevention services, encompassing both exercise and education, will be adjusted to the unique problems and issues of that group;

■ develop a competency plan to assure that staff members have the requisite knowledge and skills to work with the special groups;

■ include an assessment for special physical and psychosocial needs in the initial evaluation; and

■ identify and maintain a list of other professionals and support services that staff may need to call on to assist with implementation of secondary prevention services in special populations or with patients with special needs.

The purpose of this chapter is to provide an overview of patient-evaluation considerations and strategies to successfully implement secondary prevention services for selected subgroups of cardiac patients, with emphasis on strategies that

- maximize patient safety,
- individualize rehabilitation services, and
- optimize patient outcomes.

Older Patients

As the American population ages and the treatment of CHD improves, the number of older adults (≥65 yr) eligible for secondary prevention continues to dramatically increase. Older patients now make up the majority of cardiac patients eligible for CR programs. Patients in this group have a high degree of disability following cardiac events. Ample evidence exists that elderly people with CHD benefit from exercise training and other aspects of secondary prevention.[604,620] Unfortunately, utilization of CR by older patients with CHD has historically been poor,

especially in women.[6,8,344,621] Many older patients who would derive benefit from these interventions do not participate due to lack of recognition by health care providers, as well as by these patients and their families, of the value of secondary programming in this age group; economic and logistic considerations for those wishing to participate; and limited opportunities for safe and effective alternatives to formal programming.[6,618] Figure 9.1 summarizes suggested intervention strategies for older patients with CHD.

The clinical manifestations of CHD in older patients are the result of a combination of the disease itself and the physiologic effects of age. Elderly individuals have more extensive CAD and are more likely to have had a previous MI. Although the presentation of typical angina is common in elderly patients, an increased percentage of older patients have atypical manifestations of myocardial ischemia including dyspnea, heart failure, and non-Q-wave MI, potentially explaining the increased rate of unrecognized MI in this age group, particularly in women.[250,431,569] Reductions in functional capacity in these patients will reflect the impact not only of CHD but also that of various comorbid conditions, including COPD,

Safety	Exercise	Education
• Consider increased musculoskeletal dysfunction, decreased mobility, slower reflexes, impaired senses = extra caution; short-term memory = cognitive disorders; balance, ROM, and ≠ comorbidities • Floor surfaces require slip prevention	• Stabilize equipment; add safety accessories for mounting/dismounting (e.g., step stool for bikes, grab bar for rower); consider special pieces such as recumbent bike or stepper; adequate room to mount/dismount and move around; increase flexibility/range-of-motion activities; allow more time for progression of activity level to prevent overuse • ≠ assistance to mount/dismount • Modify rooms to accommodate preexisting problems (e.g., arthritis) • Repeat instructions; post reminders, use cue cards • Be patient • Provide age-appropriate environment • Focus on ADL, preferred recreational activities, and functional independence	• Make available materials for impaired senses, such as printed instruction for hearing impaired, large-type print for poor vision • Offer daylight times for classes as elderly are reluctant to go out after dark • Offer small amounts of information repeated often and individualized to each person • Consider social isolation by involving family members or personal caregivers • Emphasize nutrition principles adapted for this age group • Identify barriers to learning

Figure 9.1 Intervention strategies for older cardiac patients.

PAD, arthritis, and neuromuscular disorders. The absence of typical angina in this age group may merely reflect the patient's limited level of function and thus an inability to achieve an exertion-related ischemic threshold.

An increasing number of older patients are undergoing revascularization procedures, frequently as repeat procedures.[438] These patients are more likely to have severe angina, to be female, and to have hypertension, CHF, and other vascular diseases. Although outcomes for these procedures are good, in the case of CABGs, there is an increased frequency of postoperative arrhythmias, particularly atrial fibrillation, stroke, and protracted hospitalization.[67,162,416] Although frequency of complex cardiac arrhythmias increases with age (approximately 10% of individuals older than 80 yr), such findings may also be a sign of acute myocardial ischemia in the elderly.[485,568]

Secondary Prevention

Stragegies for affecting risk factors associated with secondary events in older patients with CHD are described here. Risk factors discussed include smoking, hypertension, dyslipidemia, obesity, diabetes, psychosocial dysfunction, and physical inactivity.

Smoking

Data indicate that smoking cessation reduces both morbidity and mortality rates in patients older than age 70. The reductions in relative risk of MI and death are similar to those seen in younger individuals. Smoking cessation rates in these patients range from 20% to 70% at the end of 1 yr and interventions that are effective in younger patients have also proven successful in elderly patients.[395,555] Both NRT and other pharmacological agents are safe for patients with CVD, including the elderly.[185]

Hypertension

By JNC-VII criteria, greater than 65% of people age 65 or older, especially women, are hypertensive.[304] Although the benefit of antihypertensive therapy is particularly high in patients age 60 to 80 yr, treatment and control of hypertension are suboptimal in nearly two-thirds of these patients.[81,247,355,532,609,632] Control of hypertension prevents strokes and CHF more than coronary events, but overall mortality is also reduced. Treatment of hypertension in the elderly should follow the JNC-VII guidelines.[304] Although very effective in this age group, pharmacological therapy of all types is more difficult in older patients compared to younger patients because the aging process is associated with altered pharmacokinetics

and drug responses.[118] As a result, a comparatively high incidence of symptomatic side effects, including hypotension, dizziness, and fatigue, can be anticipated. Most often, however, adverse effects of drug therapy in elderly persons are not unique but simply exaggerated responses to problems also observed in younger patients. Non-pharmacological therapy is more effective in older populations as compared to the younger age group.

Dyslipidemia

Substantial data from subanalyses of older participants within existing studies suggest the importance of lipid-lowering therapy on morbidity and mortality in elderly patients with CHD.[348,386,487] Results for older patients are similar if not better than those of younger patients. Because mortality rates increase substantially with age, the absolute risk reduction for both all-cause and CHD mortality is approximately twice as great for the older patients. Furthermore, therapy in the elderly has been projected to be cost-effective.[212] Despite these findings, clinicians should not overlook quality-of-life issues including cost of medications, concomitant illness, and life expectancy in these patients, given the potential for up to two years before any benefit is demonstrable. The NCEP-ATP III guidelines should be followed for patients of this age group.[403]

Consideration of significant dietary changes for this age group should include a consultation with a registered dietitian. The diet must maintain nutritional adequacy. A gradual change from high-fat foods to lower-fat foods is recommended. Unfortunately for those on fixed incomes, costs related to this type of supervision and to the purchase and preparation of the food itself may be higher.

Obesity

The clustering of hypertension, dyslipidemia, hypertension, and insulin resistance in older overweight people, particularly those with preferential abdominal obesity, makes obesity a risk factor for coronary events for older patients with CHD.[570,590] Unfortunately, few data are available to describe the impact of weight loss on these risk factors. The effect of exercise training on body composition in older coronary patients has suggested only minimal impact, although significant correlations between changes in body mass and lipid profile, and glucose and insulin measures have been noted.[97,343] Increasing both the frequency and the duration of exercise sessions, particularly walking, as a means to increase exercise-related energy expenditure should be implemented; calorie expenditure is otherwise generally low with either structured exercise programs, recreations, or general daily activities.[375,490] The use of hypocaloric diets in these patients has also received little attention, although in one study, significant weight reduction was accompanied by improvement in the lipid profile.[311] Because many older patients may already have poor nutrition, however, it is important to ensure the adequacy of any prescribed calorie-restricted diet.

Diabetes

Diabetes mellitus is closely associated with the occurrence of secondary coronary events in older CHD patients.[589] Exercise training improves insulin resistance and diabetic control in both healthy older persons and in middle-aged CHD patients.[159,323,483] However, some have suggested that the effect of exercise on glycemic control in older diabetic patients may relate more to its effect on fat mass or body fat distribution, and thus the treatment of obesity in these patients is particularly important.[97,343]

Psychosocial Dysfunction

Research from younger populations in general and elderly populations with noncardiac illnesses helps to define those psychosocial issues important to older cardiac patients, including socioeconomic status, psychological status, social support, cognitive function, and quality-of-life issues.[95] Assessment of these parameters is critical when designing secondary prevention programs for this age group.

Low socioeconomic status not only is a risk factor for CHD mortality but also affects participation in secondary prevention programs. As many as 15% of older patients are depressed, with 20% showing significant signs of anxiety.[168] Among those age 65 or older, 51% of women and 13% of men are widowed, and many have suffered a variety of other significant personal and financial types of losses.[211] These losses may lead to social isolation and depression. Although the presence of depression is best ascertained by a formal psychiatric interview, in the secondary prevention setting it can be detected using a brief questionnaire such as the Geriatric Depression Questionnaire.[390] Lack of a support system has also been associated with increased morbidity and mortality in patients of this age group.[335] Changes in sensory and cognitive function, which are likely to be present to some degree in this age group, may make it difficult to thoroughly read, hear, and understand health information and instructions.[211] Alcohol and drug abuse are not uncommon in older patients and should be considered and assessed.[84] Finally, providers should address end-of-life issues, including determination of patients' advance directives.[454]

Physical Inactivity

The basis for an exercise intervention in physically inactive patients includes improved functional capacity with reduced activity-related abnormal signs or symptoms.[2,3,7,343,344,618,621,622] Expected outcomes are similar to those for younger patients, although absolute levels of functional capacity in the elderly are less, and results may require longer program participation in this age group, particularly for those patients age 75 and older.[62,617,621,623] Increasing physical activity in this age group may also aid in the modification of hypertension, obesity, elevated blood glucose level, and various psychosocial parameters.[343,344,604] Whether exercise training as a part of a multidisciplinary approach to secondary prevention is associated with a reduction of events of morbidity or mortality as in younger patients has yet to be established, although one study of older patients with CHD and several others of older persons without known CHD have suggested a positive impact of physical activity on mortality.[204,255,337,596]

Methods for prescribing exercise for cardiac patients have been published and generally do not require significant modification for elderly patients.[619] The recommendations for increasing exercise participation should not be limited to structured exercise but should also employ a broader interpretation of exercise programming, including occupational and leisure activities as well as simple ADL. Rehabilitation staff should also give consideration to differences in needs between older women and men, recognizing the importance of socialization.[575] The exercise program should promote all aspects of physical conditioning, including aerobic capacity and muscular endurance, range of motion and flexibility, and muscular strength, and emphasize increasing caloric expenditure and enhancement of functional mobility. To reduce the potential for overuse injuries, increasing frequency and duration of exercise sessions should supersede increases in intensity and progression. The inclusion of strength training should improve neuromuscular function as well as muscular strength and endurance. Strength training is valuable in improving responses to the physical demands of daily living while reducing the risk of musculoskeletal injury and falls.[446]

Submaximal evaluations of the performance of specific activities such as the 6-min walk, timed stair climbing, or simulated activities of daily living in standard batteries of tests such as the Physical Performance Test or the Continuous Scale Physical Functional Performance Test can also be used to determine physical-function requirements.[129] The advantage of actually measuring responses to observed activities is that these measurements are very sensitive to change, and, unlike questionnaires, they are little affected by cultural background and educational status. An accurate determination of physical function requirements plays a crucial role in designing individualized interventions for older patients and allows for the serial measurement of progress. Strength testing is also useful in that it defines the potential to perform strength-related activities (see chapter 8, page 118). Leg strength in particular is a strong predictor of disability rates and of walking endurance.[1,249]

Young Adults

Although young adults (under 50 years of age) with CHD can exhibit a high risk-factor profile, frequently they possess normal physical functioning and skeletal muscle mass. Deconditioning during relatively brief cardiac hospitalizations is minimal, and most younger patients are capable of returning to work relatively quickly upon discharge. A major focus on risk-factor modification and return to work is warranted, and thus, baseline evaluations should emphasize these issues. Rehabilitation specialists can give the patient specific return-to-work recommendations after a baseline stress test, with low-risk patients returning to work 2 weeks after a normal stress test. Patients who return to high-intensity physical labor may benefit from a resistance training program and thus should have a strength assessment as well. When possible, it is very useful to assess work-related activities such as lifting with close monitoring to provide the patient with reassurance for specific activities. While depression is less common in younger patients, it occurs nonetheless and needs to be recognized and treated. Anxiety is a common problem that is fairly easily recognizable at the baseline interview and with standardized measurement tools.

Though it is rare to see cardiac patients in their 20s, those in their 30s and 40s are increasingly common. These patients have needs and problems different from their 60- or 80-year-old counterparts and thus present their own set of challenges. For secondary prevention services to be effective in a young adult population, professionals should recognize this age grouping as being at a distinctly different developmental stage and recognize the related tasks and priorities that occur in the young adult. Focus at this stage of life tends to be on family and job security. Most people at these ages are used to taking charge and being in control. The very possibility that a diagnosis of heart disease threatens either or both of these life priorities, and potentially decreases the patient's status in the eyes of family and peers, causes varying degrees of anxiety in these young patients. Denial is a common coping mechanism used to deal with such fear. Therefore, goals for this special population often encompass giving control back to the patient and promoting self-management and include

- facilitating return to work;
- respecting time pressures;
- involving significant others; and
- dealing with anxiety, denial, and anger.

Patients in this age group are often familiar with and have been previously involved with exercise, so getting them started in an exercise program is easier than for some other special populations. However, unlike in other groups, in young adults compliance to the exercise regime may be enhanced when similarly aged patients are grouped together. Unfortunately, because members of this age group almost universally have the need and expectation to return to work, time for exercise, either at the rehabilitation facility or at home, becomes increasingly scarce. Compliance, not just with exercise regimens but with other risk-factor management as well, quickly becomes a major issue. As young adults return to their previous jobs and social circles, they tend to return to previous lifestyle habits.

CR specialists are challenged to find ways to help this group develop and maintain healthful living as a priority in the midst of multiple life demands. Behavior specialists, who can help these young patients work on values clarification, goal setting, and other life-management strategies, are a particularly valuable resource. Also of value to a subgroup within the young adult population are vocational rehabilitation counselors. Some patients are displaced from their previous jobs as a result of their cardiac events and can benefit from job counseling or retraining.

Women

Fundamental differences exist in the profile of female cardiac patients compared with male patients in CR.[111] Women, on average, are 10 yr older than men when they initially present with symptomatic CVD. Thus, although CHD is the number-one cause of death in American women, it is more a disease of the later years than in men. In addition to the age difference, women differ from men by clinical presentation, by the frequency of cardiac risk factors, by the frequency of psychological dysfunction, by the likelihood of disability and poor physical function, and by the likelihood of participating in CR.

Clinical Presentation

Heart disease presents itself differently in women than in men, and even when MI is suspected, women frequently arrive later at the hospital.[411] Classic crushing chest pain is less common in women, and women more often experience atypical manifestations of angina or infarction such as gastrointestinal-type symptoms or epigastric pain.

Coronary Risk-Factor Profiles

The higher mortality rates after MI in women are due primarily to the older age of women at presentation. However, women are also at higher risk due to a greater prevalence of hypertension, diabetes, and CHF than men. Thus, the importance of lifestyle-related changes such as physical activity and weight loss are accentuated as they relate to hypertension and diabetic control, particularly in the presence of abdominal obesity.[443] A heightened awareness of signs and symptoms of CHF for females in secondary prevention programs is also appropriate.

Mood and Social Isolation

Female coronary patients have fewer psychosocial supports, are more likely to be depressed, and are more likely to live alone than male patients. The presence of depression predicts not only a worsened cardiac prognosis for those afflicted, but poorer physical functioning and quality of life. Though the presence of depression predicts a lower likelihood of CR participation, depression scores have been shown to improve for those who do participate when exercise is combined with group stress management.[4,350] Depression is best assessed at the baseline interview, assisted by established questionnaires such as the Beck Depression Inventory and the Hamilton Depression Rating Scale, which detail the presence of depressive symptoms.[616] Lower rates of marriage and employment at clinical presentation may also have an unfavorable impact on the physical and emotional status in women as they enter CR and secondary prevention programs.[109]

Physical Function

Women are less fit at entry to CR than men, even when the age difference is not significant.[8,109] Data from the Framingham Disability Study documents that female gender predicts significantly higher disability rates in coronary patients. Women with CHD describe a significant limitation in their ability to perform household tasks required for independent functioning.[321]

Cardiac Rehabilitation Participation

Female gender predicts a lower likelihood of CR participation, compared with age-matched males.[6,172] In two studies, this finding appears to be caused primarily by a lower physician recommendation score for participation given to women.[6,114] Other factors such as greater transportation difficulties for women and more household duties such as caring for dependent family members may also be operative.[6]

Practice Considerations

A high priority for physicians and other clinicians is to increase the number of female patients participating within secondary preventive services. The biggest barriers appear to be physician-related and patient-related reluctance to consider participation in structured exercise and lifestyle modification. When transportation or home obligations limit onsite participation, consideration of a home program is necessary. Risk-factor differences between as well as within genders must be recognized, prioritized, and addressed. Intervention considerations for female patients are described in figure 9.2. Goals for rehabilitation staff working with female cardiac patients should include

- maximizing participation of female cardiac patients by decreasing barriers that limit participation,
- recognizing gender-related differences in depression rates and in level of social support,
- recognizing gender-related differences in coronary risk profiles, and
- collaborating with primary physicians to aggressively manage risk factors.

Figure 9.3 compares risk factors in older, postmenopausal women to those in younger female cardiac patients.

The unique medical and psychosocial needs of women and men in CR must be recognized in all aspects of program design such that positive outcomes and adherence can be maximized. Issues of social support and extent of comorbidities may alter not only the exercise component, but the education and counseling needs as well. The traditional programmatic emphasis on aerobic training may need to be reassessed, particularly as resistance training has become indicated for improving response to at-home demands, enhancing weight loss, and managing diabetes. In addition, the value of lifestyle exercise, that is, pursuing physical

Safety	Exercise	Education
• Tend to have slower recovery, more complications, more recurrences, more comorbidities	• More functional impairment and less exercise in females	• Hormone replacement therapy information
• Atypical symptoms are more frequent than in males	• The importance of weight-bearing exercise for osteoporosis must be considered	• Psychosocial concerns, including guilt regarding fulfillment of traditional responsibilities and role conflicts
• Question of gender bias against females	• Decreased muscle strength, especially upper extremities, will contribute to poorer functional independence	• Inherent dangers from birth control + smoking
		• More depression
		• Counsel re: household work, return to work, and sexuality

Figure 9.2 Intervention considerations for female cardiac patients.

Premenopausal, <age 50	Postmenopausal, ≥age 50
Insulin-dependent diabetes	Abdominal obesity
Smoking	Diabetes
Family history	Hypertension
Obesity	Dyslipidemia
History of contraceptive use	

Figure 9.3 CVD risk factors in pre- and postmenopausal women.

activity during daily activities such as climbing stairs or walking to work or the market, may be especially important to achieving health-related goals. CR specialists need to recognize the unique physical and psychological issues related to female cardiac patients and to employ special strategies to address them. Creative programmatic options should be explored, such as

■ one-on-one program orientation;

■ a women-only exercise group;

■ a female drivers' group to encourage participation of nondrivers;

■ a greater emphasis on low-intensity, longer-duration exercise; and

■ a women's support group.

Racial and Cultural Diversity

Cultural diversity refers to the differences between people based on a shared ideology and valued set of beliefs, norms, customs, and meanings evidenced by a particular way of life.[526] More than 30% of all U.S. residents are presently people of color; by the year 2050, this proportion is expected to reach more than 50%. The African American population is expected to double in size and make up 22% of the total population. Hispanics and Asian Americans, the two most rapidly growing populations in the United States, are predicted to make up 18% and 10% of the total, respectively.[139] Health care providers must be prepared to meet the cultural, linguistic, and educational needs of this ever-changing mix.

CVD and Cultural Disparities

Despite differences in racial and ethnic backgrounds, CVD (primarily CHD and stroke) kills nearly as many Americans as all other diseases combined and is among the leading causes of disability in the United States.[31] According to the AHA 2003 Heart Disease and Stroke Statistics Update, the death rates from and prevalence of CVD for black males and females far exceed those for their white counterparts. The estimated age-adjusted prevalence of CVD in white adults is 30% for men and 24% for women. In contrast, it is 41% for black men and 40% for black women while it is 29% and 27% for Mexican American men and women, respectively.[31]

The prevalence of modifiable cardiovascular risk factors also varies significantly among different racial groups. A greater prevalence of CVD risk factors exists among black and Mexican American women than among white women of comparable socioeconomic status (SES). Among adult women the age-adjusted prevalence of obesity continues to be higher for black women (50%) and Mexican American women (40%) than for white women (30%). In addition, the cholesterol screening rates show that only 50% of American Indians/Alaska Natives, 44% of Asian Americans and 38% of Mexican Americans have had their cholesterol checked in the past 2 yr. Among American Indians/Alaska Natives who are age 18 and older, 64% of men and 61% of women have one or more CVD risk factors (hypertension, smoking, hypercholesterolemia, obesity, or diabetes). It was reported that had physical inactivity been included in this analysis, the prevalence rate would have been significantly higher.[31]

In addition to these morbidity and mortality levels, the effects of disparity also result in poorer functional ability, decreased quality of life, personal loss, pain, suffering, and difficulties for families and loved ones. SES has been shown to be an important and independent factor in the etiology and progression of CVD. When SES is described in terms of education, employment, and income, a consistent inverse relationship exists between these indicators and risk factors for CVD. But even after controlling for SES, health insurance, and clinical factors, racial and ethnic inequalities in health status and care exist.[463]

Health Care Disparities

Major disparities exist among population groups in terms of access to care, processes of care, and outcomes between whites and racial/ethnic minority groups in the United States.[183] Minority Americans lag behind on nearly every health indicator. Some striking examples include the following:

1. Nearly twice as many Hispanic as white adults are likely to die from diabetes, and an equal number report not having a regular physician.

2. African Americans are less likely to be hospitalized for chest pain. They also have

significantly fewer CABGS and angioplasty procedures than whites despite at least one report where blacks were shown to have better short-term and equivalent intermediate survival rates when compared with whites.[13,18,181,182,228,299,437,439,610]

3. Nearly 25% of our country's 43 million uninsured Americans are Hispanic. Many of these people work in low-wage, seasonal, or temporary jobs, unable to purchase health insurance because basic needs (food, shelter, clothing) are their first priority. Often health care consists of home remedies or over-the-counter medications and drugs and emergency room visits when needed.[322]

CR programs nationwide have strikingly low rates of nonwhite participants. The Racial and Cultural Diversity Task Force of AACVPR conducted a survey of all of its members in 1999 with 394 responses.[458] Both staff and client race is predominantly white. Fewer than 25% of respondents indicated that they serve any nonwhite populations at all. For those who do, less than 20% of their population is nonwhite, the largest of those being blacks and Hispanics. Issues of major concern to survey respondents regarding nonwhites in CR included language barrier; transportation problems; lack of culturally appropriate information on nutrition, lifestyle modification, and other educational topics; lack of understanding of the learning styles; and values and beliefs relating to adherence, need to return to work, and funding for people in financial need. Dropout rates among both black and Hispanic women are higher than for whites. Reasons cited included work conflicts, child care, and domestic issues.[110]

Eliminating Disparities: Primary and Secondary Prevention

A central goal of Healthy People 2010 is to eliminate health disparities among different segments of the population. These include differences by gender, race or ethnicity, education or income, disability, and sexual orientation. The Surgeon General challenges all individuals, communities, states, and national organizations to become involved in improving health, education, housing, labor, justice, transportation, agriculture, and the environment. To reduce health disparities, the major thrust of Healthy People 2010 is to empower individuals to make informed health care decisions and to promote community-wide safety, education, and access to health care.[179]

The U.S. Department of Health and Human Services, Office of Minority Health, recently published national standards on assuring cultural competence in health care. Based on an analytical review of key laws, regulations, contracts, and standards currently in use by federal and state agencies, these guidelines were developed with input from a national advisory committee of policy makers, providers, and researchers.[512] The 14 recommended standards address competencies for administrative, clinical, and support staff; signage; proficiency of interpreter services; outcome data management; and annual progress reports. The final version of the standards and a complete report on the project can be found online at www.omhrc.gov/clas/frclas2.htm.

Programs of primary prevention for minorities are critical if disparities are to be addressed in earnest. These programs have been shown to be most successful when undertaken through local schools, churches, and community centers because these places provide a sense of trust and safety to most minorities. Research agendas must be formulated and studies conducted by minority scientists in order that the problems be appropriately addressed to meet community health needs. The Hispanic Health Council in Hartford, CT, for example, has developed a unique research program based on identified community needs among the Puerto Rican population.[527]

On a larger scale, the Jackson Heart Study, sponsored by the National Heart, Lung, and Blood Institute and the Office of Research on Minority Health, was initiated in the fall of 2000 and plans to investigate both conventional risk factors and new or emerging factors that may be related to CVD among 6,500 African American men and women. Few large, prospective epidemiologic studies such as this have examined CVD in the African American community.

In addition to research, more affordable CR services must be made available to those with inadequate insurance coverage. Creative, safe community programs can be initiated and conducted at local YMCAs if telemetry monitoring is not deemed essential. Also, local social services agencies may be contacted by the patients themselves or by someone involved in their care to see if special funds are available for those without the means to participate.

General Strategies for Providing Culturally Competent Care in a Diverse Society

Guideline 9.2 describes specific considerations for patients of racial, ethnic, cultural, and socioeconomic diversity.

Guideline 9.2   Racial, Ethnic, Cultural, and Socioeconomic Diversity

Providers must strive to deliver the very best care possible to all patients regardless of background and remain astutely aware of how background may influence the care they provide. They must also consider socioeconomic factors when assessing cardiovascular status and outcomes, particularly with regard to race and ethnicity.[18] The following suggestions are provided to assist CR professionals in the development and provision of care for culturally diverse patients and their families.[99,220,307,351,526,583]

Getting Started

- Recognize your own cultural values and biases.
- Open your mind and learn at least basic information about the history, cultural values, health beliefs, and practices of the people you serve.
- Be respectful of, interested in, and creative in your approach to other cultures and practices.
- Establish trust and allow some time for social interaction before beginning education, screening, or treatments and procedures.

Communication Tips

- Make no assumptions relative to patients' beliefs and practices based on their culture, ethnicity, or religious affiliation. There is variation within all ethnic groups. Don't stereotype.
- Determine the patient's level of fluency in English and arrange for an interpreter if needed. The interpreter serves as a bridge between people of different cultural and linguistic backgrounds.

- Use qualified, medically trained interpreters so that medical information is conveyed in its proper context. Avoid using the patient's family or friends whenever possible.

- Miscommunication can lead to the wrong diagnosis and poor patient outcomes if the patient does not clearly understand medication and treatment goals.

- In general, an older, mature interpreter is preferable.

- Have a brief interview with the interpreter both before and after each session.

- Speak directly to the patient even when the interpreter is present.

- Keep statements short and simple.

- Some patients may be able to read English better than understand the spoken word. Determine the patient's reading ability before using written materials in the teaching session.

- Speak slowly and clearly, without raising your voice, when speaking to someone having difficulty understanding English.

- Address all adults as Mr., Mrs., or Miss, as doing otherwise is discourteous and inappropriate for anyone other than a close friend or family member. Ask how the patient prefers to be addressed.

- When addressing others, avoid using terms such as "boy," "girl," or "gal," which may be construed as derogatory.

- Sign languages of various cultures are not mutually understandable.

- Identify the primary decision maker in the family and include him or her when making major treatment choices.

- Avoid using gestures when communicating. Examples that may be offensive include the following:
  - Beckoning with the finger to come closer, which in some cultures is used only for calling animals
  - Keeping your hands in your pockets when talking to a patient, which may be considered impolite in many cultures
  - Using the thumbs-up, victory, or okay signs, which are insulting gestures in some cultures
  - Placing your foot on a stool when facing the patient as you speak to him or her, which may be considered offensive because the feet are seen as the lowest part of the body

- Avoid slang, technical jargon, idioms, and complex sentences.

- Use open-ended questions and try phrasing them in several different ways to maximize understanding.

- Check frequently for the patient's level of understanding and acceptance of instructions.

- Avoid sentences or questions with negatives, because this often increases confusion. Ask, "Have you used a treadmill before?" instead of "You haven't used a treadmill before, have you?"

- Write out the full date, year, and month; calendar date sequences can differ in other countries.

- Be sensitive when translating matters that are of a private or sexual nature, using same-sex interpreters when possible. To maintain patient confidentiality, do not use family members to translate discussions of these matters.

- Respect modesty, which most cultures value highly. Explain clearly why you need to ask personal questions, as they may not see the relevance to their medical problem and may view you with suspicion.

- Do not dismiss any health beliefs or practices as silly or old-fashioned, because many ethnic groups have deeply ingrained beliefs. Minimizing the importance of these beliefs may cause

(continued)

(continued)

the patient to stop listening to anything else you say. As long as any herbal or folk remedies used cause no harm to the patient, incorporate them into the treatment regimen.

■ If hospital clergy routinely visit, explain this to the patient before the visit. Some cultures associate clergy visits with imminent death.

Tips for Teaching Patients

■ Plan the teaching session to last longer than usual.

■ Use simple sentences when giving instruction or explanation.

■ Speak clearly and avoid technical terms.

■ Sequence the material; present it in the order in which it is to be carried out.

■ Have the patient give a return demonstration on any skill you teach.

■ Include one or more significant family members in the teaching process.

■ Partner with faith-based organizations whenever possible, because many cultures incorporate spirituality and prayer when confronted with illness.

■ Use health care providers from the patient's culture where possible.

Revascularization and Valve Surgery

The number of patients undergoing procedures to optimize coronary blood flow or to correct damaged valves continues to grow. Procedures include traditional open-chest CABGS and valve replacement or repair as well as newer minimally invasive procedures that involve small incisions or thorascope without cardiopulmonary bypass. Cardiac catheterization laboratory procedures include PTCA with or without stent placement, and atherectomy (directional, artery swab, or laser). A summary of special considerations for patients who have undergone these procedures are described in figures 9.4 and 9.5.

CABGS

- Whether the procedure resulted in complete vs. incomplete revascularization
- Whether the procedure included bypass of previous CABGS graft occlusion
- Precautions for upper-extremity exercise and sternal healing
- Patient minimization of seriousness of CHD and that patient has been "cured"
- Importance of comprehensive services for secondary prevention of CHD

PTCA/Stent

- Potential for restenosis at PTCA/stent sites
- Patient minimization of seriousness of CHD and that patient has been "cured"
- Importance of comprehensive services for secondary prevention of CHD

VHD

- Importance of anticoagulation therapy and precautions for exercise-related injuries and bleeding
- Precautions for upper-extremity exercise and sternal healing
- Avoidance of resistance-type exercise with severe valvular stenosis or regurgitation

---

Figure 9.4 Special considerations for revascularization/valve repair patients during CR. VHD = valvular heart disease.

Intervention Strategies for Revascularization/Valve Patients

- The common goal for each patient is the prevention of reocclusion.
- The common problem for rehabilitation staff is to get patients to understand that the disease has not been cured by the procedure.

CABG With Midline Sternotomy

Safety	Exercise	Education
• Incision care, infection prevention	• Avoid heavy arm exercises until healed; upper body stretches/flexes and light resistance exercises are appropriate to promote mobility	• "Normal" postoperative signs/symptoms • Cerebral anoxia = temporary memory loss

MIDCAB and PTCA (and other transcatheter procedures, e.g., stent, atherectomy)

Safety	Exercise	Education
• Risk of reocclusion	• Less deconditioning at outset may allow greater activity level	• Antiplatelet, anticoagulation • Early recognition of signs and symptoms of reocclusion

Valve Surgery

Safety	Exercise	Education
• Long-term anticoagulant therapy for mechanical valves	• More deconditioned = low start at outset; may result in conservative exercise prescription	• Medications, motivation, and encouragement to become more active

Figure 9.5 Intervention strategies for revascularization/valve patients. MIDCAB = minimally invasive direct coronary artery bypass.

Revascularization

The number of revascularization procedures performed each year continues to increase, with CABGS leading the way. In 2000, an estimated 519,000 CABGS were performed on 336,000 patients in the United States.[31] Seventy-two percent of these procedures were performed on men and 55% of the patients were 65 years of age or older. CABGS typically uses a section of saphenous vein or an internal mammary artery as a conduit to circumvent significant atherosclerotic lesions in major epicardial coronary arteries. Gastroepiploic or radial arteries may also be used for this purpose. Between 3% and 12% of saphenous vein grafts occlude within the first month following surgery and, by 10 yr postsurgery, only 60% of vein grafts are still patent.[398] Because of these patency-rate issues, redirected internal mammary arteries are the preferred conduit for CABGS.

Minimally invasive direct coronary artery bypass (MIDCAB) involves access to the heart via a left anterolateral thoracotomy through the fourth intercostal space and is performed without cardiopulmo-nary bypass. The application of MIDCAB is restricted to a proximal lesion in the left anterior descending (LAD) coronary artery using the left internal thoracic artery as the bypass conduit. Because no cardiopulmonary bypass is used during this procedure, it is performed on a beating heart. The main advantage of MIDCAB is the decreased surgical trauma, resulting in a shorter recovery time. The primary disadvantage is the limited application to individuals with proximal LAD disease that can potentially result in incomplete revascularization or the use of MIDCAB plus complementary percutaneous cardiac interventions (PCI) to achieve complete revascularization. A similar technique called thoracoscopic coronary surgery does use cardiopulmonary bypass with peripheral cannulation. Yet another emerging surgical technique using the minimally invasive thoracotomy approach is transmyocardial laser revascularization.

The other major revascularization procedure is PTCA. An estimated 561,000 PTCA procedures were performed in this country in 2000 (64% on men and 50% on persons 65 yr of age or older).[31] From 1987 through 2000, the number of PTCA procedures performed on an annual basis has increased 262%. Restenosis rates after PTCA range from 25% to 40% within the first 6 months, but these rates decrease by approximately 30% when stenting is used in conjunction with angioplasty.[474] To date, PTCA/stent remains the PCI procedure of choice.

Practice Considerations for Patients Who Have Undergone CABGS

CABGS is a recognized indication for referral to CR and secondary prevention services.[58,160,189] During hospitalization for CABGS, exercise is indicated to help avoid the deleterious effects of bed rest, including decreased functional capacity, hypovolemia, and thromboembolic complications. The recommended exercise intensity for inpatient exercise postsurgery is an HR less than or equal to the resting HR plus 30 bpm.[195] The typical length of stay for an uncomplicated CABGS patient is 4 to 6 d, which minimizes the opportunities for comprehensive CR services as an inpatient.

The rate of recovery for CABGS patients is dependent on age, gender, and the surgical techniques employed. Exercise testing 2 to 5 weeks postsurgery is indicated to help assess the results of revascularization, determine functional capacity, develop an exercise prescription, and provide advice on other physical activities. Outpatient rehabilitation can be started within a week of hospital discharge in some patients as appropriate. Exercise-prescription methodology is generally the same as that used with MI patients. Initially, some patients may need lower-intensity or modified exercise because of musculoskeletal discomfort or healing issues at the incision sites. Patients should not engage in upper-extremity resistance training using moderate to heavy weights for the first 3 months following surgery because of concerns about the stability of the sternum and sternal wound healing.[195]

Staff should assess sternal and vein harvest site wound healing in all new patients referred postsurgery. Signs of wound infection include redness, swelling, and drainage; patients with an infected wound need a sterile dressing to avoid cross-contamination of other patients in the program. Because of the possibility of graft closure, program staff should also be alert for new patient complaints of angina pectoris or angina-equivalent symptoms, signs and symptoms of exercise intolerance, and new ECG signs of myocardial ischemia, and they must educate patients to be alert for these as well.

Related to the assessment of possible ischemic signs and symptoms in CABGS patients is the importance of knowing whether the revascularization was complete or incomplete. Complete revascularization (patent bypass grafting of all significant atherosclerotic lesions) should alleviate all associated signs and symptoms of myocardial ischemia. Vessels that have smaller-than-expected coronary artery diameter or those that are diffusely diseased are more likely to result in incomplete revascularization. This increases the likelihood of postsurgical signs and symptoms of residual myocardial ischemia during exercise.

It is very important that patients take secondary prevention steps to help minimize the progression of the atherosclerotic process in native coronary arteries as well as in vein grafts. Of note, lipid values may be falsely low for several weeks following surgery, so the need for lipid reduction should be based on values obtained before surgery.

Practice Considerations for Patients Who Have Undergone PTCA

PTCA is also included in the list of indications for patient referral to CR.[58,189] Because PTCA patients are generally out of the hospital within 12 to 24 h of the procedure, opportunities for inpatient CR services are limited. It is a good strategy to link these patients at the time of discharge with outpatient CR services in order to have adequate time to provide them with information regarding an optimized plan for secondary prevention.

Exercise testing may be performed as early as 2 to 3 d after PTCA, but more routinely, exercise testing is conducted 2 to 5 weeks and again at 6 months post-PTCA. The 6-month test may be important because of the restenosis rates discussed earlier in this section, particularly if the patient develops nonspecific signs and symptoms. In addition to assessing for possible restenosis, exercise test data can also be used to develop an exercise prescription, assess functional capacity, and provide advice concerning physical activity restrictions.

PTCA patients can begin exercise training as outpatients almost immediately after hospital discharge. If the groin was used for catheter access, care should be taken to insure that the access site is healing appropriately before the patient undertakes lower-extremity exercise. Incomplete revascularization is also possible with PTCA, which increases the possibility of exercise-induced signs and symptoms of residual myocardial ischemia. Exercise-prescription methodology is the same as with MI and CABGS patients. Compared to patients who have had CABGS or PTCA with an acute event, patients who underwent PTCA in a nonacute setting may be able to progress at a faster rate because they have not sustained myocardial damage. Secondary prevention issues for PTCA patients are similar to those stated for CABGS patients, especially in patients without a previous MI or angina pectoris who may deny or significantly minimize the need for behavior modification and risk reduction.

Valve Replacement Surgery and Repair

According to the American Heart Association, valvular heart disease (VHD) accounted for 18,520 deaths in 1998 and an estimated 89,000 hospital discharges.[31] Of the total mortality, approximately 63% and 14% were from aortic and mitral valve disease, respectively. Also, nearly 96% of all hospital discharges for VHD were related to aortic and mitral valve disease.

VHD may involve either stenosis or regurgitation and can affect any of the four cardiac valves. Valvular stenosis is a narrowing or obstruction of the valve orifice, resulting in the valve not opening adequately. The causes of stenosis include degenerative calcification, rheumatic disease, or congenitally malformed valves (e.g., bicuspid aortic valve). Regurgitation is the result of an incompetent valve that allows retrograde flow through the valve and may be caused by rheumatic heart disease, infections, or congenital diseases (e.g., Marfan's syndrome). In the case of the mitral valve, regurgitation can also be the result of mitral valve prolapse or ruptured chordae or papillary muscles.

Surgical interventions for valvular dysfunction consist of annuloplasty or valve replacement. Annuloplasty tightens the annulus of a valve in an effort to restore the competence of that valve. Prosthetic heart valves are divided into two main categories: bioprostheses and mechanical prostheses. Bioprosthetic valves are further classified as heterografts, homografts, and stentless heterografts. Types of mechanical prosthetic heart valves include the caged-ball, tilting-disk, and bileaflet valves.[387]

VHD can sometimes involve multiple valves that require combined surgical or interventional management. Common combinations of VHD include mitral stenosis and tricuspid regurgitation, mitral stenosis and aortic stenosis, and aortic stenosis and mitral regurgitation. VHD can also coexist with CAD, especially in elderly patients.

Practice Considerations

Published guidelines of indications for referral to CR programs include patients with VHD.[58,189] From an exercise-testing perspective, aortic stenosis is considered the most problematic VHD because of the increased risk for ventricular tachyarrhythmias, ventricular fibrillation, and exertional syncope. Severe symptomatic aortic stenosis is an absolute contraindication, whereas moderate stenotic VHD is a relative contraindication for exercise testing.[195] However, meta-analysis has concluded that complications during testing were rare when the testing was performed with appropriate caution and monitoring.[205] Furthermore, it was suggested that emphasis should be placed on choosing an appropriate low-level testing protocol, use of a 2-min cool-down following the test, and minute-by-minute monitoring of blood pressure, symptoms, HR slowing, and premature ventricular and atrial arrhythmias.

The exercise prescription and training of VHD patients following valve replacement would be very similar to that used with CABGS patients. However, the physical activity of some VHD patients may have been very restricted for an extended period because of symptoms prior to repair or replacement. The resulting low functional capacity would require these patients to start and progress slowly during the early stages of an exercise training program. Rehabilitation professionals should use standard exercise-prescription methodology with these patients but should take care to avoid upper-extremity exercise (including resistance training involving the upper extremities) until the sternum is stable and there are no sternal wound healing issues postsurgery. Resistance training is contraindicated in any patient with existing severe valvular stenosis or regurgitation.[446]

Patients who have undergone valve replacement surgery are not cured of VHD but instead have exchanged native valve disease for prosthetic valve disease. Prevention of infections at prosthetic valve sites and management of anticoagulation medications are important issues for the postsurgical patient. Patients who have undergone combined valve replacement and CABGS have the same secondary prevention issues regarding reducing CAD risk profiles as stated earlier for the CABGS-only patients.

Patients with VHD but without valve repair or replacement may also be referred for CR. In these patients, critical aortic stenosis is a contraindication for both inpatient and outpatient CR.[195] Patients with less-severe aortic stenosis can exercise but may develop symptoms (e.g., dyspnea, angina, or syncope) during exercise. Exercise training intensity should be kept under the threshold that precipitates the onset of symptoms because these symptoms indicate that the cardiac output is not capable of meeting the demands of the exercise. Dyspnea during exercise is the primary symptom of exercise intolerance with mitral stenosis. A worsening of any of these symptoms over time may indicate a worsening of the valve disease and should be closely monitored.

Ventricular Arrhythmias, Pacemakers, and ICDs

The goals of exercise for patients with ventricular arrhythmias, pacemakers, and ICDs vary widely. Therefore, baseline evaluation and treatment plans need to be individualized. At one extreme, patients with nonsustained ventricular arrhythmias with normal myocardial function may require only several sessions of ECG-monitored exercise with subsequent serial assessments before embarking on a nonmonitored or home exercise program. At the other extreme, some patients with ICDs are physically disabled by the presence of severe myocardial dysfunction and psychologically disabled by a history of sudden cardiac death and the potential for conscious defibrillation. These patients often require more formal and prolonged ECG-supervised exercise programs (see page 65 in chapter 5).

Baseline evaluation at program entry should include a clear description of the arrhythmia, the hemodynamic consequences of the arrhythmia, possible inciting factors such as exercise or cardiac ischemia, and potential therapies should the arrhythmia recur.[317,428] Details about programmed pacemaker or ICD rates, detection parameters, and algorithms should also be obtained. The results of Holter monitoring or electrophysiological stimulation studies should be reviewed and the response to exercise assessed with the patient on the most current medical regimen. For patients with a cardiac pacemaker, exercise testing is used to guide the adjustment of the pacemaker settings and is particularly useful in active patients with rate-responsive pacemakers to ensure appropriate rate responses. Testing also will help identify presence of an angina threshold.

Cardiac pacemaker technologies have advanced substantially in recent years. As a result, the physiology of exercise for patients with pacemakers is essentially the same as for other patients. Increasing HR during exercise is the single most important factor for increasing cardiac output and oxygen uptake. For patients who cannot provide an appropriate intrinsic HR response to exercise, a cardiac pacemaker will increase HR, and thus cardiac output, to meet changing physiological demands.

Atrioventricular (AV) (dual-chamber) pacing is common and allows for physiological pacing, which refers to the maintenance of the normal sequence and timing of the contractions of the upper and lower chambers of the heart. AV synchrony provides a higher cardiac output without dramatically increasing myocardial oxygen uptake. A dual-chamber pacemaker senses the sinus node and incomplete heart block and sends an impulse to the ventricle following an appropriate AV timing interval.

The development of adaptive rate pacing (also called rate-responsive or rate-modulated pacing) has markedly changed the application of pacing with regard to exercise. The adaptive rate function is applied when the native sinus node cannot increase HR to meet metabolic demands. Adaptive-rate pacemakers can sense the body's need for more energy and produce an appropriate cardiac rate in patients with chrontropic incompetence. Sensors have been developed to detect motion and physiological and metabolic changes that occur with increased exercise. Based on computer algorithms, the sensors drive the pacemaker to appropriately pace the heart to meet energy demands. Some of the functions that are monitored are motion during physical activity, minute ventilation, body temperature, and ECG waveform intervals. Fixed-rate ventricular pacing is still prescribed for patients with rare episodes of bradycardia who have an underlying heart rhythm that appropriately increases with exercise and other stimuli.

Personnel working with patients with implanted defibrillators should know the HR at which the ICD is set to discharge, although newer devices that now sense specific changes in QRS width and QT intervals reduce the threat of ICD discharge simply with elevated HR. Baseline exercise testing can help determine whether exercise is likely to cause a discharge and will assist in determining whether exercise brings on ventricular arrhythmias. Subsequent adjustments of antiarrhythmic medications may be necessary. In any case, exercise prescription HR should be set at least 10 to 15 beats below the ICD discharge heart rate.

Practice Considerations

A common goal in the management of arrhythmias, pacemaker rhythms, and rhythms or rates that lead to ICD discharge is the early recognition of the ECG abnormality or signs and symptoms associated with the abnormality in order to prevent and treat these disorders. CR professionals frequently are the first to identify rest or exercise arrhythmias. CR staff who note any new cardiac arrhythmia or change in severity of a cardiac arrhythmia must bring such a change to the attention of the program physician and referring physician for both evaluation and management.

CR professionals can play an important role in the overall evaluation of the patient with a cardiac pacemaker by providing feedback to the physician about HR, BP, and symptomatic responses to exercise. This information will allow the pacemaker to be programmed to more closely match the needs of the patient. Among the key settings that are adjustable are the slope of the HR increase and decline and the sensitivity of the sensor. In many cases, adjustments can improve exercise capacity and reduce symptoms.

Because the type and potential consequences of rhythm disturbances will vary among patients, the CR specialist is faced with the challenge of understanding the significance of the arrhythmia, the corresponding hemodynamic consequences, and the resulting impact on the exercise physiology. Additionally, staff must have a clear knowledge of the various rhythm-management devices, that is, pacemakers and ICDs, to work with these patients and teach them about their particular disturbances. Standing orders must provide direction to individual staff members for responding to various rhythm disturbances and for providing limits to exercise levels in those patients whose arrhythmias are exercise related or who have ICDs. Figure 9.6 describes common dysrhythmias, including atrial fibrillation, and their corresponding implications for exercise and education.

For patients with pacemakers, the exercise prescription depends on the type of pacemaker that is implanted. As an example, with fixed-rate pacemakers, the cardiac output and arterial pressure are increased by stroke volume alone. Target HR cannot be used to guide exercise intensity. Consequently, RPE are especially helpful. Conversely, for dual-chamber and rate-responsive devices, the target HR can generally guide exercise intensity. When sinus function is normal, the pacemaker can track the intrinsic sinus rate and pace the ventricle. In all cases, the target HR must be kept below the anginal threshold in a patient with ischemia. The type of rate-adaptive sensor in the pacemaker will affect the HR response during exercise. Sensors that detect vibration during exercise may respond slowly to stationary cycling and increased treadmill slope because little vibration occurs in relation to the metabolic demand of the work. Here, the RPE and METs are extremely useful in guiding exercise intensity. In patients with normal sinus function and intermittent heart block, the exercise prescription can be written the same as for most other patients. Regarding HR monitoring, the use of dry-electrode HR monitors that transmit a signal to a monitor such as those worn on the wrist has no adverse effect on pacemaker function.

Heart Failure

Heart failure is a condition characterized by a reduction in cardiac output that is often insufficient to meet the demands of vital organs and physiological systems. The etiology of heart failure is caused by the impaired ability of the heart to either pump or accept blood. Inadequate delivery of blood to specific areas may be associated with a variety of physiological sequelae, as shown in figure 9.7.[106,106a] It is apparent from this table that the person with heart failure suffers from a syndrome in which pathophysiological and compensatory mechanisms act on the body in an attempt to maintain an adequate ejection of blood from the heart. However, these mechanisms may improve or maintain heart function for only a temporary period, after which heart failure will likely progress.

Recent statistics on the incidence and prevalence of heart failure indicate that almost five million Americans are affected by heart failure, with over 550,000 new cases diagnosed each year. Additionally, more than 999,000 hospitalizations each year are caused by heart failure.[31,405] Heart failure will likely continue to be a major health concern in the future and managing its clinical manifestations will require repeated hospitalizations and numerous physician visits. The estimated annual expenditure for the management of heart failure exceeds $24 billion.[31] Therefore, methods to decrease the clinical manifestations and disablement resulting from heart failure are receiving great attention. The next section of this chapter reviews the clinical manifestations of heart failure as well as discusses recommendations for rehabilitation efforts.

Clinical Manifestations of Heart Failure

The clinical manifestations of heart failure are listed in figure 9.8. Identification of the signs and symptoms of heart failure can provide important information about the severity of heart failure as well as the domain of disablement most effected by heart failure.[106] Evaluation of quality of life and disability in heart failure can be made using disease-specific questionnaires such as the Minnesota Living with Heart Failure Questionnaire, the Chronic Heart Failure Questionnaire, and the more recent Kansas City Cardiomyopathy Questionnaire, as well as general health status questionnaires such as the Medical Outcomes Short Form (SF-36).[242,252,461,597]

The primary domains of disability caused by heart failure are identified in figure 9.9. This figure also provides general interventions to deal with the various domains of disability. Although limited in scope, research has demonstrated the important role that measurement of specific impairments, functional abilities, disabilities, and quality-of-life issues may

Intervention Strategies for Patients With Cardiac Dysrhythmia

Atrial Fibrillation

Safety

- Uncontrolled atrial fibrillation is a contraindication since it may result in hemodynamic instability
- Patients with chronic atrial fibrillation are usually on coumadin which can result in bleeding problems should an exercise injury occur
- use of digitalis can cause ST segment depression that mimics cardiac ischemic response

Exercise

- For controlled atrial fibrillation use target heart rate range rather than a speciifc target heart rate due to heart rate variability
- Proceed carefully until exercise response is recognized and stable

Education

- Safety precautions with coumadin
- Causes and treatments of atrial fibrillation
- Alternatives to pulse taking (e.g., RPE, signs/symptoms)

PVC/Bigeminy/Short Runs VT

Safety

- Frequent PVCs may cause coronary perfusion which in turn may result in ischemic signs/symptoms including decreases in cardiac output and blood pressure
- Ischemia caused by exercise may result in ventricular arryhthmias due to coronary perfusion

Exercise

- Increased risk suggests ECG monitoring; document and report new or different rhythm presentations to physician
- Treat exercise-induced arrhythmias by reducing intensity or stopping exercise

Education

- Recognition of signs/symptoms associated with ventricular arrhthmias (e.g., palpitations, dizziness)
- Behavior changes that may help reduce frequency of extra beats: nicotine, caffeine, stress management

Pacemaker

Safety

- Identify rhythm and conduction history that resulted in need for pacemaker
- Device placement may limit some activities

Exercise

- Exercise prescription and method of monitoring exercise response must be tailored to characteristics of the device and the patient

Education

- Recognize/respond to signs/symptoms of pacer malfunction (e.g., dizziness, fainting, slow pulse)
- Description of what a pacemaker is and how it helps patient's heart

ICD

Safety

- History of sudden cardiac death predisposes future events
- Know how device works, heart rate settings, number of shocks available, external defibrillation requirements
- Know antiarrhythmic medications actions and side effects

Exercise

- Establish upper limit of exercise heart rate below ICD trigger point (10-15 beats below)
- Risk stratification: high risk; close rhythm monitoring with telemetry; brief VT is harbinger of future events
- Use conservative levels of exercise intensity to avoid overshooting heart rate limits; use RPE to gauge increase as tolerated
- History of restricted activity may require low, slow progression

Education

- Understand how the device operates
- Reassure patient that exercise is not likely to result in ICD discharge; people near or touching patient when device fires will not be harmed
- 1:1 counseling for fears and anxiety; use of support group

Figure 9.6 Intervention strategies for patients with cardiac dysrhythmia.

From 317, 428.

Pathology	Effects
Cardiovascular	Decreased myocardial performance, with subsequent peripheral vascular constriction to increase venous return (attempting to increase stroke volume and cardiac output)
Pulmonary	Pulmonary edema because of elevated cardiac filling pressures resulting from poor cardiac performance and fluid overload
Renal	Water retention resulting from decreased cardiac output
Neurohumoral	Increased sympathetic stimulation that eventually desensitizes the heart to beta-1 adrenergic-receptor stimulation thus decreasing the heart's inotropic effect
Musculoskeletal	Skeletal muscle wasting and possible skeletal muscle myopathies as well as osteoporosis resulting from inactivity or other accompanying diseases
Hematologic	Possible polycythemia, anemia, and hemostatic abnormalities resulting from a reduction in oxygen transport, accompanying liver disease, or stagnant blood flow in the heart's chambers resulting from poor cardiac contraction
Hepatic	Possible cardiac cirrhosis from hypoperfusion resulting from an inadequate cardiac output or hepatic venous congestion
Pancreatic	Possible impaired insulin secretion and glucose tolerance as well as the source of a possible myocardial depressant factor
Nutritional/ biochemical	Anorexia that leads to malnutrition (protein-calorie and vitamin deficiencies) and cachexia

Figure 9.7 Physiological consequences of congestive heart failure.

Adapted from *Essentials of cardiopulmonary physical therapy*, L.P. Cahalin, p. 132, Copyright 1994, with permission from Elsevier.

- Dyspnea and fatigue
- Tachypnea
- Paroxysmal nocturnal dyspnea
- Orthopnea
- Peripheral edema
- Cold, pale, and possibly cyanotic extremities
- Weight gain
- Hepatomegaly
- Jugular venous distention
- Crackles (rales)
- Tubular breath sounds and consolidation
- Presence of a third heart sound (S3)
- Sinus tachycardia

Figure 9.8 Clinical manifestations of congestive heart failure.

Adapted, by permission, from L.P. Cahalin, 1996, "Heart Failure," *Physical Therapy* 76:516-533.

have in the rehabilitation of persons with heart failure.[106,585] Measurement of these parameters is critical not only to determining the extent of individual patient benefit derived from participation in CR but also to identifying overall outcomes of the program in general. Objective documentation of progress can (1) alert a rehabilitation specialist to maintain or modify the current regimen and (2) serve as a basis for database development either in an individual program or on a larger scale through local, regional, or national oversight.

The clinical parameters that may be used to measure the role of exercise training for patients with heart failure appear to be

- the response of cardiac output to an exercise bout (exercise testing), that is, increasing, maintaining, or decreasing ejection fraction;

Signs and symptoms	CR interventions
Dyspnea	Supplemental oxygen, pursed-lips breathing, breathing exercises, ventilatory muscle training
Fatigue	Supplemental oxygen, rest, proper diet and nutrition, pharmacological agents, individualized gradual progressive exercise training program, patient education
Decreased exercise tolerance	Supplemental oxygen, rest, proper diet and nutrition, pharmacological agents, individualized gradual progressive exercise training program, pursed-lips breathing, patient education
Functional limitations	**CR interventions**
Walking	Gait training, strength and aerobic exercise training, balance training
Climbing stairs	Functional exercise training (stair climbing)
Housework and yardwork	Functional activity training
Lifting boxes	Functional activity training
Recreational pastimes and hobbies	Recreational/hobby training
Quality of life	**CR interventions**
Unable to do things with family or friends	Patient and family/friend education, functional exercise, and activity training
Being a burden to family or friends	Patient and family/friend education, functional exercise, and activity training
Traveling away from home	Patient and family/friend education, functional exercise, and activity training
Working to earn a living	Occupational therapy, vocational rehabilitation, social services, patient and family/friend education, functional exercise, and activity training
Paying for the costs of medical care	Social services, patient and family education

Figure 9.9 Primary domains of disablement in heart failure.

- the response of HR and systolic BP response to an exercise bout (exercise testing), that is, increasing, maintaining, or decreasing levels of each;
- a significant increase in peak HR with exercise testing;
- adequacy of exercise test duration; and
- presence or absence of myocardial ischemia, that is, ST segment analysis, left ventricular wall motion, perfusion score, and symptoms of angina.[72,380,611,627]

Inpatient, Home, and Outpatient Rehabilitation

The efficacy of CR in patients with New York Heart Association (NYHA) class II-III heart failure has been well described.[105,604] The major areas discussed in this section include aerobic exercise training, strength training, breathing exercises, left ventricular assist devices, and heart failure.

Inpatient and Transitional Care

Several studies have revealed the safety of exercise training in the inpatient and transitional care settings and the potential significant improvements in many cardiovascular and symptomatic responses to exercise and functional capacity, including HR, exercise tolerance (exercise testing or 6-min walk test), and peak oxygen consumption. The exercise-training programs in these studies consisted of flexibility exercises, cycle ergometry, and treadmill ambulation for an average of 30 min total, 3 to 5 d/week for up to 2 to 4 weeks, at 50 to 70% of peak cycle ergometry work rate and a mean of 2.4 mph on the treadmill.[280,383]

Home Exercise

Heart failure patients have also safely performed home aerobic exercise training, resulting in significant improvement in functional capacity, symptoms, HR, BP, exercise tolerance, and peak oxygen consumption as well as improved quality of life. The exercise training programs in these studies consisted of cycle ergometry or walking for an average of 20 to 60 min, 3 to 7 d/week for 2 to 6 months' duration at 50 to 80% of peak HR or oxygen consumption.[64,71,119,138,336,567,611]

Outpatient Exercise

The majority of studies investigating aerobic exercise training have been performed in supervised rehabilitation centers. These studies have consistently shown that aerobic exercise training can be performed safely and result in significant improvements in symptoms, HR, BP, exercise tolerance (exercise test or 6-min walk test), peak oxygen consumption, and quality of life. Consequently, the American Heart Association has provided recommendations for exercise programming in patients with heart failure as well as for patients prior to and following cardiac transplantation and with left ventricular assist devices.[439a] The exercise training programs in these studies consisted of a variety of modes of exercise (however, cycling was the most frequent mode) for 20 to 60 min, 3 to 7 d/week for 1 to 57 months duration at 40 to 90% of peak HR or oxygen consumption.[73,146,154,171,230,234,258,313,319,456,571,572,613]

Specific Methods of Exercise Training

Figure 9.10 provides an overview of several important aspects of exercise training in patients with heart failure. Of primary concern is the degree of heart failure and whether it is compensated or decompensated.[106,604] Several clinical findings appear to suggest decompensated heart failure (figure 9.8) and identification of one or more of these findings may be sufficient to terminate exercise training until heart failure has become compensated.[106] Clinical findings suggestive of a need to modify or terminate exercise training are also listed in figure 9.10. Patients who are debilitated may require a more gradual exercise progression (gradual activity protocol), whereas patients who are less debilitated may progress more rapidly through a rehabilitation program (standard activity protocol). The progression of the patient through either activity protocol or in any setting is based on the initial patient status and subsequent responses to exercise and other components of the CR program that have been identified as necessary.[106]

Initiation of an aerobic exercise training program

- Ability to speak without signs or symptoms of dyspnea (able to speak comfortably with a RR <30 breaths/min)
- Patient is only modestly fatigued generally
- Crackles present in <one half of the lungs
- Resting heart rate <120 bpm
- Cardiac index $\geq$2.0 L/min/m² (for invasively monitored patients)
- Central venous pressure <12 mmHg (for invasively monitored patients)

Indications for modification or termination of exercise training

- Marked dyspnea or fatigue
- Respiratory rate >40 breaths/min during exercise
- Development of an S3 heart sound or pulmonary crackles
- Increase in pulmonary crackles
- Significant increase in the intensity of the second component of the second heart sound (P2)
- Poor pulse pressure (<10 mmHg difference between the systolic and diastolic BP)
- Decrease in HR or BP of >10 bpm or mmHg, respectively, during continuous (steady-state) or progressive (increasing workload) exercise
- Increased supraventricular or ventricular ectopy
- Increase of >10 mmHg in the mean pulmonary artery pressure (for invasively monitored patients)
- Increase or decrease of >6 mmHg in the central venous pressure (for invasively monitored patients)
- Diaphoresis, pallor, or confusion

Figure 9.10 Criteria for the initiation and progression of exercise training in heart failure.

Adapted, by permission, from L.P. Cahalin, 1996, "Heart Failure," *Physical Therapy* 76:516-533.

Strength Training

Several studies have suggested that strength training is an important mode of exercise training for patients with heart failure. Circuit strength training combined with aerobic exercise appears to be safe while providing improvements in peripheral muscle strength and endurance, exercise tolerance, cardiorespiratory function, and symptoms. The strength training performed in these studies was administered to major muscle groups at 60 to 80% of maximum voluntary contraction or of the 10-repetition method (10RM) for 2 to 6 months. The number of repetitions and the duration of the strength-training sessions were slowly progressed and varied among studies. No major complications were observed in the studies.[142,260,357,360,381,452,455]

Breathing Exercises

Five studies have investigated the effects of breathing exercises on the clinical manifestations of heart failure. Four of the five utilized an inspiratory muscle-training device. Inspiratory muscle training was performed daily for an average of 15 to 30 min at 15 to 60% of maximal inspiratory mouth pressure for 2 to 3 months. One additional study investigated the acute and chronic effects of slowing the respiratory rate through yoga breathing. Threshold inspiratory muscle training appears to consistently improve ventilatory muscle strength and endurance and dyspnea. Yoga breathing appears to have both acute and chronic benefit, including improved oxygen saturation, exercise tolerance, cardiorespiratory function, and dyspnea.[79,300,364,601]

Left Ventricular Assist Devices

Left ventricular assist devices (LVADs) are becoming more common yet have received very little clinical rehabilitative investigation. Exercise training of patients with LVADs appears to be safe but requires gradual progressive ambulation that can lead to treadmill or cycling exercise. Treadmill or cycle ergometry exercise often begins after patients become independent with hallway ambulation and is performed in the pump-on-full mode. Some researchers have observed improved functional status and exercise tolerance and optimized recovery before heart transplantation with the mobilization and progression of such patients (see *Patients With Left Ventricular Assist Devices* section on page 157 of this chapter).[46,396]

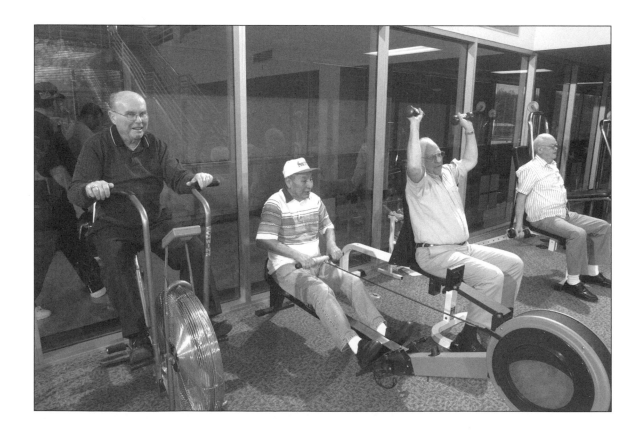

Practice Considerations

CR programs are becoming increasingly involved in the comprehensive care of patients with heart failure. This includes not only the delivery of a quantified exercise stimulus but also the optimization of medication use, monitoring of daily weights, compliance with sodium restriction, and surveillance for potential exacerbations that can be managed preferentially in the outpatient setting. CR exercise and education and counseling interventions in the heart failure population are designed to

- increase exercise tolerance,
- decrease symptoms,
- improve quality of life, and
- reduce acute problems.

To achieve these goals, CR specialists should work in close communication with physicians to report patient progress and help monitor the overall medical plan, including compliance with diet and medications. Additionally, exercise program visits provide an opportunity for sign and symptom assessment and therefore early recognition of decompensation.

Heart failure patients present a challenge to CR professionals due to pathological limitations and pathophysiologic limitations, including limited exercise capacity and the potential for decompensation, as well as the need for extensive education about and assistance with medication regimens, dietary changes, symptom recognition, and emotional support. To determine appropriate CR services for patients with heart failure, staff should consult a detailed history, results of medical and psychological tests, and results from disease-specific and general health status questionnaires.[106,604] Exercise-test results often provide important information about the severity of heart failure, the safety of exercise training, and exercise prescription. Patients with a peak oxygen consumption less than 10 to 14 ml/kg/min appear to have a poorer prognosis and are often considered candidates for cardiac transplantation. Exercise test results can provide

- an indication of complications that could potentially arise during exercise training, such as peak oxygen consumption, HR and BP response, ECG, and symptoms; and
- patient-specific exercise training parameters.

In general, a weight gain of 5 lb or more over 1 to 3 d, as well as changes in symptomatology such as an increase in dyspnea or the onset of nocturnal dyspnea, should be reported to the treating physician. The increased risk of exertional hypotension resulting from flattening or decreasing cardiac output during exercise is also of concern in these patients. Several potential causes, alone or in combination, include exercise-induced ischemia, increased volume overload, increased left ventricular end-diastolic pressure, and chronotropic incompetence (inability of the HR to increase appropriately to maintain cardiac output as stroke volume flattens or drops) with increasing activity level. Consequently, staff should evaluate BP response more frequently during exercise in these patients, particularly early in the exercise program or when workloads are significantly increased. This is especially true for patients who may be eligible for and participating in resistance training.

Figure 9.11 outlines how secondary prevention interventions can be modified for the heart failure population. In addition to expanding their education and exercise strategies, CR staff who work with the heart failure population need expanded assessment and communication skills. CR professionals need to become expert in assessing patients for early signs of failure, including listening for heart sound and lung sound changes, inspecting for edema, monitoring weight gain, and so forth. They also need to establish strong communication links with attending physicians, home health nurses, CHF clinics, and other health care providers with a role in managing the patient's total care. Clear communication of how secondary prevention achieves these goals and contributes to successful patient outcomes sets the stage for future referrals.

Heart Failure Clinics

Heart failure clinics provide comprehensive heart failure management, frequently through a physician and nurse team. Teams have often followed specific patient-care pathways that ensure timely performance of specific tests and measures as well as allocation of a variety of services. Heart failure clinics are becoming more popular because of favorable economic and patient outcomes, including a reduction in hospital admissions, readmissions, days, and costs as well as an improvement in quality of life and morbidity.[147,190,259,329,341,365,466,502,503,515,541,607]

Patients With Left Ventricular Assist Devices

For end-stage CHF patients who are candidates for heart transplantation but refractory to maximized inotropic therapy, implantation of an LVAD

Safety	Exercise	Education
• Uncompensated heart failure is a contraindication to initiating an exercise program; decompensation is reason to discontinue the exercise program	• Exercise stress tests should include, where possible, metabolic assessment utilizing a carefully progressing protocol (e.g., 1 MET per stage)	• Priority: sign/symptom recognition and response, including fatigue, weakness, SOB, DOE, orthopnea, edema, weight gain
• Thorough patient assessment should be part of pre-exercise vital signs with each rehabilitation visit	• Patients are at high risk for ventricular arrhythmias and decompensation	• Nutrition consult: low sodium diet (e.g., 2 gm; low fat)
• As part of the initial evaluation, patients should be asked about advance directives; copies of such decisions should be placed in the patient's chart	• Exercise protocol: longer warm-up and cool-down; use interval exercise (1-6 min) and careful progression; encourage weight bearing for ADL	• Drug regimen: medication education and compliance monitoring, diuretics, digitalis, ACE inhibitors, beta-blockers
	• Light resistance training as appropriate	• Psychosocial consult for depression symptomatology; CHF support group and individual counseling
	• ECG monitoring: extended period; BP: check exercise BP often—drop or failure to rise can be significant for impending failure; use subjective RPE and dyspnea scales	• Basic information regarding disease processes
	• Common side effect: fatigue for rest of the day	
	• Due to more slowly progressing exercise program and high-risk nature of patients, period of closely supervised exercise may need to be extended	

Figure 9.11 Intervention strategies for patients with heart failure. DOE = dyspnea on exertion.

From Keteyian SJ, Brawner CA, Schairer JR, et al. Effects of exercise training on chronotropic incompetence in patients with heart failure. *Am Heart J* 1999;138: 233-240; and from Meyer K, Samek L, Samek L, et al. Interval training in patients with severe chronic heart failure: Analysis and recommendations for exercise procedures. *Med Sci Sports Exerc* 1997;29:306-312.

has proved to be a viable alternative to maintain adequate hemodynamics while the patient awaits transplant. Available evidence suggests that the use of these devices has proved to be an effective bridge to transplant and, possibly, a clinical alternative to transplantation.[201,202,500] The LVAD permits end-stage CHF patients to participate in more assertive exercise therapy, which appears to be both safe and beneficial.[93,201,293,397]

There are several versions of LVADs; the device described here reflects the design of the Thermo Cardiosystems, Inc. (TCI) HeartMate devices. In brief, the LVAD pump is implanted intra-abdominally or in a preperitoneal pocket external to the abdominal viscera. The left ventricle is cannulated at the apex of the heart for inflow to the pump; a pusher-plate mechanism drives blood flow through an outflow circuit anastomosed to the ascending aorta. The chamber

capacity of the device is approximately 85 ml with a pumping frequency that can increase to provide a maximal mechanical cardiac output of approximately 11 L/min. The LVAD rate can increase automatically as the device senses the volume of blood in the pump chamber, or rate may be controlled manually. The pump operates in a fill-to-empty mode so that with increases in blood flow, as in exercise, the LVAD rate responsively increases. The native left ventricle continues to contract during LVAD operation. At rest the LVAD contributes virtually all of the cardiac output, but during exercise the native left ventricle contributes a varying amount of the total cardiac output. In the limited number of studies to date, it appears that the LVAD provides an adequate cardiac output for modest daily physical demands. The degree to which the native left ventricle contributes to total cardiac output likely is dependent on the degree of left ventricle dysfunction. A more detailed discussion of the exercise physiology of the LVAD is available.[286]

Considerations for Exercise Testing

The abdominal location of the externalized drive line makes cycling and stair climbing somewhat problematic. Thus, treadmill exercise is a preferred mode for exercise testing and is well tolerated. Given the limitations in cardiac output, 1-MET increases in exercise intensity or a gradual ramping protocol is preferred to more aggressive protocols. In the automatic mode the LVAD operates with a rate that is independent of native sympathetic drive, so the native HR and the LVAD rates will differ. As such, pulse or ECG assessment of the native HR response to exercise must be done and not inferred from the LVAD console, which reflects the LVAD rate. However, both rates increase in a linear fashion with exercise. BP response to exercise is somewhat variable at the outset, probably secondary to adjustment of fluid volume, and this may be reflected in the initial evaluation. This variability is reduced as fluid volume normalizes over time. Perceived exertion appears unaffected by LVAD implantation.[397] Reassessment usually yields only a modest increase in measured oxygen consumption, but submaximal responses are considerably improved.

Exercise Training Considerations

The largest published experience describing submaximal training in LVAD patients has suggested that exercise training was tolerated by 82% of patients, with an improvement in submaximal training workloads over 6 to 8 weeks, at which time patients were able to achieve modest workloads for 20 to 30 min.[397] Although ambulation and upper-extremity exercises are well tolerated, patients should be assessed for cycling ability on an individual basis because of the location of the external drive. Additionally, because hip flexion may be somewhat limited, it is important to include activities that prevent disuse so that a return to functional activities, such as stair climbing or stooping, is facilitated.

Educational Considerations for LVAD Patients

Patients with LVADs should participate in the education program designed for heart failure and transplant patients. In addition, LVAD patients typically receive comprehensive training regarding the mechanical operation of the device, power supply, and expected values that are displayed on the control panel, so they may inform the nursing staff when they suspect a device problem. Patients should also receive education to correlate signs and symptoms, especially those associated with hypotension, to device operation. Although the trained staff members make routine checks, patients should be instructed to report signs and symptoms of infection, because infections can occur in the area of the drive line insertion. Patients, especially smaller patients, are more likely to experience gastrointestinal symptoms and should be advised to eat smaller, frequent meals. Abdominal pain may occur secondary to the device pushing on the lower ribs.

Ongoing psychological monitoring and intervention is advisable in that LVAD patients with essentially normalized low-level left ventricular function frequently become "too well" to be hospitalized. At present, the devices are a bridge to transplantation, and as such, LVAD patients must be assured that they remain the highest priority for transplantation and that "sicker" patients are not moving past them on the transplant list. LVAD patients may develop feelings of being trapped in the hospital environment and should be encouraged to engage in a variety of activities, including exercise rehabilitation. During exercise training, patients should be well educated about reporting symptoms of light-headedness or dizziness. Although the device has an internal sensor that increases the flow rate as needed during exercise, this sensor may ultimately fail, in which case the flows can be manually increased. This can be easily accomplished during exercise depending on the patient's symptomatic response.

Cardiac Transplantation

For patients with end-stage heart failure, cardiac transplantation is the accepted form of therapy, with 1-yr and 5-yr survival of 81% and 68%, respectively.[281] Approximately 220 centers perform cardiac transplantation worldwide (9 centers in Canada, 146 centers in the U.S.), with nearly 3,500 operations reported to the Registry of the International Society for Heart and Lung Transplantation for 1999. Unfortunately, the number of potential candidates for cardiac transplantation far exceeds the available supply of donor organs.

Orthotopic transplantation is the usual surgical technique, with excision of the recipient's diseased heart and anastomosis of the donor heart to the great vessels and atria of the recipient. In the extremely rare circumstance of excessively elevated pulmonary vascular resistance in the recipient or a significant donor-recipient body weight mismatch, the heterotopic technique may be employed, in which the recipient's diseased heart is left in place and the donor heart is implanted parallel to the existing heart.[549] Five-yr survival after heterotopic transplantation is approximately 44%.

The vast majority of patients who require transplantation (approximately 90%) suffer from CHF caused by either CAD (ischemic left ventricular dysfunction) or idiopathic dilated cardiomyopathy, although hypertension, valvular heart disease, myocarditis, alcohol abuse, chemotherapy, acquired immunodeficiency syndrome, complex congenital heart disease, infiltrative diseases of the myocardium, pericardial disease, and peripartum may also be causes of terminal heart failure. The age range of transplant recipients is from newborn to the eighth decade of life, although the majority of recipients are between 35 and 65 yr of age. The average age of the donor is approximately 30 yr. The median waiting time for an organ is dependent on blood type and the degree of medical urgency. Typical wait times vary between 75 and 335 days.[312]

After transplantation, most patients report a reasonably favorable quality of life. Many patients return to work, school, or their usual avocational activities. In one series of patients under age 60 yr, the rate of return to work at 1 and 5 yr (for survivors) was nearly 70%.[315]

Immunosuppressants, Acute Rejection, and Infection Risk

Immunosuppressant medications, typically cyclosporine, azathioprine, and prednisone, are given after transplantation to prevent acute rejection of the donor heart. Tacrolimus may be used in place of cyclosporine.[435] In addition, mycophenolate mofetile may be used in place of azathioprine.

Acute rejection is characterized by T-lymphocyte infiltration of the myocardium, which may result in myocyte injury and necrosis if not detected early in its course and adequately treated. Patients are most susceptible to acute rejection during the first several months after transplantation, and most patients will experience one or more episodes during the first year after surgery. Periodic endomyocardial biopsies are performed to detect acute rejection early in its course. Rejection is graded from mild to severe, based on biopsy tissue sample analysis. Acute rejection is treated with increased amounts of immunosuppressants and may require hospitalization.

Immunosuppressants enable the patient to tolerate the donor heart but are associated with several common side effects. For example, cyclosporine may result in renal dysfunction and has general vaso-pressor effects, resulting in hypertension requiring drug treatment in approximately 67% of patients.[499] Prednisone is particularly bothersome. It alters body-fat distribution with resultant truncal obesity and a "moon"-faced appearance for many patients. Prednisone may also cause mood swings as well as skeletal muscle atrophy, weakness, and osteoporosis and usually worsens the blood lipid profile. If at all possible, the supervising physician will taper and stop the prednisone during the first 1 or 2 yr after transplantation. Skeletal muscle cramping is another common patient complaint.

As with any immunosuppressant regimen, transplant patients are at higher risk for opportunistic infections and malignancy than the general population of cardiac patients. At 5 yr after surgery, approximately 10% of recipients have experienced a malignancy.[281] CR program staff must take precautions to minimize the chances of exposure of a transplant patient to another patient or staff member with an active infection. Most transplant patients are encouraged by program staff to wear a surgical mask in public places as a barrier to infectious organisms.

Accelerated Graft Coronary Artery Disease

Accelerated graft CAD, also called cardiac allograft vasculopathy or graft vessel disease, constitutes the major limiting factor in long-term survival after transplantation and is the major cause of mortality in patients 1 yr or more after surgery. Approximately 50% of transplant recipients have angiographic evidence of the disease 5 yr after surgery. It is characterized by an unusually accelerated form of CAD, diffusely affecting epicardial and intramyocardial coronary arteries and veins.[602] It may lead to MI, CHF, or sudden cardiac death. The pathophysiology is believed to begin with repetitive endothelial injury from the immune system's response to the graft, ischemia-reperfusion injury, viral infection, immunosuppressant medications, and traditional coronary risk factors such as dyslipidemia, insulin resistance, and hypertension. Following injury, the repair response of the vessel wall results in intimal thickening that may become obstructive.

Annual coronary angiography is routinely performed for detection of CAD. Revascularization with catheter-based techniques or CABGS may be effective in patients with discrete, focal lesions. However, because of the usual diffuse nature of the lesions, retransplantation is the most common treatment, although survival is not as favorable as after the initial transplant.

Use of HMG Co-A reductase inhibitors (statins) and possibly fibric acid derivatives (such as gemfibrozil) may slow progression of accelerated graft CAD and improve survival.[534,602,606] In addition, statins have been shown to reduce the incidence of episodes of acute rejection and to improve left ventricular function.[213,294,326] These benefits appear to be independent of the effects of the statin drugs in improving the blood lipid profile.

Psychological Factors

The psychological reaction to the transplant process is understandably intense for most patients and their significant others. During the period of waiting for the operation after being accepted as a transplant candidate, emotions range from relief and happiness to anxiety (indefinite waiting time) and thoughts of death. Patients who require continuous hospitalization while waiting for an organ may find the environment supportive or overwhelmingly tedious and boring. Immediately after transplantation, patients are usually joyous at the prospects for living a longer, higher-quality life. As the period of postoperative convalescence continues, patients must adjust to the tedium of appointments and procedures. The first episode of acute rejection may result in heightened anxiety and possibly transient depression. As recovery progresses and the degree of medical surveillance decreases, patients generally shift their attention from transplant-related activities to becoming more independent and resuming family activities as well as avocational and vocational pursuits. The readjustment to life after transplantation generally requires months, and the first anniversary after surgery is an important milestone in this process.

Abnormal Responses to Acute Exercise

The responses of cardiac transplant patients to acute exercise is unique and related, in part, to the following factors:[410]

- The transplanted heart is denervated at the time of organ harvesting and receives no direct efferent activity from the autonomic nervous system and provides no afferent input to the central nervous system. Months after transplantation, some patients exhibit signs of partial cardiac reinnervation; this is discussed later in the chapter (see page 162).

- The donor heart has undergone ischemic time and reperfusion.

- There is no intact pericardium.

- The donor heart may have suffered various amounts of myocyte necrosis as a result of episodes of acute rejection.

- Diastolic dysfunction may be present.

- Abnormal skeletal muscle histology and biochemistry may be present.

- Peripheral and coronary vasodilatory capacity may be impaired.

As a result of the loss of parasympathetic innervation with transplantation, the HR at rest is elevated to approximately 95 to 115 bpm and represents the theoretical inherent rate of depolarization of the sinoatrial node.[530] With graded exercise, the HR typically does not increase during the first several minutes, followed by a gradual rise with peak HR slightly lower than normal (approximately 150 bpm). Many transplant recipients achieve their highest exercise HR during the first few minutes of recovery from exercise rather than at the time of the highest exercise intensity. HR may remain near peak values for minutes during recovery before gradually returning to resting levels. Humoral regulation of the HR during exercise occurs via circulating catecholamines.

With orthotopic transplantation, it is possible that the sinoatrial node of the recipient's heart may be left intact. The depolarization wave will generally not pass through the suture line in the right atrium, but the ECG may show two distinct atrial "p" waves (one from the recipient and one from the donor sinoatrial nodes).

BP at rest is usually mildly elevated, even though most patients receive antihypertensive medications. During exercise, blood pressure increases appropriately, although peak exercise BP is usually slightly lower than expected for normal persons.[318] Intracardiac and pulmonary vascular pressures are generally elevated in transplant patients.[308] Systemic vascular resistance is generally elevated as well.

Left ventricular systolic function, as measured by ejection fraction, is in the normal range at rest and during exercise in most patients.[308] However, diastolic function, as measured by end-diastolic volume, is impaired. This results in a below-normal increase in stroke volume during exercise. This impaired rise in stroke volume coupled with the below-normal HRR mentioned previously results in an impaired exercise cardiac output.

Several skeletal muscle structural and biochemical abnormalities develop during the clinical course of chronic heart failure, such as a reduced aerobic metabolic enzyme activity, lower capillary density, impaired vasodilation during exercise, and conversion of some slow-twitch motor units to fast-twitch motor units with a greater reliance on anaerobic metabolic energy production. These abnormalities generally persist after transplantation with partial improvement after several months in some patients.[339,543]

The efficiency of ventilation is below normal during the first several months after transplantation. This is demonstrated by an elevation in the ratio of minute ventilation to carbon dioxide production (the ventilatory equivalent for CO_2, VE/VCO_2). This excess ventilation results in a heightened sense of shortness of breath during exercise. The increase in tidal volume during exercise is blunted, probably due to respiratory muscle weakness, deconditioning, and the effects of corticosteroids.[102] Diffusion impairment is present in 40% or more of transplant recipients.[531]

Arterial saturation with oxygen at rest and during exercise is normal for the vast majority of patients, however.[529] A few patients with pretransplant diffusion abnormalities will experience mild arterial saturation (approximately 90%) with exercise.[91] Azathioprine may cause anemia in some patients that may reduce arterial oxygen content.

Extraction of oxygen from the arterial blood by body tissues, as indicated by the arterial-mixed venous oxygen difference, is normal at rest. However, during graded exercise the arterial-mixed venous oxygen difference does not increase in a normal manner and reflects abnormalities with both the delivery of capillary blood to the exercising skeletal muscle and impairment in the oxidative capacity of the muscle.[308]

As a result of an impaired rise in both cardiac output and arterial-mixed venous oxygen difference with exercise, the rate of increase in $\dot{V}O_2$ (oxygen uptake kinetics) is slower.[377] Peak exercise oxygen uptake is considerably below average for age and gender (typically 60%-70% of predicted).[318] However, considerable diversity in $\dot{V}O_{2peak}$ is seen in transplant patients, with some individuals exhibiting above-average cardiorespiratory fitness and some with severely impaired capacities.[529] Patients with a greater chronotropic reserve generally exhibit a higher $\dot{V}O_{2peak}$.[156]

Partial Cardiac Reinnervation

The occasional cardiac transplant patient with graft vessel disease with resultant myocardial ischemia will report anginal symptoms, suggesting at least partial cardiac afferent reinnervation.[314] It also appears that partial cardiac sympathetic efferent reinnervation occurs in many patients over the first several months to years after surgery. The evidence for this statement is based on neurochemical evaluation as well as the observation of improved HR responsiveness to exercise.[316,498] The HRR, or chronotropic response, to graded exercise increases during the first 6 weeks after transplantation in most patients. In a subset of patients, there is a further improvement in the HRR over the next 6 to 12 months. In addition, a more rapid return of HR to baseline after exercise, 1 to 2 yr after transplant, has been reported. In a subset of patients, a partial normalization of the HR response to graded exercise occurs with a linear increase in HR, with the peak HR occurring at the highest exercise intensity and a linear decrease in heart rate during the recovery period.

Graded Exercise Testing

Exercise testing is useful after cardiac transplantation in determining the exercise capacity, prescribing exercise intensity, and counseling patients regarding the timing of return to work or school or resumption of avocational activities. Because of the recovery and healing processes that take place after surgery and the patient's usually deconditioned state before surgery, it is best to wait 4 to 8 weeks after surgery before performing graded exercise testing to maximal effort. In patients with complicated postoperative courses, a longer period of recovery is necessary before graded exercise testing occurs.

Treadmill or cycle ergometer protocols, with continuous exercise (2- to 3-min stages) or ramp tests, may be used. Arm-cranking protocols may also be employed, after adequate sternal healing, for a specific upper-extremity fitness evaluation or upper-extremity exercise prescription.[318] The initial exercise intensity should be approximately 2 METs, with 1- to 2-MET increments in intensity per stage.[314,318] Continuous ECG monitoring with BP measurement and RPE for each exercise stage is recommended. For precise determination of aerobic capacity and the ventilatory anaerobic threshold, direct measurement of $\dot{V}O_2$ and associated variables is highly desirable. The endpoints of graded exercise tests should be maximal effort (symptom-limited maximum) or signs of exertional intolerance.

Responses to Exercise Training

Cardiac transplant patients respond to aerobic exercise training in a relatively similar fashion to that of other cardiac patients.[314,318,529] Peak oxygen uptake generally improves by approximately 25% after 2 to 6 months of training. Potential additional benefits of regular exercise training include the following:

- Improved submaximal exercise endurance
- Increased peak cycle power output or peak treadmill exercise workload
- Increased maximal HR
- Decreased exercise HR at the same absolute submaximal workload
- Increased ventilatory anaerobic threshold
- Decreased submaximal exercise minute ventilation
- Lessened symptoms of fatigue and dyspnea
- Reduced rest and submaximal exercise systolic and diastolic BP
- Decreased peak exercise diastolic BP
- Reduced submaximal exercise RPE
- Improved psychosocial function
- Increased lean body mass

The increased peak exercise HR is probably an important factor in the improvement in aerobic capacity. Rate-responsive pacing increased the chronotropic reserve and $\dot{V}O_{2peak}$ by 22% in a group of eight patients.[90] Both supervised training programs and self-directed home programs have been demonstrated to improve $\dot{V}O_{2peak}$ in transplant patients. However, more structured, supervised programs generally improve fitness to a greater extent than less-supervised approaches to training. At the end of early outpatient rehabilitation (phase II), aerobic capacity of transplant patients is similar to that of CABGS patients of similar age. However, over the next several months transplant patients do not improve fitness as much as do CABGS patients. At 1 yr after surgery, transplant recipients are generally less fit than other types of patients who have undergone cardiothoracic surgery.[137]

Exercise training improves mitochondrial function in transplant patients but does not apparently increase capillary density as in healthy people.[340] Resistance exercise training improves skeletal muscle strength and partially reverses corticosteroid-related myopathy, which is common among transplant recipients. In addition, strength training has been shown to improve bone mineral density and to reduce the potential for development of osteoporosis associated with corticosteroid use.[92] Importantly, exercise training does not compromise immune function.[639]

Intervention in CR programs

The types of interventions provided by the rehabilitation staff to transplant patients are similar to those provided for the more typical CR patient with CHD, including patient and family education, psychosocial evaluation and counseling, CVD risk-factor management, early mobilization, and outpatient exercise training. Different from these interventions is the inclusion of inpatient exercise training necessary because of a lengthier inpatient stay.

Patient and Family Education

Specific topics for transplant patients and families include the following:

- Medications: purposes of the drugs, potential side effects, importance of strict compliance with recommended dosing, and schedule for taking medications
- The risk of acute rejection, infection, and accelerated graft CAD: symptom recognition and appropriate response
- Postoperative management schedule: appointments, biopsies, blood work, other periodic tests
- Diet low in fat, cholesterol, and sodium to help prevent body-fat gain associated with prednisone use and to help prevent hypertension
- The importance of regular exercise in promoting functional capacity and the feeling of well-being

Psychosocial Intervention

As discussed previously, most patients and loved ones experience some challenges in making the adjustment to posttransplant living. Patients in general will need to rebuild family relationships and reestablish friendships and business or professional contacts. CR programs can provide ongoing emotional support and encouragement. Group discussion or support sessions that include the patient, the family, and group leaders are particularly helpful in helping patients and loved ones develop coping skills, stress-management techniques, and practical skills to deal with the multitude of issues involved in posttransplant life. An occasional patient may experience severe anxiety or other symptoms of psychological distress. CR professionals may assist the transplant team and primary physician in identifying patients who require psychiatric referral.

Coronary Risk-Factor Management

The relationship of classic coronary risk factors, such as cigarette smoking, dyslipidemia, hypertension, and a sedentary lifestyle, and accelerated graft vessel disease or longevity in cardiac transplant patients is not well established. However, most transplant programs strongly encourage optimal control of all modifiable risk factors. In particular, transplant patients should receive all the necessary help required to stop all tobacco use should they resume the habit after surgery.

As discussed previously, use of statin medications after transplantation has been demonstrated to reduce the incidence of acute rejection and graft vessel disease and to improve 1-yr survival. The beneficial effects are not necessarily related to the power of the drugs to improve blood lipid profile. Nonetheless, a goal for LDL-C of less than 100 mg/dL is generally recommended.

Control of BP is a major concern given the high prevalence of hypertension after transplantation. The combination of proper diet and regular exercise is crucial to maintenance of an acceptable body weight.

Early Mobilization and Inpatient Exercise Training

After surgery, patients are extubated as soon as possible, usually within 24 h. Passive range of motion for the upper and lower extremities, sitting up in a chair, standing, and slow ambulation may begin and gradually progress after extubation.[372] Ambulation and cycle ergometry may gradually increase in duration to 20 to 30 min. Exercise intensity is guided using RPE of 11-13 (fairly light to somewhat hard) with a frequency of two or three sessions per day. Typically, patients who do not develop postoperative complications remain hospitalized for 7 to 10 d. During this stage of rehabilitation, as well as in the post-hospitalization period, episodes of acute rejection of moderate or greater severity may require alteration of the exercise plan. If the rejection is rated as moderate, the patient may continue activity at the present level but may not progress until after the rejection has resolved with treatment. Severe acute rejection necessitates suspension of all physical activity, with the exception of passive range-of-motion exercises.

Outpatient Exercise Training

Transplant patients may enter an outpatient CR program as soon as they are dismissed from the hospital. The transplant team generally requires patients to remain near the transplant center for approximately 3 months for close follow-up, and ideally, patients should exercise in both a supervised program (up to 3 sessions/week) and independently (at least 3 sessions/week).

Continuous ECG monitoring during the first few exercise sessions is standard practice. It is not necessary to perform graded exercise testing before the patient begins the outpatient exercise program. However, graded exercise testing should be performed by 8 weeks after surgery (for patients with relatively uncomplicated courses), when the patient has recovered sufficiently from surgery, to assess the cardiopulmonary response to exercise and to refine the exercise prescription.

Exercise prescription for cardiac transplant recipients is similar to the methods used with other patients who have undergone cardiothoracic surgery. The one exception is not using a target HR unless the patient has a normalized response caused by partial reinnervation, as discussed previously (see page 162). The typical denervated heart increases rate slowly during submaximal exercise, and HR may drift gradually upward during steady-state exercise or may plateau after several minutes.[529] RPE (Borg scale) of 12 to 14 (somewhat hard) may be used to prescribe exercise intensity. The exercise prescription includes standard warm-up and cool-down activities and a gradual increase in aerobic exercise duration to 30 to 60 min, with a frequency of 3 to 6 sessions/week. Modes of aerobic exercise commonly used during the early outpatient recovery period include walking outdoors or in shopping centers or schools, treadmill walking, cycle ergometry, and stair climbing.

The sternal incision necessitates a special emphasis on upper-extremity range-of-motion exercises. After 6 weeks from the surgery date, when sternal healing is nearly completed, rowing, arm cranking, combination arm-leg ergometry, outdoor cycling, hiking, jogging, and swimming are additional exercise options. The patient may engage in sports such as tennis and golf as early as 6 weeks after surgery if his or her fitness is adequate (directly measured $\dot{V}O_{2\,peak}$ of approximately 5 METs or greater) and sternal healing is nearly completed.

Skeletal muscle weakness in transplant patients is very common and relates to the following factors:

- Chronic heart failure may cause skeletal muscle atrophy.

- Before transplantation, patients may become very deconditioned.

- After surgery, patients take corticosteroids as part of the immunosuppressant drug program.

Muscle-strengthening exercises should be incorporated into the exercise rehabilitation program. For the first 6 weeks after surgery, bilateral arm lifting is restricted to less than 10 lb (4.5 kgs) to avoid sternal nonunion. After 6 weeks of satisfactory recovery from surgery, patients may be started on weight machines, emphasizing moderate resistance, 10 to 20 repetitions per set, one to three sets of exercises for the major muscle groups, on a two- to three-session-per-week basis.[318]

Diabetes

Diabetes mellitus is a complex metabolic disorder characterized by impaired uptake of glucose by the tissues caused by insufficient pancreatic insulin production (type 1) or loss of peripheral insulin sensitivity (type 2). Type 1 diabetes is usually manifest at a much younger age than type 2, is generally not associated with obesity, and is less responsive to exercise as therapy. Exercise will nonetheless increase glucose disposal and diminish insulin requirements on exercise days. Type 2 diabetes usually has its onset in adulthood and is often associated with obesity, hypertension, abnormal lipids, and clotting abnormalities. Type 2 diabetes affects approximately 85 to 90% of the 16 million people with diabetes. Weight loss and exercise have been shown to diminish the insulin resistance of people with type 2 diabetes, although in the patient with heart disease, comprehensive treatment often involves oral hypoglycemic, antihypertensive, and lipid-lowering medications.

The risk of a heart attack is 50% higher in men with diabetes and 150% higher in women with diabetes than in their nondiabetic counterparts. The risk of death from cardiovascular causes is doubled in men with diabetes and is four times higher in women with diabetes compared with patients without diabetes. Among patients with diabetes, CHD, stroke, hypertension, and peripheral arterial disease are the major causes of morbidity and mortality.[186]

One of the biggest challenges patients with diabetes face is how to comply with complex treatment regimens. CR professionals are in a key position to help monitor and motivate patient compliance with medications as well as with diet and exercise routines. CR program staff must work closely with the patient's primary care physician or endocrinologist to optimize management of the diabetes.

Benefits of Regular Exercise in Patients With Type 2 Diabetes

The benefits of exercise for the patient with type 2 diabetes are substantial, and recent studies strengthen the importance of long-term exercise programs for the treatment and prevention of this common metabolic abnormality and its complications (see figures 9.12, 9.13, and 9.14). Regular exercise improves diabetes management, reduces the risk for CVD and its com-

plications, and improves overall health and wellness in patients with type 2 diabetes and prevents or delays the onset of type 2 diabetes in patients prone to the disease.[25,26,593] The improvement in many of the risk factors for CVD has been linked to a decrease in plasma insulin levels and the improved insulin sensitivity associated with exercise.[484]

Exercise and Type 1 diabetes

Exercise is not considered a component of treatment per se in type 1 diabetes to lower blood glucose. Several studies have failed to show an independent effect

- Improved sensitivity to insulin in the peripheral tissues
- Improved blood glucose control
- Reduction in the dosage or need for insulin or oral hypoglycemics
- Decrease in plasma insulin levels
- Improvement in glucose tolerance
- Lower hemoglobin A1c levels

Figure 9.12 The role of exercise in improving diabetes management.

- Improved functional capacity
- Improvement in lipid profile (decrease in triglycerides, VLDL, and small dense subclass of LDL-C)
- Weight loss, loss of intra-abdominal fat, and improved waist:hip ratio
- Lowering of systolic and diastolic BP
- Increased fibrinolytic activity
- Decreased susceptibility to serious ventricular arrhythmias

Figure 9.13 The role of exercise in reducing the risk for CVD and its complications.

- Lower incidence of depression and anxiety
- Improved quality of life
- Better management of life, family, societal, and work stressors

Figure 9.14 The role of exercise in improving overall health and wellness.

of exercise training on improving glycemic control as measured by HbA1c in patients with type 1 diabetes. Rather, those with type 1 diabetes are encouraged to exercise to gain the benefit of exercise in improving known risk factors for atherosclerosis. CR professionals need to advise patients with type 1 diabetes about safe and enjoyable physical activities that are consistent with their lifestyle and culture.[13]

Risks of Exercise in Patients With Diabetes

Most patients with diabetes can exercise with a high level of safety. But exercise is not without risks for patients with diabetes, and health care professionals should be keenly aware of these risks when working with this patient population (see figures 9.15 and 9.16).[232]

Screening Patients With Diabetes for Exercise Programs

The recommendation that people with diabetes participate in an exercise program is based on the premise that the benefits of such a program outweigh the risks. To maximize the benefits and minimize the risks of exercise in this patient population, it is nec-

essary to provide appropriate screening of patients, program design, monitoring, and patient education. The chronic hyperglycemia of diabetes is associated with long-term damage, dysfunction, and failure of various organs, especially the eyes, kidneys, nerves, heart, and blood vessels.[175] In screening patients for an exercise program, Schneider and colleagues found the prevalence of undiagnosed disease as follows: ischemic heart disease, 6%; peripheral arterial disease, 14%; hypertension, 42%; proteinuria, 8%, and background retinopathy, 16%.[494] Effective screening of patients with diabetes before they begin an exercise program should include screening for vascular and neurological complications including

- peripheral arterial disease,
- retinopathy,
- nephropathy,
- peripheral neuropathy, and
- autonomic neuropathy.

Screening patients for their knowledge level and how they currently control their diabetes should also be performed, including discussion of

- insulin and oral hypoglycemics,
- self-monitoring of blood sugar levels,

Cardiovascular risks

- Cardiac dysfunction and arrhythmias caused by ischemic heart disease (often silent ischemia)
- Excessive rises or falls in BP or HR caused by autonomic neuropathy
- Postexercise orthostatic hypotension due to autonomic neuropathy
- Cardiomyopathy caused by long-standing diabetes

Metabolic risks

- Worsening of hyperglycemia and development of ketosis
- Hypoglycemia in patients on insulin or oral hypoglycemic agents

Musculoskeletal and traumatic risks

- Foot ulcers (especially in the presence of neuropathy)
- Orthopedic injuries related to peripheral neuropathy
- Accelerated degenerative joint disease

Microvascular risks

- Retinopathy: Patients who have proliferative diabetic retinopathy should avoid anaerobic exercise and exercise that involves straining, jarring, or Valsalva-like maneuvers.
- Nephropathy: There is no reason to limit low- to moderate-intensity activities, but high-intensity exercise is discouraged.
- Neuropathy: Peripheral neuropathy is an indication to limit weight-bearing exercise (refer to figure 9.16 on page 167)

Figure 9.15 Risks associated with exercise in patients with diabetes.

Contraindicated	Recommended
Treadmill	Swimming
Prolonged walking	Bicycling
Jogging	Rowing
Step exercises	Chair exercises
	Arm exercises
	Other non-weight-bearing exercises

Figure 9.16 Exercise for diabetic patients with loss of protective sensation.

- dietary habits, and
- current level of regular physical activity.

Exercise Testing in Patients With Diabetes

The prevalence of premature CAD is high in patients with diabetes, but a majority of cases occur in the absence of typical signs and symptoms.[635] Thus, formal exercise testing is often advisable if previously sedentary diabetics are to undertake an exercise program. In patients with diabetes who are planning to participate in low-intensity forms of exercise (<60% of maximum HR) such as walking, the health care professional should use clinical judgment in deciding whether to recommend an exercise stress test. It is recommended that the following patients undergo a graded exercise test with ECG monitoring as part of the medical evaluation before beginning a moderate- to high-intensity exercise program:[13,195]

- All people with known or suspected (on the basis of symptoms) CAD, irrespective of age
- Patients who have any microvascular or neurological diabetic complication (i.e., retinopathy, nephropathy, peripheral arterial disease, autonomic neuropathy, peripheral neuropathy)
- The following asymptomatic patients:
  - patients who have had type 1 diabetes for longer than 15 yr
  - patients with type 1 diabetes who are older than 30 yr
  - patients with type 2 diabetes who are older than 35 yr
  - patients who have had type 2 diabetes for longer than 10 yr

The exercise stress test should be performed with such patients for evaluation of ischemia, arrhythmias, abnormal hypertensive response to exercise, or abnormal orthostatic response during or after exercise. The stress test also provides information regarding initial levels of working capacity, specific precautions that may need to be taken, and target HR used to prescribe activities.

Education, Monitoring, and Management of Patients With Diabetes

Various suggestions for providing appropriate education, monitoring, and management for patients with diabetes are included here. Figure 9.17 describes precautions and special instructions for these patients.

Foot care is an important consideration for patients with diabetes who exercise. Complications involving the feet are common in those with diabetes. Problems most often develop when blood flow is poor or when nerve damage exists in the legs and feet. Such problems can include very dry skin that may peel or crack; the buildup of calluses that may ulcerate; and foot ulcers, particularly at the ball of the foot or on the bottom of the big toe. Staff should routinely inspect diabetic patients' feet, and strongly encourage these patients to bring any sores, infections, or inflammation to the immediate attention of the staff. In addition, assessment for peripheral neuropathies and pulses should be performed. Staff should instruct patients on the following procedures for care of their feet (see figure 9.18).[347]

Exercise Prescription for Patients With Diabetes

The exercise prescription for people with diabetes must be individualized according to medication schedule, presence and severity of diabetic complications, and goals and expected benefits of the exercise program. Food intake with exercise must also be considered. The goals of patients participating in an exercise rehabilitation program should include

- normalization of blood sugar levels,
- minimalization of diabetic complications,
- management of weight, and
- incorporation of daily physical activity into their lifestyle.

The formulation and components of an exercise prescription for a patient with diabetes (figure 9.19) are very similar to the standard exercise prescription methodologies, with a few key exceptions.[231,232]

- Exercising late in the evening increases the risk of nocturnal hypoglycemia.
- Avoid strenuous exercise until diabetes is under control.
- Know the signs, symptoms, and management of hypoglycemia: confusion, weakness, fatigue, loss of consciousness, and convulsions. Episodes of hypoglycemia may occur as late as 24-48 h after exercise.
- Certain medications tend to mask or exacerbate the effect of hypoglycemia with exercise:
  - Beta-blockers
  - Coumadin
  - Calcium channel blockers
  - Diuretics
  - Nicotinic acid
- Carry a carbohydrate source during exercise.
- Avoid exercising at time of peak insulin effect, or do one of the following:
  - Consume a carbohydrate snack 30 min before exercising.
  - Decrease insulin or oral hypoglycemic dosage before exercising.
- Test blood glucose frequently; glycemic responses to different circumstances vary with each individual.
- Schedule exercise 1-2 h after meals, not at peak insulin time.
- Drink plenty of water before, during, and after exercise.
- Use caution when exercising in hot weather. Be careful of overheating. Heat loss is less efficient in many patients with diabetes because of poor peripheral circulation and failure of the sweating mechanism.
- Monitor blood pressure for hypertension during exercise and hypotension after exercise.
- Carry identification that indicates you have diabetes.
- Carry change for a phone call or have a cell phone available.
- Extremities to be used during exercise should not be used as insulin injection sites.
  - Inject insulin into the abdomen if exercise will begin within 30 min after injection.
  - When insulin is injected into the active muscle, muscle glucose is used rapidly and the elevated insulin levels will inhibit glucose production, resulting in hypoglycemia.
- Oral antidiabetes agents such as metformin and rosiglitazone do not increase insulin secretion and thus do not increase the risk of hypoglycemia. These agents are best described as insulin sensitizers.
- Neuropathy in patients with diabetes
  - Patients with peripheral neuropathy will require an alternative method to pulse taking (e.g., RPE).
  - Patients with autonomic neuropathy will exhibit abnormal pulse rates and BP responses.
  - Caution patients with autonomic neuropathy not to make rapid changes in position in conjunction with their exercise.
  - Patients with peripheral neuropathy must be extremely careful with their feet and hands because of loss of sensation to touch, heat, cold, and other potential irritants.

Figure 9.17 Precautions and special instructions for patients with diabetes.

From Gordon NF. The exercise prescription. In: *The health professional's guide to diabetes and exercise.* Alexandria, VA: American Diabetes Association, 1995. pp. 70-82.

Guidelines for Monitoring Diabetic Control and Patients' Response to Exercise

When patients with diabetes begin an exercise program, blood glucose levels associated with exercise may need to be monitored systematically.[51,551] Monitoring and recording a patient's blood glucose level before and after exercise is very important for the following reasons:

- Many patients report that their diabetes is under good control, but it is not.
- Checking blood sugars before and after exercise helps a patient identify the immediate risk of becoming hypoglycemic or hyperglycemic.

- Inspect feet daily for blisters, cuts, and scratches and report to health care provider if problems with healing.
- Wash feet daily. Dry them carefully, especially between the toes.
- Avoid bathing in extreme temperatures.
- If the feet feel cold at night, wear socks.
- Do not walk barefoot, especially on hot surfaces such as sandy beaches or pool decks.
- Do not use chemical agents for the removal of corns and calluses.
- Do not use adhesive tape on the feet.
- Inspect the insides of shoes daily for rough areas.
- Have a family member inspect feet daily and trim nails and calluses if necessary.
- Do not soak feet.
- To relieve dry skin on the feet, apply baby oil after bathing and drying feet.
- Wear properly fitting stockings, such as socks, pantyhose, and so on. Avoid mended stockings and stockings with seams that may irritate the feet. Change stockings daily.
- Do not wear garters.
- Buy comfortable shoes made of leather.
- Do not wear shoes without socks.
- Do not wear sandals with thongs between the toes.
- Wear wool socks and protective footwear in the winter.
- Cut toenails straight across.
- Do not cut corns and calluses.
- Make sure that your physician examines your feet at each visit.
- Notify your physician at once if you develop a blister or sore on the foot.
- Have two pairs of shoes to wear while exercising, and alternate them to keep feet dry.

Figure 9.18 Instructions for foot care for patients with diabetes.

- Checking blood sugars provides the basis for progressing the exercise prescription.
- Monitoring of blood sugars provides positive feedback regarding the effects of exercise.

Guidelines for Monitoring Patients With Diabetes

It is understood that clinical judgment should be used in conjunction with all finger stick blood glucose values described in figure 9.20. The following considerations are also important:

- The type of insulin or oral medication the patient takes
- The time the patient takes the insulin or oral medication
- The time the patient last ate
- The time of exercise session
- The level of exercise to be performed

Unless ketosis, hyperglycemia, hypoglycemia, or diabetes-related symptoms are present, it is acceptable to allow a patient to continue his or her exercise program while at the same time developing a specific plan in conjunction with the patient's physician to optimize blood sugar control. Measures of HbA1c provide a useful approximation of long-term glucose control, which helps in regulating dosing of medications, exercise, and weight-loss goals. A desirable HbA1c reflecting good long-term glucose control and a low likelihood of complications is <7.0 mg/dL. The combination of exercise as therapy, appropriate adjustment of medications, and proper monitoring of blood glucose levels before and after exercise in a CR setting may maximize the benefits and minimize the risks for patients with diabetes who participate in exercise training.

Pulmonary Disease

The coexistence of cardiac and pulmonary disease is rising. Many people who have significant CVD,

Mode of exercise

- Avoid or limit high-impact exercise to limit risk of musculoskeletal injuries.
- Patients with neuropathy should not perform activities that cause excessive jarring or a marked increase in BP.
- High-resistance exercise using weights is not acceptable for older patients or those with long-standing diabetes. Nearly all patients with diabetes can engage in moderate weight-training programs.

Frequency of exercise

- The duration of glycemic improvement after the last bout of exercise in patients with diabetes is >12 h but <72 h
- 3-5 d/week
- Obese patients and patients on insulin may need to exercise daily.

Intensity of exercise

- Patient should exercise at the minimal threshold needed to improve functional capacity but below a level that may elicit undesirable responses.
- Higher-intensity exercise is associated with greater cardiovascular risk, greater chance of injury, and lower compliance than lower-intensity exercise.

Duration of exercise

- 20-60 min
- 700-2,000 kcal/week for health benefits
- Longer exercise sessions may result in a higher incidence of musculoskeletal injury and lower long-term compliance.

Rate of progression

- Increase frequency or duration initially instead of intensity.
- Do not allow beginning exercisers to perform too much exercise too soon.
- Closely monitor the patient's signs, symptoms, and response to exercise.

Figure 9.19   Components of the exercise prescription for patients with diabetes.

such as CHD, cerebrovascular disease, or peripheral arterial disease, also have significant pulmonary disease, and in many instances, it is the latter that limits exercise ability. Given the prevalence of smokers and the significant lag time (often several decades) leading up to the development of symptoms related to such smoking, it is not surprising that many patients are diagnosed with concomitant cardiac and pulmonary disease. It is important to consider the possibility of the presence of pulmonary impairment for any patient entering into a CR program because as many as 20% of these patients will have a pulmonary disease symptomatology.[432]

Patients with coexistent pulmonary impairment are likely to present with undue shortness of breath (either at rest or with exercise), cough, or sputum production. The patient may have an increased respiratory rate, wheezing, a hyperinflated chest, or significant muscle wasting. In patients with undiagnosed pulmonary disease, several simple tests can help to clinically clarify the signs and symptoms. First, a chest roentgenogram may show signs typically associated with airway obstruction (lung hyperinflation, diaphragmatic flattening). Pulmonary function tests can help differentiate whether an obstructive (e.g., emphysema, chronic bronchitis), a restrictive (e.g., interstitial fibrosis), or a vascular (e.g., primary pulmonary hypertension or chronic thromboembolic pulmonary hypertension) lung disease process is present. Finally, an arterial blood gas can be helpful to determine whether hypoxemia or impairment of gas exchange exists. This can be indirectly assessed during exercise and pulse oximetry. The measurement of arterial blood gases is a helpful guide to the necessity for the administration of supplemental oxygen.

Cardiopulmonary exercise testing can be helpful in determining the causes for exercise limitations. Exercise testing of a patient with significant pulmonary impairment will often indicate exercise limitations secondary to lung disease manifested as a decrease in ventilatory reserve, an increase in dead space ventilation, and hypoxemia. In some instances, pulmonary disease may be the limiting factor to the

Basic procedure for checking patient fasting blood glucose (FBG) levels:

1. Patients with diabetes who are taking an oral hypoglycemic agent or are on insulin for control of their diabetes will have FBG performed before and after exercise for six exercise sessions to establish the patient's level of glucose control and subsequent response to exercise. Pre- and postexercise checks of FBG will continue if values of 90 mg/dL or ≥300 mg/dL are recorded.

2. A dietitian will be alerted when patients are in poor diabetic control to facilitate reinforcement of dietary aspects of self-care.

3. When patterns of diabetes control show change (improvement or worsening), a staff member will contact the patient's physician to provide data so that the primary care physician or endocrinologist can adjust medications as needed.

Procedure for managing FBG: Measures:

1. If pre-exercise FBG is ≥300 mg/dL, a urine sample will be checked for ketones. The patient must not exercise if ketones are present. The patient's physician will be informed.

2. If FBG ≥300 mg/dL but no ketones are present, the patient may exercise unless the following conditions exist:

   - Type 1 (insulin-dependent)

     If FBG ≥300 mg/dL: NO EXERCISE*

   - Type 2 (on oral agent/insulin-requiring)

     If FBG ≥300 mg/dL and symptomatic: NO EXERCISE*

   - Type 2 (on oral agent/insulin-requiring)

     If FBG ≥300 mg/dL and asymptomatic: EXERCISE*

   *In all of these cases the patient's physician will be contacted.

3. If pre-exercise FBG is 100 mg/dL, a snack will be provided and the staff will evaluate the patient for the presence of symptoms. Patients will NOT be allowed to exercise during a period of symptomatic low blood sugar. After a snack and reevaluation of symptoms, a patient may, at the discretion of the staff, be allowed to exercise. The patient will be allowed to exercise only if his or her blood glucose level has elevated sufficiently to eliminate symptoms. If the decision is made not to allow a patient to exercise, a snack and reevaluation of the patient's FBG and symptoms will be made before the patient's departure.

4. If postexercise FBG is 90 mg/dL and the patient is symptomatic, a snack will be provided.

5. Patients should be encouraged to test their FBGs 1 h after exercise at home or work and be made aware of potential hypoglycemic responses for 24-48 h after an exercise session. Patients may need to bring their own glucose measuring devices to ensure adequate technique and equipment operation and to cross check with devices used in the rehab setting.

6. Snacks appropriate for abnormal pre- or postexercise FBG measures should contain 15-30 g of carbohydrate:

   - 4-8 oz of fruit juice (not tomato juice)
   - 4 glucose tabs
   - 1/2 to 1 banana
   - 1 cup milk

Figure 9.20 Guidelines for assessment and evaluation of fasting blood sugar assessment.

attainment of maximal exercise, thus preventing the manifestation of evidence of underlying CHD, such as the occurrence of angina or ST-segment abnormalities. Although exercise testing with the measurement of expired gases need not be performed in every patient who is entering a CR program, it can be extremely helpful for those people who have concomitant cardiac and pulmonary disease to determine the cause for the exercise limitation as well as to determine an effective exercise prescription for the training program.

COPD is the most common type of pulmonary disease present in patients who have cardiac disease. Obstructive lung disease refers to the inability of the patient to expire air normally; it comprises the diagnoses of asthma, emphysema, and chronic bronchitis. The increase in the work of breathing is secondary to the increase in the mechanical load placed on the respiratory muscles, causing muscle fatigue and hypoxemia and eventually resulting in exercise limitation.

Optimal management for a patient who has COPD frequently includes the administration of supplemental oxygen; medical management, including pharmacotherapy as indicated; and the cessation of smoking (see *Smoking* in chapter 8, page 96).[432,566] The use of supplemental oxygen has been shown to reduce mortality by 50% in patients who have COPD and resting hypoxemia (defined as an arterial PaO_2 less than 55 torr or an arterial oxyhemoglobin saturation less than 89%). Oxyhemoglobin saturation can easily be measured during exercise testing with the use of a cutaneous pulse oximeter and should be performed whenever pulmonary disease is suspected. Oxygen can also be titrated to the specific needs of the patient during the rehabilitation sessions to maintain an oxyhemoglobin saturation above 90%.

A variety of medical therapies may be used for the patient with COPD. The effective use of various medications, including inhaled beta adrenergic agonists and anticholinergics, oral and inhaled corticosteroids, and theophyllines, is important in the management of such patients. In some instances, certain medications such as theophylline or beta-blocker agents may aggravate an underlying cardiac problem, and thus knowledge of the potential side effects of each medication is important. Techniques of bronchial hygiene, including bronchial clearance of secretions, and postural drainage are frequently necessary. Finally, psychosocial counseling with particular attention to the patient's underlying COPD may be indicated for appropriate patients.

Other modalities of treatment are helpful in the management of such patients, particularly adequate instruction of breathing-training exercises. Pursed-lip breathing and diaphragmatic breathing should be taught and measures of energy conservation should be reviewed, especially for those patients who have extreme exercise limitation. If the patient has a cough with significant sputum production, the CR professional should address measures for deep breathing and postural drainage

Standard exercise-prescription regimens can often be used for most patients, as noted in chapter 8. In many patients with cardiac and pulmonary disease, exercise limitation is caused by a combination of both diseases. In those patients who have exercise limitation due primarily to pulmonary disease, an exercise prescription regimen based on symptom-limited endpoints can be used. Weakness of the upper extremities is less frequently a significant component

of exercise limitation in patients with isolated CHD than in patients with pulmonary disease. Specific upper-body exercises, including potentially light resistance training, should be included as part of the patient's rehabilitation program; careful attention should be placed on the excess ventilatory response that may be exacerbated in these patients.

Peripheral Arterial Disease

Most vascular rehabilitation programs focus on peripheral arterial disease (PAD), one form of peripheral vascular disease. PAD most often presents first in the lower extremities as leg pain during walking, a symptom called intermittent claudication. This exercise limitation presents a unique challenge to CR specialists in that it will often have a significant impact on the rehabilitative process. Typically, patients are often older, so modifications previously described are applicable to them.

Evaluation of Claudication

Because leg discomfort is not an uncommon complaint, particularly among older patients, it is helpful to identify some characteristics of claudication that differentiate it from other causes of leg pain. By definition, intermittent claudication is simply pain or profound fatigue in a muscle brought on by exertion and relieved by a few minutes of rest. Typically, a patient with PAD will experience pain in a calf, thigh, or buttocks, exacerbated by walking. The distance to onset of claudication depends on the severity of the disease. The pain subsides after a variable period of rest and the patient may resume walking, often for the same distance. The symptom is consistent and reproducible and is associated with a *chronic* arterial occlusive disease process. It should not be confused with the severe pain due to a sudden occlusion or thrombosis of an artery in the lower extremity. *Acute* occlusion of an artery causes pain that is severe, constant (even at rest), and associated with other exaggerated signs of obstructed blood flow such as a cold, pale, or bluish extremity without pulses below the area of obstruction.

Claudication should also be differentiated from two other frequent causes of leg aches and pains in the older population: arthritis and chronic venous insufficiency. Arthritis differs from claudication in that it causes pain in the joints, may vary from day to day or with changes in the weather, and may occur with or without activity. Chronic venous insufficiency in the lower extremities results in blood pooling in the extremities and is associated with leg or ankle edema. The symptom is aggravated by standing or sitting for long periods. It is described as an ache or full sensation in the legs, is typically worse at the end of the day, and is relieved by resting with the legs elevated.

Specific findings on physical assessment help confirm the diagnosis of PAD and claudication. Peripheral pulses are diminished or absent by palpation. Color changes include pallor of the extremity, especially if elevated above heart level, or dependent rubor, a bright reddish color occurring in the affected limb when it is placed in the dependent position. Diminished arterial flow results in a cooler extremity when compared to the unaffected leg. Mild claudication is not a limb-threatening condition and is best treated through exercise and risk-factor modification. If claudication becomes severely limiting and interferes with the ability to work, revascularization may be necessary.

When PAD becomes severe, patients may develop the more serious condition of rest pain. The patient experiences this symptom as a burning pain in the toes, and it occurs most often when the patient is in bed or has the affected limb elevated. Patients may get some relief by hanging the foot over the side of the bed or by sitting up in a chair. Even narcotics provide only minimal relief. Ischemic pain may progress to paresthesia and paralysis of the toes and foot. Rest pain is a limb-threatening condition and must be referred immediately for further evaluation and revascularization.

Evaluation of Functional Status

The comprehensive assessment of the PAD patient must focus on the impact of claudication on ADL. Improving the functional capacity of the patient becomes a central goal of the vascular rehabilitation. A baseline of functional disability documented at the beginning of the program can then be used to measure therapeutic outcomes of treatment. Disease-specific questionnaires, such as the Walking Impairment Questionnaire and the PAD Physical Activity Recall Questionnaire, have been found to be beneficial in documenting the functional status of patients before and after participation in a rehabilitation program.[274]

Assessing Cardiac Status in the PAD patient

The risk of CAD is 3 to 10 times greater in patients with PAD.[130,408] Because claudication limits their activity, many patients may not experience any cardiac symptoms. Before beginning any rehabilitation program, these patients should undergo appropriate cardiac stress evaluation. A bicycle instead of a treadmill may permit increased myocardial work before peripheral limitations occur and therefore allow more accurate assessment of cardiac risk. Although pharmacological stress testing such as dobutamine stress echocardiography and sestamibi or thallium scintigraphy with adenosine may be considered for the patient with claudication, an exercise study should always be done before program participation.

Walking Capacity

Once cardiac risk has been determined, the effects of claudication on walking capacity should be assessed. A treadmill is useful in evaluating the extent of claudication, as well as to evaluate the effectiveness of any treatment. Historically, claudication distance and maximum walking distance were evaluated using a fixed speed and grade. Two graded protocols are suggested for use with claudication patients. The same speed, 2 mph, is used in both protocols. The Gardner-Skinner protocol increases the grade by 2% every 2 min. The Hiatt protocol increases the grade by 3.5% every 3 min. Both protocols are widely accepted and have proven effective and accurate in evaluating onset of claudication and maximum walking distance.

Doppler Evaluation

Before beginning the exercise program, patients with PAD should be evaluated in the vascular laboratory by noninvasive Doppler arterial testing of the lower extremities. A complete study begins with segmental systolic arterial pressures. These are obtained using BP cuffs placed in four locations on the leg: the upper thigh, above the knee, below the knee, and at the ankle. A Doppler ultrasound stethoscope is used to measure systolic pressures at all four levels. Generally, these pressures should be equal to, or slightly higher than, the brachial systolic pressure. Leg pressures that are lower than brachial pressures by 20 mmHg or more indicate arterial insufficiency.

To reproduce the symptom of claudication, the patient is asked to walk on a treadmill until the claudication forces cessation of exercise. Immediately after the patient stops, ankle pressures are recorded again. In the absence of PAD, ankle pressures will not decrease with exercise. A postexercise drop in ankle systolic pressure confirms the diagnosis of arterial disease. Subsequent ankle pressures are recorded at 1-min intervals for 10 min or until the return to pre-exercise levels. In addition to estimating the location and severity of the disease, this testing provides baseline information for subsequent progress evaluations. Follow-up testing should be performed upon completion of vascular rehabilitation and should include a resting ankle brachial index (ABI) calculation, a treadmill walk at the same settings as the baseline evaluation, and postexercise ankle pressures with recovery time. Though the ABI may actually change very little in response to exercise training, improvement is noted by a delayed onset of claudication, increased maximum walking distance, and shorter recovery time of ankle pressures.

Cardiovascular Disease Risk Factors

The same risk factors that contribute to cardiac disease also cause PAD and should be treated just as aggressively. Strong evidence indicates that smoking is the most significant controllable risk factor for PAD.[214] Aside from its contribution to the development of atherosclerosis, cigarette smoking increases the severity of claudication pain, reduces peripheral circulation, and negatively affects cardiopulmonary responses with exercise. These effects further reduce the exercise capacity of patients with claudication. Strict adherence to an exercise program will be of marginal benefit if patients, particularly those who have undergone revascularization procedures, continue to smoke. Please refer to *Smoking* on page 96 of chapter 8 for information related to this intervention.

Skin and Foot Assessment

Impaired arterial flow to the extremities contributes to poor skin perfusion, making skin more fragile and susceptible to injury and infection. Many PAD patients also have diabetes and suffer from neuropathy, which decreases their ability to feel pain or irritations to the feet until damage is severe. When the protective barrier of the skin is broken, the arterial system is unable to meet the extra demands required for healing. Unfortunately, at this point revascularization may be the only alternative. Foot care should follow the recommendations described in the *Diabetes* section of this chapter (figure 9.18, page 169). If ulcers are present on the extremity, delay rehabilitation until the ulcers are healed.

Practice Considerations

Efforts to provide greater structure to rehabilitation of the vascular patient have increased since the mid-1980s. These efforts have taken two directions: the development of dedicated vascular rehabilitation programs, and the incorporation of vascular

protocols within existing CR programs to accommodate the patient with both cardiac disease and PAD.[166] Unfortunately, due to a lack of consistency in reimbursement policies, these programs have not proliferated. In January 2001 the current procedural terminology (CPT) editorial board approved a code for PAD rehabilitation. This code, 93668, is a major step toward providing structured vascular rehabilitation to patients with PAD. Unfortunately, reimbursement remains inconsistent.

Exercise Prescription

For the patient with both cardiac disease and PAD, aerobic training equipment choices should focus on those that are more sparing of the calf muscle so that claudication will not limit the activity. However, to attempt to improve walking capacity that is limited by claudication, treadmill walking should be the primary modality. At a minimum, it should be utilized at the beginning and the end of the exercise session directed at improving symptoms. Interval training may prove to be a helpful variation in the training regimen. An exercise log kept by the patient provides a record of walking progress at the center or at home, documenting the onset of claudication, the maximum walking distance, and the recovery time needed for claudication to subside—all markers of improvement. Knowing that the staff will review the home exercise record every week also seems to improve patients' compliance with home exercise.

Exercise intensity should be guided by pain ratings (see figure 6.11, page 81) and should be at a level well below that at which any signs or symptoms of cardiac disease develop. Encouraging patients to continue walking after the initial onset of claudication will provide valuable information and increase the progress they make in the program. Some experience a crescendo type of claudication pain, which may require discontinuing exercise, whereas other patients experience claudication pain that plateaus, which can be tolerated during continued walking. Still others have described the phenomenon of "walkthrough claudication," where the pain actually begins to subside as they continue walking.

Post-Revascularization Considerations

The length of time after surgery until rehabilitation may begin will depend on the procedure and the overall condition of the patient. Generally, patients who have a minimally invasive procedure, such as peripheral angioplasty, will be ready for a rehabilitation program relatively quickly, within a week or two. Conversely, abdominal aortic surgery carries a much longer recovery period (generally 6-8 weeks).

Lower-extremity bypass procedure patients may recover more quickly but are limited more by groin and knee incision soreness. Any graft placement that crosses the knee joint requires the avoidance of any prolonged, sharp flexion of the knee joint, which could cause a kink in the graft. Cycles are usually permissible with proper seat height adjustment, but such patients should probably avoid rowing machines.

Pharmacological Treatment

Medications used to control atherosclerotic risk factors (lipid-lowering agents, antihypertensives, NRT, etc.) are part of the regimen for patients with PAD. Patients who have thromboembolic disease may also benefit from antithrombotic agents such as anticoagulants, antiplatelet medications, or thrombolytic therapy. Medications specifically targeted at treating the symptoms of claudication are very few. Pentoxifylline has been used for the treatment of claudication. This agent is said to increase red cell flexibility and reduce blood viscosity, thereby increasing the delivery of oxygenated blood to ischemic extremities. Some patients have noted improved walking tolerance, whereas others have not. A newer medication, cilostazol, has been shown to improve pain-free walking distance and increase maximum walking distance in claudication patients.[394] The exact mechanism of action is unclear, though it seems to exhibit a peripheral vasodilating effect. Other beneficial effects are a decrease in triglycerides and an increase in HDL cholesterol. Several other drugs are currently under investigation. When using any medication for claudication, it is important to inform patients that it does not cure atherosclerosis and should not be used as a substitute for a regular walking program. Perhaps the greatest role of these medications is as an adjunct to rehabilitation, because they lessen the severity of claudication symptoms and enable patients to comply with the all-important daily exercise regimen that helps them achieve and maintain cardiovascular health.

Summary

Although the process of providing secondary prevention to patients with CHD requires a general organizational structure, it is clear that such programming must be individualized to specific groups of patients as well as to a particular patient's needs. Consideration of various groups of patients with specific needs and the implementation of strategies to meet these needs is critical to the success of the secondary prevention intervention. Some, but not all, of the potential groups of patients involved in the secondary prevention of CHD are discussed here, but the rehabilitation specialist is reminded to continue to work to identify other specific group characteristics that may assist both staff and patients in the process of secondary prevention.

Administrative Considerations

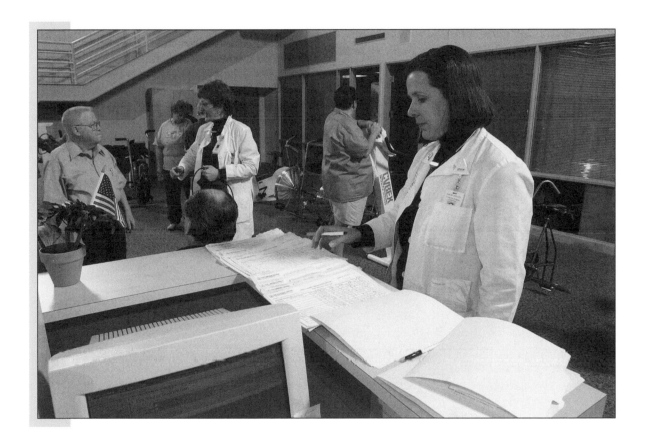

The evidence supporting the clinical importance and scientific efficacy of CR programs is widely accepted.[604] The application of standards and guidelines to improve both clinical efficacy and cost-effectiveness requires a somewhat sophisticated approach to management and administration. Effective administration requires knowledge of clinical practice guidelines, personnel management, budget, policy and procedure formation and implementation, productivity, utilization, insurance and managed-care contracting, and quality and performance-improvement issues.

This chapter addresses recommendations for the establishment of the program administration.

Administrative Structure

The administrative structure of a program is multifactorial, and each area requires specific attention. These areas, as well as the regulatory functions required, are discussed here.

Organizational Policies and Procedures

All health care providers come under the purview of regulatory bodies, including state regulatory boards, the JCAHO, or other accrediting organizations such as the American Public Health Association, the Commission on Accreditation of Rehabilitation Facilities (CARF), and the National Committee for Quality Assurance (NCQA).[301,404] In the case of the JCAHO, this accrediting organization evaluates health care organizations based on services provided and reimbursement criteria from federal agencies. The facilities that come under review include

- hospitals,
- long-term-care organizations,
- home care organizations,
- ambulatory care organizations,
- organization-based pathology and clinical laboratory services, and
- health care networks.

An operational design integrating the directives of the originating health care organization, as well as the requirements of state, regional, and national licensing and accreditation organizations, is required. Policies and procedures become standard operating procedure for all aspects of patient care, facility operations, and administrative considerations (guideline 10.1).[145]

Policies and procedures must conform to these regulatory standards and should be approved by appropriate channels within the parent organization.[270] In many cases, department-specific policies for those areas mentioned previously may be required. The policy and procedural guidelines and standards of the institution should address the following topics:

- Infection control and hazardous waste
- Human resource management
- Nursing practice
- Performance improvement
- Emergency and disaster response
- Administrative policy and procedures
- Safety

A number of previously published organization statements, policies, and guidelines are available that can serve as a basis for the development of program policies and procedures. A list of some of these appears in figure 10.1.

Leadership

Giving excellent service to patients requires effective leadership. Effective leadership provides for the processes of planning and designing programs, facility utilization, staff growth and assignments, and all other areas of program development. Program leaders are responsible for directing, integrating, and coordinating program services.

Institutional leadership usually establishes business policies and practices, whereas program leadership is responsible for communicating and implementing decisions and recommendations from upper administration. An organizational chart should be included in the policies and procedures manual (guideline 10.2 and figure 10.2).

Guideline 10.1	Availability of Policies, Procedures, and Guidelines

A central location should be created for all policies, procedures, and guideline references.

Guideline 10.2	Organizational Chart

An organizational management chart should be accessible to all staff.

- Agency for Health Care Policy and Research cardiac rehabilitation guideline[604]
- Agency for Health Care Policy and Research guide for smoking cessation specialists[579]
- American College of Cardiology/American Heart Association guidelines for the evaluation and management of chronic heart failure in the adult[22]
- American College of Cardiology/American Heart Association guidelines for the management of patients with acute MI[23]
- American College of Cardiology/American Heart Association/American College of Physicians/American Society of Internal Medicine guidelines for the management of patients with chronic stable angina: Executive summary and recommendations[24]
- American College of Sports Medicine guidelines for exercise and prescription, 6th ed.[195]
- American College of Sports Medicine health/fitness facility standards and guidelines[557]
- American Diabetes Association clinical practice recommendations: Summary of revisions for the 2001 clinical practice recommendations[27]
- American Heart Association and the American College of Cardiology guidelines for preventing heart attack and death in patients with atherosclerotic cardiovascular disease—2001 update: A statement for healthcare professionals[517]
- Joint National Committee on Prevention, Detection, Evaluation, and Treatment of High Blood Pressure, 7th report[304]
- National Cholesterol Education Program (NCEP) executive summary of the third report of the expert panel in detection, evaluation, and treatment of high blood cholesterol in adults (Adult Treatment Panel III)[403]
- National Institutes of Health clinical guidelines on the identification, evaluation, and treatment of overweight and obesity in adults: The evidence report[176]
- U.S. Department of Health and Human Services and the Centers for Disease Control and Prevention physical activity and cardiovascular health[575]
- World Health Organization rehabilitation after cardiovascular diseases with special emphasis on developing countries[631]

Figure 10.1 Published standards and guidelines.

The medical director is responsible for assisting with establishing and approving all clinical practice guidelines. The program director (department head, manager, coordinator) is responsible for the overall development, planning, and operation of the program and ensuring that all policies and processes are appropriately implemented. The AACVPR minimum and preferred qualifications for medical and program directors are as follows:

I. Medical director
A. Minimum qualifications
1. Cardiologist, internist, or other physician with interest and experience in the program; licensed to practice in the jurisdiction and with special competence in cardiovascular care
2. Experience in exercise testing, prescription, and counseling
3. Successful completion of an AHA Advanced Cardiac Life Support (ACLS) course or experience and knowledge in emergency procedures
B. Preferred qualifications
1. Board-certified cardiologist

2. Experience in medical supervision of cardiovascular and rehabilitation services

II. Program director
A. Minimum qualifications
1. Bachelor's degree in an allied health field, such as exercise physiology, or licensure in the jurisdiction, for example, as a registered nurse or physical therapist
2. Advanced knowledge of exercise physiology, nutrition, risk-factor modification strategies, counseling techniques, and uses of education programs and technologies as applied to cardiovascular rehabilitation and secondary prevention services
3. Experience in staff coordination and delivery of secondary prevention services to patients
4. Successful completion of an AHA Basic Life Support (BLS) or ACLS (if eligible to provide such services) courses
5. Certification, experience, and training equivalent to those specified for an Exercise Specialist™ by the ACSM, certification through the American Nurses Credentialing Center (ANCC), or the advanced specialty

Organizational chart

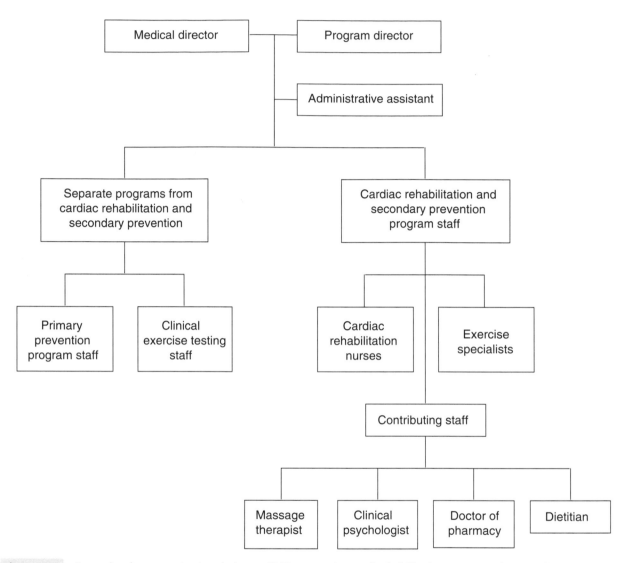

Figure 10.2 Example of an organizational chart—CVD prevention and rehabilitation program (freestanding center).

in cardiopulmonary rehabilitation of the American Physical Therapy Association (APTA)[34,35,195]

    B. Preferred qualification

        1. Successful completion of ACLS course

Effective leaders develop a program that fosters continuous patient service and quality improvement, with specific health-related issues within the community in mind. Leadership also ensures that all services are integrated, of high quality, provided in a safe environment, and in concurrence with the most recent established scientific literature on secondary prevention of CVD.

Environmental Concerns

Policies and procedures regarding the management of the facility are aimed at providing a safe, functional, and effective environment. Many of the requirements for providing program services are stringently regulated by federal, state, and local agencies. Hospital-affiliated programs must meet Occupational Safety and Health Administration regulations for safety of personnel. In addition, these facilities fall under the purview of state and local fire safety codes and, in some instances, state program facilities accreditation and guidelines.[557] Many of these procedures may be found within the institutional policies. The components of these policies should include

- planning of space utilization,
- maintenance of equipment,
- reduction and control of environmental hazards and risks,

- maintenance of safe conditions, and
- climate control.

Facilities and Equipment

The AACVPR further delineates these issues to better ensure safe and effective facilities and equipment. As such, guidelines are organized into four areas:

- General; these apply to all rehabilitation service facilities and equipment.
- Inpatient; these specifically address the needs of inpatient services.
- Outpatient; these specifically address the needs of outpatient rehabilitation, both early and long-term services.

- Stress testing; these are specific to programs that provide stress-testing services.

Inpatient Facilities and Equipment

Inpatient areas should comply with guidelines 10.3 and 10.4. The environment should allow safe and easy patient movement. Exercise services may be conducted in patient rooms, hospital hallways, and stairwells. Where utilized, hallways should be free of obstruction, with access to handrails, and distances should be measured. Equipment depends on the services provided. The following exercise equipment is recommended: portable step benches, 1- to 3-lb dumbbell weights, cycle ergometers, and treadmills with low speed capabilities.

Guideline 10.3 General Facility Considerations

- Space must meet the requirements for the activities and services provided and the unique needs of patients. There must be emergency access to all patient areas, and floor space must allow easy access of personnel and equipment. Floor space should be approximately 40 to 45 sq ft (3.7-4.2 sq m) per patient.
- All areas should provide temperature and humidity control that allow for a comfortable environment. Humidity should be approximately 65%; temperature 65 to 72 °F.
- Sound levels should be kept at a level comfortable for all participants.
- Ceiling height in exercise areas must allow for full, unrestricted activity with a minimum height of 10 ft (3 m).
- A water source should be immediately available to all exercise areas. Food and drink should not be allowed on or near exercise or monitoring equipment.
- All facilities must provide for confidentiality of patient records and patient privacy.
- A regularly tested telephone and emergency call system should be available in all exercise areas and an emergency phone list available at all phones. Emergency delivery system guidelines are described in chapter 11. Basic first aid should be available to all exercise areas.

Guideline 10.4 General Equipment Considerations

- Equipment requirements may vary depending on the patient population and the staff training.
- All equipment should be commercial grade, with stringent maintenance guidelines to ensure patient safety.
- Scheduled maintenance and cleaning programs for all exercise equipment should be documented.
- All equipment that is not functioning appropriately or is damaged and may cause a hazard should be designated as out of order until repairs are complete.
- Equipment such as treadmills or cycle ergometers should be regularly calibrated and maintained as recommended by the manufacturer.
- Staff should be thoroughly trained in the use of all equipment, and information for correct use, calibration, and troubleshooting should be readily available.

(continued)

(continued)

- A chair and an exam table or a cart suitable for supine and recumbent positions should be available in the area.

- Equipment for patient assessment including a quality stethoscope, portable sphygmomanometer, ECG surveillance capabilities, pulse oximeter, portable oxygen, and a posted and clearly visible RPE scale is required for exercise areas.

Outpatient Facilities and Equipment

Outpatient areas should also comply with guidelines 10.3 and 10.4. To conduct safe and effective programming, facilities should provide separate space for patient reception and waiting, patient consultation, exercise, education, confidential chart storage, space for safekeeping of valuables, and an easily available restroom. Outdoor exercise areas may also be included. Outpatient facilities should provide for the following:[557]

- Program and safety information that is accessible and clearly posted

- Hard, nonslip floor surfaces, which, if carpeted, should be antistatic and treated with antifungal and antibacterial agents

- Exercise floor space of 20 to 25 sq ft (1.8-2.3 sq m) per person for aerobic conditioning, resistance training, and stretching activities

- Six sq ft (0.6 sq m) of space for individuals using equipment, in addition to the manufacturer's listed space requirements

- A patient-consultation area with adequate space, privacy, and amenities for interviewing, counseling, teaching, and physical examination

- Separate toilet and shower facilities

- Showers equipped with nonslip surfaces that are cleaned and disinfected on a regular basis

- A regularly tested emergency call system in locker rooms and shower rooms

- Locker and shower rooms with adequate space, approximately 15 sq ft (1.4 sq m) per person.

Specific equipment selection depends on individual program preference, available space, and budget. Exercise equipment should provide multiple modalities for safe and effective aerobic conditioning. Motorized treadmills with speed and grade control; calibrated cycle ergometers; calibrated upper-body ergometers; and mechanical or computerized step machines, rowing machines, or elliptical trainers that display work units are examples of such equipment. Other potential exercise equipment includes resistance training equipment with adjustable benches; individual dumbbell weights in pairs, which are easily accessible and safely stored; and elastic bands. Individual step benches, floor mats, and sport balls provide for an increased variety of activities, and an outdoor or indoor walking track (or other space) free of obstruction and wide enough for easy passage is attractive and effective in exercise programs. Additional facility and equipment (materials) recommendations for program operations include

- emergency equipment (see chapter 11);

- rating scales for anginal pain, shortness of breath, or other discomfort;

- a clock with a sweep second hand, easy to read from all exercise areas;

- a blood glucose meter and glucose supplements (e.g., fruit juice) in programs where persons with diabetes are included;

- a body-weight scale and protocols for determining body composition (e.g., BMI) or other necessary equipment (e.g., skinfold calipers or measuring tapes); and

- an education area with a chalkboard, white board, or flip chart; a conference table with comfortable chairs; access to audiovisual equipment; a resource library; and anatomical models or diagrams.

Stress-Testing Facility and Equipment

Areas used for exercise testing should comply with guidelines 10.3 and 10.4. The following equipment should be present in the stress-testing facility:

- Examination table with supine and semirecumbent positions

- Ergometer: cycle, treadmill, other (with measurable workload and able to be calibrated)

- Electrocardiographic monitoring equipment (including 12-lead ECG)

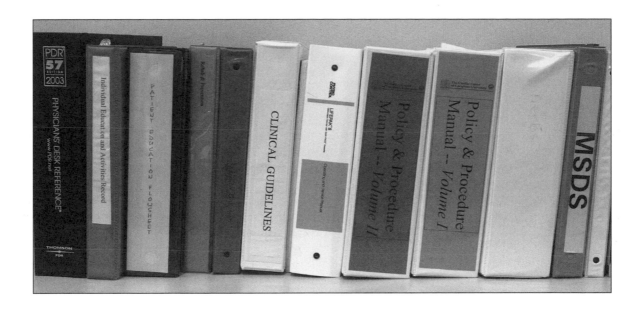

- Skin-prep items including alcohol swabs, gauze pads, razor, abrasion equipment, and gloves
- Sphygmomanometer
- High-quality stethoscope
- Basic first-aid materials
- Emergency resuscitation equipment and crash cart (consistent with institutional standards)
- Sharp-object disposal container
- Clearly visible rating scales of perceived exertion, dyspnea, and angina
- A calibrated weight scale

Patient selection, safety, and financial considerations should influence decisions concerning facilities and equipment for programming. Staff training is essential for patient safety.

Program Performance

Program success is dependent on the staff delivering excellent services; implementing new and innovative techniques; and applying the must current, scientifically based interventions aimed at producing positive outcomes. Patients, providers, and payers are increasingly demanding continuous assessment of resource utilization, cost-effectiveness, and overall justification of the appropriateness and benefits of care. One mechanism for continuous evaluation is assessing program efficacy through outcomes tracking. Outcomes tracking should continue for a minimum of 1 yr in order to document long-term cost-effectiveness. Continuous quality improvement should mirror the parent organization plan (guideline 10.5).

Regulating agencies such as JCAHO, CARF, and NCQA that are involved in accrediting organizations require the organization and individual departments to demonstrate continuing evaluation of the quality

Guideline 10.5 Continuous Quality Improvement

Program staff should develop a process for ongoing
- review of policy and procedure manuals to assure that they are comprehensive and accurate;
- evaluation of performance dimensions, such as timeliness, effectiveness, continuity, safety, and efficiency;
- evaluation of client satisfaction; and
- continued scrutiny of related research to compare outcomes with national, regional, and local programs.

of care.[120,301,302,404] Additionally, each of the regulatory agencies has established outcome measures that organizations must follow related to

- comprehensive care, for example, advising smokers to quit, beta-blocker treatment after a heart attack;
- access to and availability of care: adult access to preventive and ambulatory health services;
- satisfaction with the experience of care: customer satisfaction survey;
- health plan stability;
- use of inpatient and ambulatory care services;
- cost of care;
- informed health care choices; and
- health plan descriptive information.

The JCAHO mandates a process of "total quality improvement," or a mechanism for studying outcomes and processes. Consequently, regular review of outcomes assessment parameters is required. The value of the program is determined by measuring outcomes and identifying the cost of achieving those outcomes.

Outcome Assessment

The primary reasons for including outcome assessment within programs are to assess the effectiveness in providing patient care and using the information to guide quality-improvement activities. Traditionally, outcomes measured within individual programs have focused on physiological responses whereas assessments of changes in morbidity and mortality associated with CR participation have been described in large trials or through meta-analyses. Together, these data have suggested that CR and risk-factor interventions result in improved functional status after MI and significant reduction in mortality.[414,418] More recently, psychosocial and quality-of-life indices have been measured, and improvements in these parameters have also been demonstrated (see guideline 10.6).[417]

Figure 10.3 illustrates a model for outcome evaluation consistent with the services provided in contemporary CR and secondary prevention programs.[55] The model provides measurement options for evaluating patient outcomes within the traditional health, clinical, and behavioral domains. A new domain, the service domain, provides measurement options for assessing other aspects of program effectiveness related to overall patient satisfaction and financial and economic considerations. Optimal outcome evaluation reflects the ability to assess (1) the individual patient's progress toward health, clinical, and behavioral goals for each relevant component of care, and (2) the program's effectiveness in providing all the components of care.[55] Program staff can select a battery of outcome measures that are most appropriate for the patient population, setting, and resources.

Assessment categories can be measured using one or more of the examples within each domain and should be determined at regular intervals of program participation for individual patients as well as groups of patients, for example, at baseline, 3 months, and 12 months. Everyone involved in the program should recognize the importance of careful measurement to reduce the variability in the assessment of these outcome domains.

Health Domain

Assessment of program-related and non-program-related levels of morbidity and mortality can be identified using descriptive statistics and is helpful in ascertaining potential areas of need in overall patient care. Unfortunately, meaningful data require large numbers of participants and thus, many programs will have difficulty with this particular outcome. Nonetheless, the collection of such information can be used to contribute to larger databases on a state, regional, or national level.

Quality of life (QOL) assessment can be more easily measured within individualized programs, identifying a number of potential variables that may be described with various measurement tools. Examples of variables that might be assessed are also identified in figure 10.3. In addition, other important areas in the evaluation of QOL should include sexu-

---

Guideline 10.6 **Outcome Assessment**

Program professionals should uniformly measure outcomes in a variety of domains within the core components of care. The resulting data provide valuable information for quality improvement, accreditation, and reimbursement.

ality, coping skills, and self-control and self-reliance, although in some cases these may be more difficult to measure per se. It is important to include the patient's previously set goals as a part of QOL assessment. Progression toward these goals and how they might be modified throughout the program is a part of the assessment process. A sample of tools for assessing QOL is listed in figure 10.4.

Clinical Domain

Within this domain are the categories of physical, psychological, and medical utilization, all of which can be assessed by various tools such as those listed within each category. The physical category includes measurement of resting and exercise parameters including functional capacity but also focuses on

Health	Clinical	Behavioral	Service
Morbidity	*Physical*	*Compliance to medical regimen*	*Patient satisfaction*
• Program exercise	• Weight	• Medications	• Satisfaction with care received
• Session-related events	• Heart rate and blood pressure	• Exercise sessions	*Financial and economic*
• Non-program-related events	• Food records	• Progress toward goals	• Reimbursement
Mortality	• Functional capacity	• Smoking-cessation classes	• Deductibles
• Program exercise	• Lipids	• Home exercise program	
• Session-related deaths	• Blood glucose levels	*Recognition and reporting*	
• Non-program-related deaths	• Blood nicotine levels	• Understanding disease state and signs and symptoms of heart disease	
Quality of life	*Psychological*		
• Functional	• Anxiety	• Changes in condition	
• Social	• Depression	• Physician visits	
• Vocational status	• Stress	• Medication changes	
• Avocational status	• Perception of health status	• Medical procedures	
• Independent living status	*Medical utilization*		
	• Hospitalizations		
	• Nonroutine physician visits		
	• Emergency room visits		

Figure 10.3 Outcome domains, assessment categories, and examples of variables to be assessed.

General well-being and quality of life
- Dartmouth Primary Care Cooperative (COOP) Information[599]
- Medical Outcomes Study SF-36 (Short Form 36) Health Status Questionnaire[597]
- Sickness Impact Profile[112,224]
- Nottingham Health Profile[288]
- Quality of Well-Being Index[98]

Psychological status and well-being
- Profile of Mood States[373]
- Beck Depression Inventory[69]
- Center for Epidemiologic Studies Depression Inventory (CES-D)[457]
- Spielberger State-Trait Anxiety Inventory[528]

Figure 10.4 Tools for assessing quality of life.

assessments of levels of various risk factors associated with recurrent events and mortality. Frequency and intensity of symptoms may also be determined within this category.

Although exercise capacity is commonly used as an indicator of clinical status and many programs use some form of graded exercise testing or exercise-performance assessment as the basis for evaluating functional capacity, various other tools are available for describing functional status (figure 10.5). Physiological data including HR, BP, exercise time, exercise workload, RPE, ECG changes, and symptoms can be assessed. In addition, such measures as weekly caloric expenditure in exercise may also be useful tools for assessing functional capacity and exercise habits.

Identification of and education regarding CVD risk factors are major components of rehabilitation programs. Data regarding lipid and lipoprotein levels, smoking, stress and psychological well-being, exercise, weight control, and management of hypertension and blood glucose should be evaluated. Figure 10.6 lists some recommended outcome tools for measuring changes in risk factors, also including examples of assessment tools that should be helpful.

Psychological status and perception of health and well-being include assessment of mood, anxiety, and depression, all of which may be affected by thoughts of the future, feelings about personal relationships or critical life events, and fears associated with disability or death. Chapter 8 (p. 123) provides greater detail into evaluation and suggestions for outcome assessment of psychological status. (See figure 10.4 on page 185.)

Behavioral Domain

The ability to change behavior is the key to successful change in both the health and clinical domains. Not surprisingly, the changes that occur in the health and clinical domains are frequently emphasized as outcomes related to behavior change. Neglected are the components of the behavior domain, which directly

---

Lipids
- Measurement of change in blood levels (cholesterol screening)
- Reported adherence to medication regimen with interview or diaries

Smoking
- Self-report
- CO levels
- Cotinine (saliva or blood)

Hypertension
- BP
- Weight control
- Diet

Exercise
- Self-report/diary
- Attendance
- Borg scale
- Achievement of physiological adaptations

Weight
- Weight
- Body fat
- Waist-to-hip ratio
- BMI

Diet
- Diet Habit Survey[124]
- Harvard-Willett Food Frequency Questionnaire[614,615]
- Food Processor[170]
- Food Questionnaire[85]

Symptom recognition/disease management
- Blood levels (for example, glucose in diabetes)

Figure 10.6 Tools for measuring adherence to risk modification.

Functional capacity
- Graded exercise test
  - Exercise time
  - METs or watts
  - Metabolic studies or estimates
  - HR, BP, rate pressure product, 6-min walk test
  - Distance
- Specific Activity Scale[186]
- Functional Independence Measure[184,328,415,422]
- Duke Activity Status Index[275]
- Physical Performance Test[464]
- Return to vocation or avocation
- Borg scale

Symptoms
- Anginal index
- Mahler's Baseline Transition Dyspnea Index[358]

Figure 10.5 Tools for assessing functional outcomes.

result in many of the changes observed within the health and clinical domains. Figure 10.6 describes examples of both clinical and behavioral variables that may be used to delineate overall behavioral domain changes. These components must be evaluated and include assessment of need, identification of behavior goals, referral and entry into appropriate programming, participation, adherence, and reassessment. These components can be applied to each of those categories within the behavioral domain as follows:

- To what extent were all patients assessed for specific needs?
- To what extent were patients in need referred to or entered into appropriate interventions?
- To what extent did referred and entered patients participate (attend) in appropriate interventions?
- To what extent did patients adhere to the strategies employed in the intervention?
- To what extent did the health or clinical domain category variables change?

Program records for each patient should provide the data to evaluate the number of patients assessed and referred to and entered into appropriate interventions. The use of interviews, diaries, and attendance records will describe participation and adherence to the prescribed regimens. The reassessment of variables of concern will provide for reevaluation of goals and long-term programming.

Service Domain

Other factors affect patient outcomes that do not fit within the health, clinical, or behavioral domains but need to be considered when assessing quality of care. Patient satisfaction represents quality from an external perspective and is a strong determinant in decision making for future needs. Although many instruments have been developed, no one instrument is widely used in health care settings, and few have been tested to be reliable and valid. Programs are encouraged to include a patient-satisfaction survey that is congruent with their health organization's measures of satisfaction.

Patient outcomes are also affected by the patient's baseline characteristics, the program setting, and the processes of care, all of which need to be considered when assessing health care quality. Balancing cost and quality is imperative in today's health care environment, so it is important to include operational data (e.g., cost of services, referral, enrollment, and completion rates) with patient outcome data to help evaluate cost-effectiveness and utilization of the services provided. Outcome assessment that leads to improved quality of care must include a broader scope of measures that lead to actions designed to improve program effectiveness and efficiency.

Implementing Outcome Assessment

Outcome-assessment tools should be both reliable and valid; should place minimal burden on the patient; and should be easily administered, scored, and interpreted. Tests to measure variables within the domains generally provide relatively objective data with objective endpoints. They are both valid and reliable for assessing outcomes. Tests to measure QOL are subjective by definition, but validated tests are available. Tests to measure variables within the psychological category of the clinical domain can be either objective or subjective. Subjective forms of data collection may be less reliable. Although outcome assessment may seem a formidable task, studies show that follow-up data collected by phone, interview, or mail are reliable. In assessing outcomes over time, one can evaluate patient status across a variety of parameters throughout the secondary prevention process in order to demonstrate program effectiveness. Interpreting data, however, can be a more difficult task. Unless treatment is uniformly applied and variables carefully controlled, it is often difficult to draw valid conclusions. Typically, change over time is evaluated in groups of patients. Results may also be compared to benchmarks found in published reports.

Significance of Measuring Outcomes

The data collected from outcome studies serve as information for program evaluation, which is mandated for the accreditation by JCAHO and Medicare. The AACVPR has made available outcome domains and tools for measuring these outcomes. [429,430] Examining, redesigning, and refining secondary prevention protocols related to outcomes are essential to quality improvement, continuous or total quality improvement, or total quality management.

Empirical evidence for the efficacy of secondary prevention is crucial to the future of all clinical programs. Program efficacy can be evaluated by determining program cost and outcomes of the specific treatment in comparison with other means of treatment or no treatment at all. Unfortunately for most programs, outcome assessment performed in the clinical setting is limited by the inability to make comparisons to control groups, potentially leaving the program staff with erroneous conclusions regarding the effectiveness of the secondary prevention intervention. Program staff must recognize that many factors, including the recovery process itself, as well as the ongoing medical oversight will also affect many of the measurement variables. In evaluating outcomes, program staff should consider which outcomes are under the purview of the rehabilitation program, placing greatest emphasis on the importance and measurement of behavior change.

To carefully evaluate such outcomes, a number of issues must be addressed by the program staff before beginning to credit or discredit the role of a program on an individual basis or the impact that the program has on all its patients. For example, does the program have control over how patients are treated across all parameters? Does the program affect all types of patients in the same way? If not, which patients should be studied, and how? What are the subgroups of patients within a program? Simply providing service to large numbers of patients at low cost without assessing benefit does not describe program efficacy. Conversely, measuring various parameters without careful consideration as to the design of the outcomes-assessment process can result in misleading conclusions. For instance, physicians referring patients into the secondary prevention program will have a variety of perspectives on lipid management in specific patients, even though guidelines for such management exist. The question becomes whether it is fair to compare changes in lipids across all patients regardless of the intensity of intervention—for example, dietary counseling or conservative or aggressive pharmacological management. In this case, rather than observing the numerical change in lipids as an outcome, which is a parameter not necessarily under the control of the program, program staff might review the extent to which behavioral counseling and education were provided to patients needing reduction in lipids, a parameter that is under the control of the program. Finally, the process of outcome intervention is most important as it relates to the costs associated with various treatment or nontreatment options.

Information Management

Information management involves oversight of the storage, transmission, utilization, and tracking of information related to the operation of the program and facility. Policies and procedures related to information management should include

- patient records, patient privacy and confidentiality, and storage and outcome data;

- financial records, analysis, budget allocation, and capital and operational expenses;
- insurance billing, precertification, and reimbursement;
- provision of charity and scaled remunerative services; and
- patient or client registration and procedure scheduling.

The policies for management of information are usually developed and implemented by the institutional management team in a centralized area or department.

Documentation

The requirements for documentation of program services should specify uniform standards for evaluation, intervention, and outcome measurement. A properly documented program record shows a clear, concise, logical, and organized evaluation and intervention plan. This is essential for describing the therapy and education provided and the response to these interventions. Relevant documentation includes subjective and objective information and includes measurable indices for describing outcomes. Specific documentation requirements and formats vary. However, the following considerations should influence the design and selection of forms and the use of terminology:

- Clarity of information—information should be accessible and understandable to all staff using the document.
- Consistency of information—the type and extent of information should be consistent from patient to patient and staff member to staff member.
- Efficiency of information—essential information should be recorded accurately, without redundancies, using acceptable abbreviations and terminology.

In addition, an effective documentation system provides

- information for planning and evaluating outcomes and future care;
- a source to review, study, and evaluate patient interventions for audit, staff education, and evaluation;
- a legal record that can be used to protect involved parties; and
- a database for research.

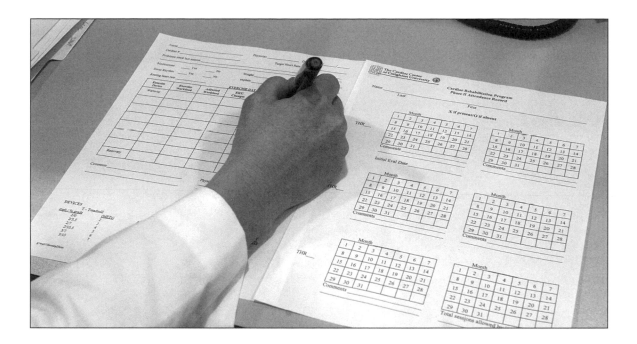

The content outlines for documentation should emphasize several primary areas, including program entry; the care plan; provisions of service, including exercise; and the discharge evaluation. These are described in guideline 10.7. The overall care plan is based on results of the intake evaluation, documen-tation of the plan for physical activity, education of the patient and his or her family and significant others, and risk-factor status and lifestyle modification and should include measurable outcomes in the health, clinical, and behavioral domains (see figure 10.3).

Guideline 10.7 Documentation

Program Entry

Documentation at program entry should include

- patient demographic and reimbursement information (outpatient services);
- various medicolegal documentation, including
  - a written, signed physician referral;
  - an informed-consent form (see appendices C, N, O); and
  - a signed release for medical information for outpatient services; and
- an initial evaluation that includes those items reviewed in chapter 6 (see page 69).

Care Plan

Documentation of the care plan should specifically include

- identification of the desired outcomes;
- a description of the mechanism for achieving the objectives and the manner in which each objective will be measured;
- the exercise prescription;
- the specifics of the risk-factor intervention and lifestyle-management programs (e.g., lipid intervention, psychosocial counseling); and
- the frequency and manner in which adjustments to the plan will be made.

(continued)

(continued)

Provision of Service

Documentation of the provision of service should specifically include

- daily progress notes (see appendices H, I, J, and K);
- progress flow sheets, education flow sheets, and a discharge summary (see appendices L and M);
- monthly reports for the patient, referring physician, and third-party payer, where appropriate;
- documentation of changes in the clinical profile, including changes in medical condition and medication regimens (see appendix H); and
- documentation of emergent interventions and subsequent hospital admission.

Exercise Training

Exercise prescription should be quantified, incorporating the general parameters of intensity, duration, frequency, and mode. Exercise can be described in terms of

- distance (feet, meters);
- grade (degrees);
- speed (kilometers or miles per hour, rpms);
- time (minutes, seconds);
- metabolic equivalents (METs);
- caloric expenditure; and
- workload (kilogram-meters, watts).

A method should exist for transforming workloads from modality to modality (e.g., rower to cycle ergometer to treadmill) so that quantification of exercise therapy can be clearly documented; for example, workloads measured in watts can be converted to kilogram-meters and speed/grade to METs. Response to exercise therapy should be quantified in terms of

- HR (bpm),
- BP (mmHg),
- cardiac rhythm,
- RPE, and
- gait and balance.

Support measures that are quantified include

- use of supplemental oxygen;
- use of nitroglycerin before, during, or after exercise; and
- physical assistance by program personnel.

Adverse responses (signs or symptoms) to exercise, including what actions were taken to remedy the adverse reaction and the result, may include

- musculoskeletal pain, discomfort, or injury;
- anginal symptoms;
- dizziness;
- arrhythmias; and
- other abnormal signs or symptoms.

(continued)

Changes in the exercise plan should reflect therapeutic response and evaluation of the results of therapy. Examples of the parameters that might change include

- intensity,
- duration,
- frequency, and
- modality.

Discharge Evaluation

Documentation of the discharge evaluation should specifically include

- a description of the extent of outcome achievement, and
- a specific plan to maintain lifestyle changes, medications, and a follow-up schedule.

All communications with physicians, other health care professionals, and families that may affect patient outcomes should be documented in compliance with general guidelines. This includes telephone conversations with physicians regarding adverse reactions to exercise therapy, progress on risk-factor modification, and formal physician letters describing the plan of care and outcomes. Any occurrences related to clinical status, including those away from the program, should be documented (e.g., changes in medical therapy, new signs or symptoms, physician visits, or other information that may affect patient outcome). The discharge summary at the termination of CR for inpatient and outpatient services should briefly describe the course, final outcomes, and future plans. In all circumstances, patient information is confidential. The program department policies and procedures manual should define the content, use, and storage of patient records. Exact specifications for forms used to collect and record patient data may vary.

Patient Rights and Confidentiality

Policies and procedures that establish guidelines to ensure that patient records and information are confidential must be in place. The delivery of patient care should improve outcomes while respecting individual rights and ethically conducting the business of the program or facility. This includes promoting consideration of patient values and preferences, recognizing the facility or program's responsibility, and comprehensive communication and record keeping. Record keeping should include informing patients and clients of risks and processes and receiving written consent to provide all aspects of the secondary prevention program.

Patient Education and Counseling

Education and counseling promote healthy behavior and thus are key functions of programming. Policies and procedures concerning these programs should be in place (see chapter 7, p. 85).

Insurance and Reimbursement

Continuous change in health care management and reimbursement patterns for CR is evident in nearly all markets across the United States. Program staff must be aware of the processes for determining the rules and regulations regarding reimbursement. Specifically, staff should verify policy, whether precertification is required, the level of reimbursement, and the number of sessions provided.

Health Insurance Companies

Health insurance companies may be divided into two distinct sectors, private and public. The private sector contracts with individuals or groups, offering a variety of plans that may provide no coverage, minimum coverage with co-pays and deductibles, through the continuum of 100% coverage with no co-pays or deductibles. The enrollee may make these contracts directly or through the employer. Private-sector insurance companies include independent insurance companies, health maintenance organizations (HMOs), and a number of other types of managed care plans such as point-of-service (POS) and preferred provider organizations (PPOs). Managed-care plans may be promulgated by integrated delivery systems, hospital systems, insurance companies, and private for-profit companies. Public-sector insurance is administered under a government-sponsored program. These programs are financed through a taxing mechanism (state and federal) and workers' compensation fees. Examples of public-sector companies are Medicare, Medicaid, Civilian Health and Medical Programs of the Uniform Services (CHAMPUS), Workers' Compensation for Medical Care, and the Bureau of Vocational Rehabilitation.

Plan Coverage

Payment for services is determined by the benefits that have been established in the contract between the insurance carrier and the enrollee. Consequently, it is important that the program reimbursement coordinator, billing department, or precertification office maintain a list of the names and telephone numbers of health plan intermediaries, case managers, and precertification officers to ascertain the extent of coverage for services prior to enrollment and application.

As of 1997, Medicare provided for services under coverage guidelines (section 3525) published in September 1982 from the Intermediary Manual part 3, claims process.[576] Section 3525 provides for services under the guidelines for patients who have had a documented diagnosis of acute MI within the preceding 12 months, have had coronary bypass surgery, or have stable angina pectoris and are considered to have a clear medical need for CR. Subsequently, several federal intermediaries for Medicare have published updated local Medicare review policies (LMRPs) that specify policies.

Though the Centers for Medicare and Medicade Services (CMS) is the governing body for establishing payment guidelines for Medicare, these guidelines are distributed to regional offices throughout the United States.[577] Each region is overseen by an intermediary, often an insurance company, that administrates the CMS guidelines. Each intermediary interprets the guidelines in the context of the region. As a result, coverage across the United States and from region to region is not uniform, because the CMS guidelines are not applied uniformly. It is in each program's interest to confer with its region intermediary regarding the specifics of the application of payment guidelines.

Programs must fulfill the specific conditions related to the facility; that is, a designated area must be established for the rehabilitation process, and healthy people must not be intermingled with patients. A physician and cardiopulmonary emergency equipment must be readily available. The staffing must consist of qualified personnel. The program is applied as reasonable and necessary for up to 36 sessions provided 3 times/week in a single 12-week period. Medicare mandates that therapy end when

- the patient achieves a stable level of exercise tolerance without ischemia or dysrhythmia,
- symptoms of angina or dyspnea are stable at maximal exercise level,
- resting BP and HR are within normal limits, and
- the stress test is not positive during exercise.

Reimbursement

Reimbursement policies discussed here are specific to obtaining Medicare reimbursement and other fee-for-service payments. Patients may be eligible for program services if they meet the diagnosis coding in figure 10.7. Should CMS expand coverage to other specific diagnoses, it will be important to obtain both a diagnosis from the physician and the diagnosis code followed by the procedure code. In addition, program directors need to work closely with their billing offices or accounting departments to ensure proper coding, clarifications, and billing efforts. Though newly approved diagnoses may be added to this list, this does not necessarily mean that diagnosis codes for billing have been added, thus effectively limiting reimbursement for those diagnoses.

To reduce the likelihood of claim denial and better ensure complete patient records for reimbursement review, a comprehensive outpatient file should include the following:[378]

- Physician referral
- Plan of treatment
- Functional goals
- Educational goals
- Estimated number of visits
- Physician signature and evidence of physician involvement in therapy
- Authorization where required
- Daily progress notes
  - Identifying short-term gains
  - Compliance with plan of care
  - Where necessary, ECG recordings
- Discharge summary

Professional staff should do the following:

- Obtain a signed physician order from the referring physician with appropriate diagnosis for establishing medical necessity. (See appropriate diagnosis codes acceptable for Medicare reimbursement.)

- Obtain the *Current Procedural Terminology,* known as the CPT-4 Code Book, which is a listing of all outpatient procedures applied within the services of medicine. Review the established numerical code for each procedure. As part of the 2003 CPT-4 Code Book, the following two codes are appropriate to the program:

  - 93797—physician services for outpatient program without continuous ECG monitoring; note that the use of the 93797 code is subject to regional interpretation and not accepted by all intermediaries

  - 93798—physician services for outpatient program with continuous ECG monitoring

- Identify the appropriate diagnosis code that must accompany the procedure change. The diagnosis code is obtained in two steps: (1) the physician must denote the diagnosis on referral, and (2) the diagnosis is coded using the *International Classification of Disease,* also called the ICD-9 Code Book. Current acceptable diagnoses and codes for reimbursement are as follows:

Stable angina	413.9
CABGS	414 and then V45.81
Anterolateral AMI	410.02
Anterior AMI	410.12
Inferior lateral AMI	410.22
Inferior AMI	410.42
Lateral AMI	410.52
Unspecified AMI site	410.92

- Where required, obtain preadmission for precertification for services, recording the

  - insurance policy, managed care plan, and coverage benefits;

  - appropriate contact person; and

  - precertification confirmation, notation of number of visits, time of service, copayments, and amount of reimbursement.

Figure 10.7 Medicare guidelines for obtaining reimbursement and other fee-for-service payments.

Human Resources

Qualified health care personnel, including a program medical director, acting on the referring physician's individual treatment plan, provide the services for a successful program (guidelines 10.8 and 10.9). The collective knowledge, skills, and clinical experience of the professional staff must reflect the multidisciplinary competencies necessary to effect the desired treatment outcomes. The clinical skills and medicolegal authority required for patient safety must be ensured by appropriate requirements for individual staff positions.

Guideline 10.8 Human Resources

Policies and procedures should include provisions for the following:

- A competency-based job description

- Required education, continuing education, experiences, licenses, and certifications

- An orientation checklist, a competency assessment, and a regularly performed (at least annually) performance appraisal

Guideline 10.9   Medical Director

Each program should have a licensed physician serving as medical director. Physicians should

- have special competence and ongoing experience in cardiovascular care and may include an internist, family practitioner, or cardiologist (mandated by CMS);
- be available for medical consultation;
- assist in program development;
- approve all clinical policies and procedures; and
- be regularly involved in the therapeutic aspects of the program (mandated by CMS).

The knowledge and technical skills required for optimal care are derived from several disciplines and health care professions. No particular combination of staffing defines a minimum guideline for program competence. Given the multidisciplinary nature of the program, applying these staffing principles allows enough flexibility for even small clinical facilities to meet program-competency guidelines.

The number of staff members and professional specialists may vary from one facility to another. Each program and facility should select the personnel with professional specialties that fit the model and policies of the institution and the human resource department. Additionally, title and level of positions are a function of the institution and program. Nevertheless, the collective knowledge base of the staff should include a comprehensive understanding of CVD, cardiovascular emergency procedures, nutrition, exercise physiology, pharmacology, behavior-modification strategies, health psychology, and medical and educational strategies for CAD risk-factor management. Both licensed and nonlicensed health care professionals may be included on the rehabilitation team. The professions most frequently represented in the essential staff positions include specially trained registered nurses, exercise physiologists, dietitians, health educators, health psychologists, vocational rehabilitation counselors, physical therapists, occupational therapists, pharmacists, and physicians. It is important for staff to participate in multidisciplinary patient-care continuing educational activities. Ongoing education and certification of staff will also assure the maintenance of competence.

The competency guidelines for program personnel specified here agree with standards previously published by other organizations and government agencies and are summarized in the AACVPR Core Competencies Document.[524] In addition, guidelines for professional education and minimal competencies expected for certification of Exercise Specialists™ have been developed by the ACSM. Specialty prac-

tice roles have been defined by the ANCC and the APTA.[34,35,195] Furthermore, guidelines from AACVPR-affiliated associations are often available through the offices of the current presidents of these associations (for information, write to AACVPR, 401 N. Michigan Ave., Suite 2200, Chicago, IL, 60611).

Core Functions

Core functions for secondary prevention programs include the provision and coordination of a broad range of services and adequate emergency response capability. In addition, each program professional should possess a common core of professional and clinical competencies regardless of academic discipline. The following delineates the basic core competencies of all rehabilitative care professionals.

I. Minimum qualifications

A. Bachelor's degree in a health field such as exercise science, or licensure in the jurisdiction

B. Experience or specialty training in cardiovascular rehabilitation and secondary prevention

C. Basic knowledge of exercise physiology, nutrition, risk-factor and behavior-modification strategies, counseling techniques, and uses of educational programs and technologies as applied to cardiovascular rehabilitative services

D. Successful completion of BLS course

II. Preferred qualifications

A. Successful completion of ACLS course

B. Certification by a professional organization that documents core competencies

The following delineates staffing recommendations and basic core competencies for providing emergency services.

I. Minimum qualifications

A. At least one person who has successfully completed an ACLS course and has the medicolegal authority to provide such care shall be present whenever directly supervised rehabilitative exercise is provided for high- and intermediate-risk patients.

Chapter 11 provides further clarification of the personnel requirements and performance expectations needed to provide appropriate emergency cardiac care in the rehabilitation setting.

B. The early posthospital discharge outpatient program should have a maximum patient-to-staff ratio of five to one. Nevertheless, a second staff person should be available in case of emergency. Intermediate and maintenance programs that do not involve continuous ECG monitoring should have a maximum patient-to-staff ratio of 15 to one. Even lower patient-staff ratios and intensified monitoring techniques may be necessary if a greater proportion of the participants are intermediate-risk patients. When high-risk patients participate in structured exercise sessions, a supervising physician should be immediately available.

Program Personnel

Although basic administrative, medical-consultation, case-management, and emergency functions can be offered by as few as one qualified provider, adding a variety of specialists to the secondary prevention team can enhance treatment services. Such additions may be full-time or part-time staff or consultants. Regardless of the specific linkage, coordination of the treatment plan is essential. Outlined here are specific personnel and associated core competencies typically found in program settings for all rehabilitative providers.

I. Registered nurse
  A. Minimum qualifications
    1. Licensed to practice as a registered nurse in the jurisdiction
    2. Successful completion of an ACLS course is a minimum qualification if care is provided by a single nurse.
  B. Preferred qualifications
    1. ACLS certification
    2. Certification, experience, and training equivalent to those specified for an ANCC program nurse or an ACSM Exercise Specialist™
II. Exercise specialist
  A. Minimum qualifications
    1. Bachelor's degree in exercise science or related field
    2. Certification, experience, or training equivalent to that specified for an ACSM Exercise Specialist™
    3. Experience in exercise program planning, supervision, and counseling with cardiovascular rehabilitation patients
  B. Preferred qualifications
    1. Master's degree in exercise science or related field

    2. ACSM Exercise Specialist™ certification
III. Registered dietitian
  A. Minimum qualifications
    1. Registered dietitian status with the American Dietetic Association
    2. Experienced in practicing therapeutic dietetics in a clinical or community setting, particularly in areas of lipid disorders, obesity, diabetes, and hypertension
  B. Preferred qualifications
    1. Master's degree in nutrition
    2. Registered dietitian with the American Dietetic Association
IV. Mental health professional
  A. Minimum qualifications
    1. Licensed to practice in the jurisdiction
  B. Preferred qualifications
    1. Licensed for practice in the jurisdiction as a clinical social worker, counselor, psychologist, or psychiatrist
    2. Experienced in psychological assessment, administration of behavioral health interventions, and counseling with cardiovascular rehabilitation or chronic disease patients
V. Health educator
  A. Minimum qualifications
    1. Bachelor's degree in health education or related field
    2. Experience in providing individual and group educational programs for patients and family members to reduce CHD risk factors and promote health self-maintenance
    3. Experience in the wide range of available technologies to provide individual health self-monitoring and promote positive health behaviors
  B. Preferred qualifications or related field
    1. Certification as a health education specialist
    2. Master's degree in health education
VI. Vocational rehabilitation counselor
  A. Minimum qualifications
    1. Rehabilitation counselor with professional education or in-service training in meeting cardiac patient needs
    2. Experience in vocational counseling with cardiovascular rehabilitation patients
  B. Preferred qualifications
    1. Master's degree in vocational rehabilitation counseling
VII. Physical therapist
  A. Minimum qualifications
    1. License to practice physical therapy in the jurisdiction
    2. Experience in the identification and physical remediation of various musculoskeletal

limitations that may be present in cardiovascular rehabilitation patients

        3. Experience in exercise-program planning, supervision, and counseling with cardiovascular rehabilitation patients

        B. Preferred qualifications

        1. Certification, experience, or advanced specialty in cardiopulmonary rehabilitation training equivalent to that specified for the APTA advanced specialty certification or the ACSM Exercise Specialist™

VIII. Occupational therapist

        A. Minimum qualifications

        1. Bachelor's degree in occupational therapy

        2. License to practice as an occupational therapist in the jurisdiction, if applicable

        3. Registered with the American Occupational Therapy Association

        4. Experience in providing occupational therapy in CVD patients or related field

        B. Preferred qualification

        1. Master's degree in occupational therapy

  IX. Pharmacist

        A. Minimum qualifications

        1. Graduate of an accredited school of pharmacy

        2. License to practice pharmacy in the jurisdiction

        3. Experience in providing medication counseling to patients with CVD

Staff Education and Performance Review

A requirement of JCAHO is that staff members receive continuing education. There should be policies regarding the number of continuing education hours, in-services, and educational experiences that are required of staff. JCAHO and most other surveying organizations require documentation of monthly emergency education and skill in-services, department meetings, agendas, education programs, and completed certifications and certificates. The policies and procedures manual should describe this process.

Continuum of Care and Services

Policies delineating the integration of all activities directly or indirectly related to the continuum of care from entry through exit should be in place. The needs of patients should be matched with the appropriate appraisals, programs, and services. Policies in this section should establish the process by which the patient is able to move through the secondary prevention program, affording a minimum of difficulty and excess time involvement, with a clear understanding of the process, and address

- appointment scheduling,
- parking,
- registration,
- insurance pre-authorization and enrollment,
- informed consent,
- program evaluation,
- intermittent progress evaluations, and
- discharge planning and follow-up.

The Impact of Limited Resources

Establishing a program does not require a large facility with state-of-the-art equipment, a large staff, and the most expensive monitoring equipment. There are opportunities for developing programs in existing facilities such as high school and elementary school gymnasiums, YMCAs, Jewish Community Centers, and other fitness facilities. Innovative programs should include such designs as one-on-one counseling and follow-up; daylong workshops with telephone follow-up; a 3-h initial session and monthly hourly sessions; a full 5-d, 8 h/d intensive education week with telephone and face-to-face follow-up every 3 months thereafter; or a model that is completely managed by telephone.

Summary

Regardless of the model, emphasis should be placed on smoking cessation; dietary management; behavior and lifestyle education and support; adherence to the prescribed medical regimen; and an introduction to the concepts and importance of regular exercise, whether it is done in the home, around the neighborhood, or in the community or hospital-based fitness center. The potential for success of any secondary prevention programming model is based on long-term compliance to the interventions, and thus follow-up must be an integral part of each of these models. It is the responsibility of the patient to assume ownership of the prevention course to be taken, but clearly it is essential the program staff provide ongoing support along the way wherever possible.

Management of Medical Problems and Emergencies

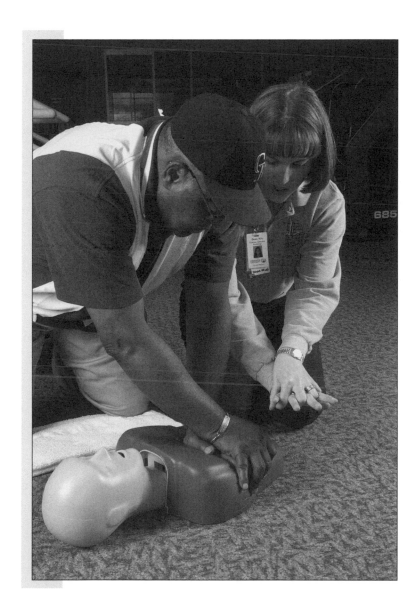

A critical responsibility of the CR service is to offer patients a safe environment in which to exercise while at the same time anticipating and preparing to provide patient care in situations involving medical problems. This responsibility is of paramount importance regardless of whether the site of service is a hospital, freestanding center, community-based facility, or home.

OBJECTIVES

This purpose of this chapter is to

- describe the potential risks of medical emergencies in secondary prevention programming;

- identify procedures for assessment and screening for potential problems;

- identify procedures for medical intervention for emergencies, including the use of emergency equipment and standing orders;

- delineate staff training requirements;

- describe documentation procedures; and

- identify considerations for alternatives for service delivery, including transtelephonic ECG monitoring, home health, and community-based programming.

Potential Risks in Outpatient Cardiac Rehabilitation

The safety of CR exercise programs is well established, with very low mortality and infarction rates during exercise training.[580] However, although patients are thoroughly screened at program entry and on each day before beginning exercise participation, the potential for the unpredictable occurrence of complications before, during, or after exercise is ever present, particularly as more patients at increased risk of events are entering programs.[467]

Services offered in hospitals and some other facilities that have been accredited by the JCAHO must meet the standards as identified by the institution for emergencies, availability and administration of medications, and safety.[302,303] Minimum guidelines described in this chapter for the management of medical problems and emergencies do not supersede JCAHO standards but rather complement and further detail the preparation for and delivery of care in these particular circumstances.

Advance Directives

Advance directives are documents that patients prepare to direct their future health care should they become unable to make such decisions. When a patient enrolls in CR, the staff should ascertain if advance directives exist and if so, these should be communicated to all staff members. In accordance with the Patient Self Determination Act, all institutions serving Medicare and Medicaid patients are required to provide information to patients and train health care providers about advance directives. The outpatient CR setting provides an opportunity for doing so.[267,268]

Patient Assessment and Screening

Although patients have been evaluated before entering the CR program, the clinical status of a patient may well change. In addition, risk-stratification models and routine diagnostic procedures, such as treadmill stress testing, may not identify all patients at risk for exercise-related events, particularly when they use modes of exercise other than treadmill walking. Consequently, it is important to observe patients carefully during a variety of exercise situations and modes.

The staff must be prepared to anticipate and recognize impending problems by evaluating a change in the patient's condition and providing appropriate intervention. In many cases of impending emergency, patients exhibit warning signs and symptoms. A change in the usual clinical status of a patient with otherwise stable disease can alert the staff to the possibility of a developing medical problem (see guideline 11.1).

Guideline 11.2 lists clinical problems CR professionals should easily recognize and for which they should

Guideline 11.1 Routine Patient Screening and Documentation

All patients should be routinely screened before each exercise session for changes in clinical status including, but not limited to,

- recent medical history since the last patient visit,
- heart rate and rhythm,
- ECG when indicated,
- BP,
- body weight, and
- medication compliance.

All screening will be documented regardless of the findings.

Guideline 11.2 Clinical Problems Requiring Intervention

Guidelines for managing the following conditions, including standing orders for emergency interventions where appropriate, should be included in program policies and procedures:

- New or changing pattern of angina
- New or changing patterns of arrhythmias
- Decompensated heart failure
- Hypoglycemia or hyperglycemia
- Syncopal or near-syncopal episodes
- Hypotension, hypertension
- Decreased exercise tolerance
- Claudication
- Depression
- Cardiac or respiratory arrest

be prepared to provide immediate intervention. The CR program's policies and procedures and standing orders should describe specific treatment guidelines (see appendices P and Q). New or changing patterns of signs and symptoms should be reported to the program medical director and the referring physician.

Angina/Ischemia

Both quality and quantity of chest discomfort or angina equivalent (e.g., atypical chest discomfort, shortness of breath) as well as frequency, duration, and triggers for angina (e.g., physical exertion, exposure to cold, the postprandial period, emotional stressors) should be noted. If angina or ischemic changes occur during supervised exercise, the exercise workload and rate-pressure product (RPP) at which the signs and symptoms appeared should be

documented, as well as associated signs or symptoms (e.g., light-headedness, fall in blood pressure).

Arrhythmias

Frequency, duration, and type of arrhythmias, including accompanying signs and symptoms, should be noted (e.g., ECG findings of ischemia, light-headedness, near-syncopal episode). Arrhythmias to be documented should include, but are not limited to, exercise-induced ventricular ectopy, atrioventricular block, symptomatic bradycardia, atrial or ventricular tachyarrhythmias, and intraventricular conduction delays.[167,306]

Heart Failure

Signs and symptoms such as shortness of breath at rest or with usual activity, weight gain, edema, or

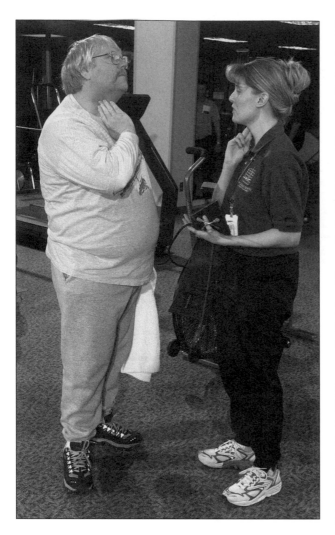

decreased exercise tolerance may indicate worsening heart failure and should be noted.

Hypoglycemia or Hyperglycemia

Note persistent pre- or postexercise hypoglycemia or hyperglycemia (in patients with type 1 or type 2 diabetes or insulin-resistant patients) as well as whether it is symptomatic or asymptomatic.

Syncopal or Near-Syncopal Episodes

Documentation should include the onset, duration, and severity of the episode, along with BP and cardiac rhythm.

Hypotension or Hypertension

Note persistent pre- or postexercise hypotension that is associated with signs or symptoms; persistent resting hypertension, or excessively high exercise BP.

Exercise Intolerance

Increasing fatigue or level of RPE at similar exercise workload and inability to tolerate usual level of activity, as well as abnormal hemodynamic responses to exertion, should be noted.

Depression

Persistent depression or changes in affect should be further assessed to determine necessity for treatment and to rule out risk of suicide. Immediate or elective referral to the patient's primary physician and a psychosocial professional may be indicated.

Intermittent Claudication

Note onset, duration, and severity of claudication as well as the exercise workload at which symptoms occur.

For each of these occurrences, follow-up should include notes verifying any interventions or changes in medical therapy. Patients involved should receive reminders about the warning signs and symptoms of these clinical findings. During assessment of a clinical problem or emergency situation, and for the general purposes of patient evaluation, CR staff should describe and document measurements of the patient's clinical status. Appropriate interventions may then be applied. Where appropriate, assessment of the patient's clinical status should include the following:

- Self-reported history describing symptoms—the degree and type, precipitating factors, and any change in pattern
- HR
- BP
- ECG monitoring (preferably diagnostic quality and more than one lead);
- 12-lead ECG if diagnostic-quality ECG monitoring is not available
- Results of the most recent exercise test or pharmacological stress test
- Auscultation of the heart and lungs
- Assessment of peripheral pulses and perfusion
- Pulse oximetry for oxygen saturation
- Assessment of level of consciousness
- Blood glucose level

Based on these assessments, interventions may include the following, as appropriate:

- Not beginning exercise or terminating the exercise session
- Assisting the patient to a comfortable sitting or lying position
- Comforting the patient
- Monitoring BP and HR/heart rhythm
- Administering supplemental oxygen
- Administering sublingual nitroglycerin
- Administering glucose orally or intravenously per institutional policy
- Establishing intravenous (IV) access and administering IV fluids
- Administering BLS
- Administering ACLS
- Transferring to cardiac catheterization laboratory, intensive care unit, emergency department, or, for freestanding center, transporting to a hospital or providing emergency services for immediate care
- Notifying the program medical director and the referring physician
- Notifying the patient's family

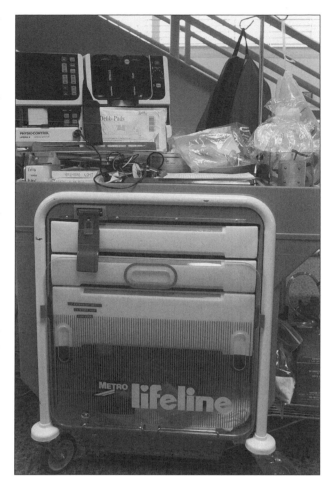

Documentation of Emergencies

Emergencies must be documented according to the standards set forth by the agency's risk-management or legal department. All incidents must be documented in the patient's chart. Other documentation may include an incident/accident form (see appendix R) and an emergency code form. The AHA recommends uniform reporting of in-hospital resuscitations using the Utstein-style form (appendix S).[133]

Emergency Equipment

Emergency equipment availability for program services is dependent on the particular site at which care is being delivered. The emergency equipment for outpatient CR and secondary prevention is presented in guideline 11.3. The emergency cart, resuscitation equipment, and medications must be checked regularly. Examples of forms found in appendices T, U, V, and W may be used to document equipment checks and maintenance.

Staff Training and Site Preparation

The AHA provides the recommended training courses for emergency cardiac care (ECC) for CR services. ECC includes treatments for sudden and often life-threatening events affecting the cardiovascular and pulmonary systems. BLS, AED, and ACLS are the typically recommended AHA training courses for adult CR depending on personnel training requirements (guideline 11.4).[30,32]

The concept of early defibrillation applies to resuscitation efforts in inpatient and outpatient CR programs. Since the advent of the AED, staff members successfully completing BLS and AED training may provide for an open airway, rescue breathing, chest compressions, and immediate defibrillation, if indicated.[56,57,134] The International Liaison Committee on Resuscitation (ILCOR) encourages nonphysician CR personnel to be authorized, trained, equipped, and directed to operate a defibrillator if their professional responsibilities require them to respond to persons in cardiac arrest when ACLS providers are not

Guideline 11.3 — Emergency Equipment and Maintenance

Emergency equipment should be immediately available to all exercise areas and should include the following:

- Code phone, medical alert signal, or other emergency signal system to call for paramedics or code team as applicable

- Portable battery-operated defibrillator with ECG printout and monitor and external pacemaker capability, each with low battery–light indicator. Direct current (DC) capability in case of battery failure should be available for the defibrillator, monitor, and ECG printout.

- Defibrillator with cardioversion and battery-check capability and automatic external defibrillator (AED) for use when ACLS personnel are not immediately available

- Portable oxygen and tubing, with nasal cannula, and face masks

- Adult airways (large, medium, and small) should be standard equipment on all emergency carts as well as bag-valve mask and pocket face masks.

- Intubation equipment and air adjuncts such as Combitube or laryngeal mask airway. If intubation equipment is available for use, personnel who are certified and licensed to perform intubation should be accessible.

- Portable suction equipment

- Intravenous access and administration equipment and fluids

- ACLS medications as noted in the AHA standards and based on community standards and medical advisory committee recommendations

- BP measurement equipment (sphygmomanometer and stethoscope(s) with a bell and a diaphragm)

- Cardiac board

- Cart or mobile storage unit for emergency equipment and medications. The emergency equipment and medications should be appropriately stored, locked, and secured out of reach of the general public when not in use.

- Biomedical engineering check of equipment for maintenance and performance should be performed every 6 months, or as JCAHO standards or state regulations require. Documentation of such maintenance is required.

- Defibrillators should be checked daily for discharge capability.

- Medications should be checked per agency policy by a pharmacist or other designated professional staff for outdates.

immediately available and until a code team arrives. (Such may be the case in early-morning or evening maintenance programs staffed by nonmedical staff.)[325] According to the ECC Guidelines for Advanced Cardiac Life Support, "All healthcare providers with a duty to perform CPR should be trained, equipped, and encouraged to perform defibrillation [guideline 11.5]. The use of defibrillation now transcends both ACLS and BLS care."[32] Because CR services, whether in-hospital or freestanding, are medical facilities and under the auspices of a physician medical director, they are not subject to public access defibrillation regulations but rather to the policies and procedures of the supervising physician and parent medical facility.

Professional staff who are qualified, appropriately licensed, and have successfully completed ACLS may administer medications to cardiovert or defibrillate patients as allowed by state licensure laws, which usually apply to physicians and registered nurses but may include other allied health or emergency personnel as well. Successful completion of either course does not imply licensure or warrant future performance. Tracheal intubation may be performed only by health care providers experienced in this skill

Guideline 11.4	Professional Staff and Emergency Care in Outpatient Cardiac Rehabilitation: Hospital-Based or Freestanding Center

- All professional staff will have successfully completed the National Cognitive and Skills examination in accordance with the AHA curriculum for BLS.

- Medical supervision for moderate- to high-risk patients will be provided by a physician, registered nurse, or other appropriately trained staff member who has successfully completed the National Cognitive and Skills examination in accordance with the AHA curriculum for ACLS and has met state and hospital or facility medicolegal requirements for defibrillation and other related practices.

- Standing orders or policies and procedures for all emergency situations will be in place and reviewed regularly by the staff and the program medical director.

- Regularly scheduled and documented emergency procedure in-services including mock codes (at least four per year) for all staff involved in patient care will be performed and documented (see appendix X).

- Regularly scheduled reviews (monthly is recommended) of emergency cart equipment, emergency medications, and supplies will be performed and appropriately documented.

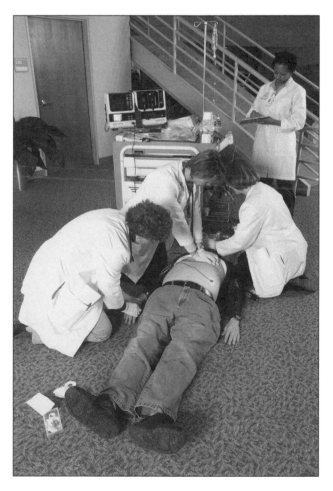

and who obtain regular experience (6-12 times per year). Therefore, most providers employed in CR programs should use alternative, noninvasive techniques for airway management, such as a bag-mask device, laryngeal mask airway, esophageal-tracheal Combitube, or pharyngotracheal lumen airway.[32]

Within a hospital facility, the emergency plan must address transportation of patients to a hospital emergency room or other destination (e.g., intensive care unit). Such a plan must include telephone access to call a code, 911, or the local emergency unit access system. For programs not operating within a hospital, staff should be familiar with the emergency transport teams in their geographic area so that access and location of the center are clearly identified. The emergency response team should be greeted at the entrance of the facility so that they can be promptly guided to the site of the emergency situation when possible, which assures that the victim remains directly supervised by an appropriate staff member at all times. A number of publications have made recommendations for staff experience and emergency care and are the basis for guidelines regarding professional staff and emergency care.[59,94,187,189,261,525,557]

Inpatient programs have a wide range of standing protocols for the treatment of medical emergencies. Because the patient is being seen on an inpatient unit, staff nurses and the code team will be available to respond to an emergency.

Transtelephonic ECG Monitoring

Transtelephonic ECG monitoring (TEM) is used primarily in patients who require monitored exercise programs but whose geographic location is not within reasonable proximity for travel to an outpatient exercise facility.[5,525] The prime example of such monitoring is its use for at-home programming, but it may be used in more typical types of exercise facilities such as community centers, health clubs, or gymnasiums. The professional staff member supervising the incoming ECG signal is responsible for recognizing impending problems, evaluating a change in the patient's condition through history and ECG interpretation, and providing direction to the patient and whoever might be with the patient to avert further problems. In cases of patients exercising in a facility where health personnel are providing direct supervision, such staff members should meet personnel requirements as described for outpatient program staff for emergency care. In situations in which patients are exercising without health care staff supervision, however, the plan for the course of action is much different (guideline 11.6).

Home Health

Secondary prevention services performed in the home may be subject to different personnel requirements inherent in the unique delivery of care. Whereas home health nurses are not typically ACLS-prepared and do not carry an ECG monitor or a defibrillator to the patient's home, those providing CR should be similarly qualified as nurses providing the care in a hospital or outpatient setting. Personnel requirements for these staff are listed in guideline 11.7. Other recommendations relative to guideline 11.7 include the following:

- The patient's family members will be taught CPR.
- The patient's home will be evaluated for ease of emergency access with a stretcher. An emergency plan will be determined and reviewed with the patient and family, including assisting the family in labeling telephones with the local EMS number, such as 911, and home address and directions to the home. This will provide accurate information for anyone needing to place an emergency call.

Guideline 11.5 — Personnel Requirements Related to Emergency Care

- All staff involved with the patient in exercise and education will have successfully completed the National Cognitive and Skills examination in accordance with the AHA curriculum for BLS and AED training.
- Medical supervision for moderate- to high-risk patients will be provided by a physician or registered nurse who has successfully completed the National Cognitive and Skills examination in accordance with the AHA curriculum for ACLS.
- All professional staff will be aware of the specific emergency procedures required by the agency for inpatients and outpatients and specific patient care units.

Guideline 11.6 — Transtelephonic Supervision of Exercise in the Absence of Onsite (in the Home or Non-Supervised Center) Health Care Providers

An open telephone line to provide access to the patient will be available not only for routine communication with the patient but also in times of an emergency situation. Previous contact with local emergency care providers will have been made, including the development of a plan for and the availability of access to emergency cardiac care to the home or non-supervised facility.

Community-Site Programming

As patients are encouraged to make their exercise program a lifelong commitment, many will use a community-site facility. The ACSM's *Health/Fitness Facility Standards and Guidelines* offers guidelines for emergencies within these facilities.[557] Guideline 11.8 is based on that document.

Summary

It remains the ultimate responsibility of the medical director and the professional staff to provide emergency care to the patient, regardless of the site of the CR service. Regular review of the plan and appropriate modifications to enhance patient outcomes is required. The foundation of emergency care in CR is continued assessment of the patient and recognition of changes in the patient's condition that may be treated to avert an emergency. The role of AED with BLS and ACLS is paramount, and defibrillation may be the first treatment administered to the patient with sudden cardiac arrest. It is important that all CR programs be prepared with an emergency plan of early recognition and activation of the plan, including providing BLS and ACLS as appropriate.

Guideline 11.7 Home Health Personnel Requirements Related to Emergency Care

- All staff involved with the patient in exercise and education will have successfully completed the National Cognitive and Skills examination in accordance with the AHA curriculum for BLS.

- All home health nurses who provide CR services will have previous experience in cardiac nursing and will have successfully completed the National Cognitive and Skills examination in accordance with the AHA curriculum for ACLS.

- All home health nurses and other professional staff providing direct patient care will be familiar with the local emergency medical service (EMS) access number (911 or other appropriate number).

Guideline 11.8 Community-Site Personnel Requirements Related to Emergency Care

All staff, including support staff, will have successfully completed the National Cognitive and Skills examination in accordance with the AHA curriculum for BLS and AED training.

- The facility will have a medical liaison—a physician, an ACLS-trained registered nurse, or an emergency medical technician (EMT)—to oversee emergency planning.

- Staff will perform and document emergency plan practice drills at least four times a year.

- Standards for such programming should comply with those for hospital-based centers but should be subject to the particular oversight of the community program medical director.

- Emergency equipment for such programming should comply with those for freestanding centers and include emergency airway supplies, AED, medications, and medication-administration supplies as determined by the community program medical director.

- Telephones will be available and labeled with the local EMS number and the address of and directions to the building and area.

Inpatient Rehabilitation
Services Record

	Imprint patient's plate here

Date	Diagnosis:
C.R.	Remarks: (day #)
	Exercise: monitored/unmonitored; O_2:
	Response: HR BP SS Assistance
	Rest:
	T1
	T2
	T3
	Comments:
	Education:
	Instructions:
	Plan:

From *Guidelines for Cardiac Rehabilitation and Secondary Prevention Programs, Fourth Edition*, by American Association of Cardiovascular and Pulmonary Rehabilitation, 2003, Human Kinetics, Champaign, IL.

B The Biology of Atherosclerosis and Acute Coronary Syndromes

The rationale for aggressive secondary prevention interventions is best appreciated by an understanding of contemporary views of CVD pathophysiology. Three decades of basic and clinical research have elucidated many primary mechanisms of the atherosclerotic process, as well as their relationships to acute coronary syndromes (ACS).[14] Over the past decade, as the basic physiology of both vascular biology and atherogenesis has been clarified, the understanding and treatment of coronary heart disease has improved markedly.

The atherosclerotic process is an inflammatory response to endothelial injury or insult to the arterial wall causing dysfunction in the endothelium and the underlying vascular wall. The endothelium undergoes many changes including self-destruction (a type of programmed cell destruction called apoptosis) and changes in vasoreactive ability, partially mediated by a reduction in or inhibition of nitric oxide, along with other substances (e.g., endothelin) produced in the endothelium. Oxidized low density lipoprotein (LDL) enters the vessel wall causing macrophage influx and further damage to both the endothelium and the vascular smooth muscle layer. Damage to the endothelium and vascular wall facilitate accumulation of plaque, begins the atherogenic process, and further complicates the vascular dysfunction caused by the original injury.[14]

Plaque exists in different "phases", some being more vulnerable to disruption than others.[208] A high lipid content and a relatively thin fibrous cap characterize the so-called vulnerable plaques. They are generally not the larger, calcified lesions (critical lesions) visualized in coronary angiography; most are less than 75% occlusive and many occupy less than 50% of the lumen. Nonetheless, it is these so-called non-critical lesions (on coronary angiography), which frequently are not associated with symptoms that result in more than 75% of ACS. Conversely, the calcified plaques are less prone to rupture and thrombus formation.[177,178,208,272] Consequently, plaque disruption and ACS are more dependent on composition and vulnerability of the lesion than the extent of stenosis. Vulnerability itself is dependent on composi-

tion and inflammatory processes within the plaque while actual disruption appears to be dependent on mechanical forces that affect the plaque and endothelial stability.[178]

Many interrelated and complex processes interact to exacerbate vascular dysfunction and facilitate atherogenesis. Among them are shear stresses from blood flow over existing plaques, infectious processes (which, in some cases, may provide the initial insult to the endothelium), inflammatory processes that accompany damage to the endothelium, oxidation of LDL, dyslipidemia, diabetes mellitus, hypertension, physical inactivity, obesity, mental stress, and tobacco use.[29,40,47,77,89,150,209,272,482,493] Macrophage activity is also found in plaques, indicating that the vulnerability of plaques is more complex than simply being stimulated by mechanical forces. The degradation of various components of the fibrous cap of the plaque, as well as other phagocytic and enzymatic changes that occur can weaken the protective cap, making the plaque vulnerable to rupture. Stabilization of the plaque is currently one goal of secondary prevention efforts. Some drugs such as lipid-lowering agents (HMG Co-A reductase inhibitors), ACE inhibitors, and beta-blockers seem to stabilize plaque and endothelial function.[49,74,203,297,366,488,497,538] It is also known that cessation from tobacco use, moderate physical activity, lowering LDL, or raising high density lipoprotein-cholesterol (HDL) acutely and chronically improve endothelial function.[29,40,47,77,89,150,209,272,284,482,493]

Plaque disruption may cause a mural thrombus, which may be occlusive, to develop within the vessel, as in ACS, or alternately a type of mural thrombus to develop on the vessel wall. The formation of a mural thrombus along the wall of the vessel may not be associated with ACS, but rather may be associated with rest or unstable angina. These thrombi are not usually totally occlusive, and are associated with rapid growth of additional plaque and remodeling of the vessel wall. This process ultimately results in complicated lesions that combine a lipid-rich core with large amounts of macrophages, foam cells, and other foreign materials that infiltrate the wall. This material and the remodeling of the vessel wall further

From *Guidelines for Cardiac Rehabilitation and Secondary Prevention Programs, Fourth Edition,* by American Association of Cardiovascular and Pulmonary Rehabilitation, 2003, Human Kinetics, Champaign, IL.

deteriorate normal endothelial function (i.e., these vessels exhibit paradoxical vasoconstriction under the influence of adrenergic stimulation). Additionally, it is thought that small coronary vessels may also be prone to vascular wall dysfunction, plaque development, and thrombus formation and, thereby also contribute to symptomatic CHD.[148,178]

These processes are important to secondary prevention, not just because of the therapeutic approaches used to ameliorate them (a variety of pharmacological therapies), but also because the life-style behavior interventions provided through secondary prevention programs are also acutely related to endothelial dysfunction, thrombus formation, and atherogenesis. That is, it has been shown that behaviors such as consumption of a single high-fat meal, little or no physical activity, having poorly controlled blood glucose, dyslipidemia, hypertension, and acute anger cause or exacerbate endothelial dysfunction. These are all related to the risk factors assessed at entry to secondary prevention programs.

From *Guidelines for Cardiac Rehabilitation and Secondary Prevention Programs, Fourth Edition,* by American Association of Cardiovascular and Pulmonary Rehabilitation, 2003, Human Kinetics, Champaign, IL.

Informed Consent for Exercise Testing of Patients With Known or Suspected Heart Disease

Name _____

1. Purpose and Explanation of Test

I hereby consent to voluntarily engage in an exercise test to determine my capacity and state of cardiovascular health. I also consent, if necessary, to the taking of samples of my exhaled air during exercise to properly measure my oxygen consumption. It is my understanding that the information obtained will help me evaluate future physical activities in which I may safely engage and aid my doctor in the determination of an appropriate medical treatment for me.

I understand that my physician has recommended the exercise test and referred me to this particular center for performance of the test. I have provided correct responses to the questions as indicated on the patient medical history form or to those of the interviewer. I understand that based on this information, it will be determined if there are any reasons that would make it undesirable or unsafe for me to take the test. Consequently, I understand that it is important that I provide complete and accurate responses to the interviewer and recognize that my failure to do so could lead to possible unnecessary injury to myself during the test.

The test that I will undergo will be performed on a motor-driven treadmill or bicycle ergometer with the amount of effort gradually increasing. As I understand it, this increase in effort will continue until I feel and verbally report to the operator any symptoms such as fatigue, shortness of breath, or chest discomfort. I have been clearly advised that it is my right to request that a test be stopped at any point and that I should immediately upon experiencing any such symptoms inform the operator.

It is further my understanding that prior to beginning the test, I will be connected by electrodes and cables to an electrocardiographic recorder which will enable personnel to monitor my cardiac (heart)

activity. During the test itself, it is my understanding that a physician or trained observer will monitor my responses continuously and take frequent readings of blood pressure, the electrocardiogram, and record my expressed feelings of discomfort or effort.

Once the test has been completed, but before I am released from the test area, I will be given special instructions about showering and the recognition of certain symptoms that may appear within the first 24 hours after the test. I agree to follow these instructions and promptly contact the program personnel or medical providers if such symptoms develop.

2. Risks

It is my understanding, and I have been informed, that there exists the possibility of adverse changes during the actual test. I have been informed that these changes could include abnormal blood pressure, fainting, disorders of heart rhythm, stroke, and very rare instances of heart attack or even death. Every effort, I have been told, will be made to minimize these occurrences by observations taken during the test. I have also been informed that emergency equipment and personnel are readily available to deal with these unusual situations should they occur. I understand that there is a risk of injury, heart attack, or even death as a result of my performance of this test, but knowing those risks, it is my desire to proceed to take the test as herein indicated.

3. Benefits to Be Expected and Alternatives to the Exercise Testing Procedure

I understand that the possible beneficial results of this test depend on my doctor's medical reasons for requesting it. It may be helpful in determining my chances of having heart disease that should be treated medically. If my doctor suspects or knows already that I have heart disease, this test may help to evaluate how this disease affects my ability to safely do certain types of physical work or exercises and how best to treat the disease.

4. Confidentiality and Use of Information

I have been informed that the information obtained from this exercise test will be treated as privileged and confidential and will consequently not be released or revealed to any person without my express written consent. I do, however, agree to the use of any information for research or statistical purposes as long as same does not provide facts that could lead to identification of my person. Any other information obtained, however, will be used only by the program staff to evaluate my exercise status or needs.

5. Inquiries and Freedom of Consent

I have been given the opportunity to ask questions regarding the procedure.

I further understand that there are remote risks other than those mentioned previously that may be associated with this procedure. Despite the fact that a complete accounting of all remote risks is not entirely possible, I am satisfied with the review of these risks which was provided to me, and it is still my desire to proceed with the test.

I acknowledge that I have read this document in its entirety or that it has been read to me if I have been unable to read same.

I consent to the rendition of all services and procedures as explained herein by all program personnel.

_____   _____
Patient's Signature   Date

_____   _____
Witness's Signature   Date

_____   _____
Test Supervisor's Signature   Date

From *Guidelines for Cardiac Rehabilitation and Secondary Prevention Programs, Fourth Edition,* by American Association of Cardiovascular and Pulmonary Rehabilitation, 2003, Human Kinetics, Champaign, IL.

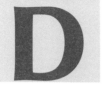

Protocol for Six-Minute Walk Assessment

1. **Equipment**—Rolling distance marker and stopwatch.

2. **Exclusion criteria** (may vary with study protocol)—Patients with musculoskeletal problems that preclude walking such as intermittent claudication, paralysis, pain, and psychiatric problems that would contribute to decreased walking performance. Uncontrolled angina, hypertension, recent history of cardiac dysrhythmia, or other forms of heart disease may also preclude testing.

3. **Protocol**—

   a. Prior to the first walk; resting HR, BP, and EG (if indicated) will be recorded.

   b. Walks should take place at least two hours following a meal.

   c. Patients may be asked to walk on a walking track, covering as much ground as possible in 6 minutes.

   d. The 6MW can be carried out on a quiet indoor hallway that is at least 100 feet in length.

   e. Three walks should be carried out with at least 15 minutes of rest between each test or on separate days

   f. The following instructions are an example for a 6MW using a hallway:

   "The purpose of this test is to find out how far you can walk in six minutes. You will start from this point and follow the hallway to the marker at the end, then turn around and walk back. When you arrive back at the starting point, you will go back and forth again. You will go back and forth as many times as you can in the six-minute period. If you need to, you may stop and rest. Just remain where you are until you can go on again. However, the most important thing about the test is that you cover as much ground as you possibly can during the six minutes.

   I will tell you the time, and I will let you know when the six minutes are up. When I say 'stop', please stand right where you are."

   Subjects will then be asked to repeat the gist of the instructions to validate understanding.

   g. During the walks, the following words of encouragement will be provided at 30-second intervals " . . . you're doing well", " . . . keep up the good work", " . . . good job", " . . . you're doing fine".

   h. Patients are told when 2, 4, and 6 minutes (Stop) have elapsed.

   i. The longest distance walked of the three trials will be recorded as 6MDW, although all distances will be documented.

   j. Immediately following completion of the walking test, patients will be asked to rate their level of perceived exertion and HR, BP, and ECG (if indicated) will be recorded. Total distance walked will also be determined for future comparisons.

Reprinted, by permission, from B. Steele, 1994. The six-minute walk. In *AACVPR Proceedings, 9th Annual Meeting, Portland, OR, 1994* (Chicago: AACVPR), 383-388.

From *Guidelines for Cardiac Rehabilitation and Secondary Prevention Programs, Fourth Edition,* by American Association of Cardiovascular and Pulmonary Rehabilitation, 2003, Human Kinetics, Champaign, IL.

Smoking History

Name: _____ Date: _____

1. Have you smoked at least one cigarette, cigar, pipeful of tobacco, or cigarillo or had one chew of tobacco in the past month?

   _____ No; do not ask any of the remaining questions on this form.

   _____ Yes; continue.

2. What type of tobacco product do you use predominantly? (Circle one.)

   1   Cigarette   3   Pipe   5   Snuff/chewing tobacco

   2   Cigar   4   Cigarillo

3. On average, in the past 6 months how many cigarettes (or other tobacco products) have you smoked per day?

   _____ # of cigarettes   _____ # pipefuls of tobacco   _____ # of chews

   _____ # of cigars   _____ # of cigarillos

4. How old were you when you began to smoke?

   _____ years of age

5. How many years have you smoked on a regular basis?

   _____ # of years

6. How many times have you made a *serious* attempt to quit smoking?

   _____ # of times (if never, go to #12)

7. What was the longest time you have been off cigarettes?

   _____ # of years   _____ # of months   _____ # of days

8. In what year did this occur?

   _____ (year)

From *Guidelines for Cardiac Rehabilitation and Secondary Prevention Programs, Fourth Edition*, by American Association of Cardiovascular and Pulmonary Rehabilitation, 2003, Human Kinetics, Champaign, IL.

9. When was the last time you made a serious attempt to quit smoking?

   _____ / _____

10. What prompted you to begin smoking after your last attempt to quit? (Choose only one.)

    1   Crisis (death, illness, loss of job, family)

    2   Chronic stress

    3   Social/party situation

    4   Withdrawal symptoms

    5   Boredom

    6   Other; please explain: _____

11. What method of stopping smoking has worked best for you in the past, if any? (Choose only one.)

1	Quit on own	6	Formal program
2	Pamphlets	7	Private therapy
3	Buddy system	8	Other medications
4	Nicotine gum/patch	9	Other: _____
5	Hypnosis, acupuncture		

12. Have you ever used any prescribed medication(s) like nicotine chewing gum or the patch to help you stop smoking?

    No

    Yes   Which medication(s)? _____

Questions 13 and 14 relate to addiction. Patients smoking within 30 minutes of waking and always/usually when ill are normally highly addicted to tobacco; pharmacological therapy may be highly beneficial.

13. How soon after you wake up do you smoke your first cigarette? (Circle only one.)

    1. When you first open your eyes

    2. Within the first 15 minutes of waking up

    3. Between 15 and 30 minutes after waking up

    4. Between 30 and 60 minutes after waking up

    5. Between 1 and 2 hours after waking up

    6. More than 2 hours after waking up

14. Do you smoke on the days that you are so ill that you are in bed most of the day? (Circle only one.)

    5   Always

    4   Usually

    3   Sometimes

    2   Rarely

    1   Never

15. Does the person you are closest to (spouse, companion) smoke?

No

Yes   Who is this? _____

16. Do you intend to stay off cigarettes, or other tobacco products, in the next month?

1	2	3	4	5	6	7
Definitely no	Probably no	Possibly no	Maybe	Possibly yes	Probably yes	Definitely yes

17. How often do you drink some kind of alcoholic beverage? (If you choose an answer other than 'never,' proceed to #18.)

_____ Daily or almost every day

_____ 3 or 4 times a week

_____ Once or twice a week

_____ Once or twice a month

_____ Less than once a month

_____ Never (go to question 23)

Questions 18-21 are the CAGE questions related to alcohol. A score of 2 or greater significantly increases the probability of alcoholism; additional screening is warranted.

18. Have you ever felt you ought to CUT DOWN on your drinking?

No

Yes

19. Have people ever ANNOYED you by criticizing your drinking?

No

Yes

From *Guidelines for Cardiac Rehabilitation and Secondary Prevention Programs, Fourth Edition,* by American Association of Cardiovascular and Pulmonary Rehabilitation, 2003, Human Kinetics, Champaign, IL.

20. Have you ever felt bad or GUILTY about your drinking?

No

Yes

21. Have you ever had a drink first thing in the morning (EYE OPENER) to steady your nerves or get rid of a hangover?

No

Yes

22. How many of these alcoholic beverages do you drink during an average week?

_____ # of 12-oz. bottles or cans of beer, ale, etc.

_____ # of 4-oz. glasses of wine, sherry, port, etc.

_____ # of shots (a shot = 1.5 ounces) of vodka, rum, Scotch whiskey, bourbon, tequila, or gin (including mixed drinks and cocktails)

_____ # of after-dinner drinks

23. How hard has it been for you not to smoke since you've been in the hospital?

1	2	3	4	5
Very easy	Easy	Moderately easy	Hard	Very hard

24. How severe have withdrawal symptoms been for you?

1	2	3	4	5
Not at all severe	Mildly severe	Moderately severe	Severe	Very severe

Question 25: A response of 5 or greater may indicate moderate problems with depression, suggesting a need for further screening or intervention; pharmacological therapy (buproprion SR) may be highly beneficial.

25. How troubled are you by feeling miserable and depressed?

1	2	3	4	5	6	7	8	9
Hardly		Slightly		Moderately		Markedly		Very severely

26. How confident are you that you will be able to stay off cigarettes once you are discharged from the hospital? (0% = no confidence, 100% = total confidence)

0%   10%   20%   30%   40%   50%   60%   70%   80%   90%   100%

From *Guidelines for Cardiac Rehabilitation and Secondary Prevention Programs, Fourth Edition,* by American Association of Cardiovascular and Pulmonary Rehabilitation, 2003, Human Kinetics, Champaign, IL.

Cage Questionnaire

___ No ___ Yes Have you ever felt you ought to CUT DOWN on your drinking?

___ No ___ Yes Have people ever ANNOYED you by criticizing your drinking?

___ No ___ Yes Have you ever felt bad or GUILTY about your drinking?

___ No ___ Yes Have you ever had a drink first thing in the morning (EYE OPENER) to steady your nerves or get rid of a hangover?

_____ TOTAL (No = 0; Yes = 1)

A total score of 2 or greater significantly increases the probability of alcoholism—additional screening is warranted.

From *Guidelines for Cardiac Rehabilitation and Secondary Prevention Programs, Fourth Edition,* by American Association of Cardiovascular and Pulmonary Rehabilitation, 2003, Human Kinetics, Champaign, IL.

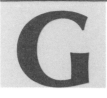

Algorhithm for Assessment of Patient Willingness to Quit Smoking

Are you willing to quit smoking now?	
No	**Yes**
• Provide strong, unequivocal advice. • Ask about knowledge of negative consequences (risks).	• Determine need for cessation or relapse prevention.
• Identify potential benefits.	**Cessation**
• Ask patient to limit # of cigarettes/tobacco products.	• Set quit date.
• Protect cardiac disease status (i.e., antiplatelet agents, beta-blockers).	• Determine method for cessation: • Cold turkey • cigarettes • Switching brands
• Provide resources regarding smoking programs, if applicable.	
• Ask about capability of follow-up.	
	• Ask patient to self-monitor.
	Relapse prevention
	• Identify high-risk situations.
	• Offer cognitive and behavioral strategies.
	• Contract to remain nonsmoker.
	• Provide counseling for the following: • Weight gain • Alcohol use • Loss/deprivation • Social support • Exercise • Depression
	• What about slips?
	• Recommend pharmacologic therapy for all eligible patients.
	• Provide medication instruction.
	• Offer instruction sheets.

From *Guidelines for Cardiac Rehabilitation and Secondary Prevention Programs, Fourth Edition,* by American Association of Cardiovascular and Pulmonary Rehabilitation, 2003, Human Kinetics, Champaign, IL.

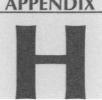

Cardiac Rehabilitation Clinical Review

Date	Diagnosis:		
	OR Date: Surgeon/Physician:		
	Summary:		
	ECG/dysrhythmia/test results:		
	Lab values:		
	Medications:		
	Activity order:		
	Plan:		

From *Guidelines for Cardiac Rehabilitation and Secondary Prevention Programs, Fourth Edition,* by American Association of Cardiovascular and Pulmonary Rehabilitation, 2003, Human Kinetics, Champaign, IL.

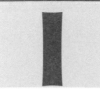

Example of Early Outpatient Program Daily Exercise Record

Name: _____ THR: _____

	Entry		Exercise 1					Exercise 2					Exit	
Date	HR	BP	Mode	HR	BP	RPE	Min	Mode	HR	BP	RPE	Min	HR	BP
Wt.														
Comments:														
							Signature:							

	Entry		Exercise 1					Exercise 2					Exit	
Date	HR	BP	Mode	HR	BP	RPE	Min	Mode	HR	BP	RPE	Min	HR	BP
Wt.														
Comments:														
							Signature:							

	Entry		Exercise 1					Exercise 2					Exit	
Date	HR	BP	Mode	HR	BP	RPE	Min	Mode	HR	BP	RPE	Min	HR	BP
Wt.														
Comments:														
Signature:														

From *Guidelines for Cardiac Rehabilitation and Secondary Prevention Programs, Fourth Edition,* by American Association of Cardiovascular and Pulmonary Rehabilitation, 2003, Human Kinetics, Champaign, IL.

Cardiac Rehabilitation Clinical Review

Name: _____

Target HR: _____

Date: _____

Problems since last session: _____

_____

Medications: ___ yes ___ no Weight: _____ Resting BP: _____

Sinus rhythm: ___ yes ___ no Explain: _____ Recovery BP: _____

Resting heart rate: _____

Exercise data						
Exercise device	Exercise workload	Adjusted workload	ECG changes	Signs/symptoms	Exercise HR	Recovery HR
Warm-up						
Recovery						
				Average ExHR		

Comments: _____

_____

From *Guidelines for Cardiac Rehabilitation and Secondary Prevention Programs, Fourth Edition,* by American Association of Cardiovascular and Pulmonary Rehabilitation, 2003, Human Kinetics, Champaign, IL.

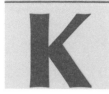

Example of Long-Term Outpatient Program Daily Exercise Record

Name: _____

Target HR: _____

Exercise prescription: _____

Date	Adjustments or comments	Meds	Rest HR	Rest BP	Warm-up	Ex HR 10 min	Ex HR 20 min	Ex HR 30 min	Post-ex BP	Weight

From *Guidelines for Cardiac Rehabilitation and Secondary Prevention Programs, Fourth Edition,* by American Association of Cardiovascular and Pulmonary Rehabilitation, 2003, Human Kinetics, Champaign, IL.

Education Flow Sheet

Topics	Teaching needs Please check	Discussed	Reinforced	Verbalized understanding	Teaching materials*	Comments
Orientation to early outpatient cardiac rehabilitation						
1. Registration						
2. Medical history—initial evaluation						
3. Risk-factor identification						
4. Orientation to staff and equipment						
5. Explanation of exercise prescription and target HR						
6. Instruction/review pulse check technique						
Anatomy and physiology						
1. MI						
2. CABGS						
3. PTCA						
4. Angina						
5. Other—please list						
Risk factors						
1. Smoking						
2. Hypertension						
3. Hyperlipidemia						
4. Diabetes						
5. Obesity						
6. Stress						
7. Inactivity						
8. Family history						
9. Age/sex						

* H = handout; AV = audiovisual; C = class.

From *Guidelines for Cardiac Rehabilitation and Secondary Prevention Programs, Fourth Edition*, by American Association of Cardiovascular and Pulmonary Rehabilitation, 2003, Human Kinetics, Champaign, IL.

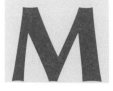

Example of Early Outpatient Program Daily Exercise Record

Date	Diagnosis:		
CR	Remarks:		
	___ Discharge instructions reviewed with patient; questions answered; phone number provided for follow-up		
	Patient received:		
	___ Specific literature		
	___ Guidelines for resuming ADL		
	___ Guidelines for modifying risk factors		
	___ Guidelines for progressing activity		
	___ Home exercise program		
	Week	Walk min × day Bike min × day Other	
	1		
	2		
	3		
	4		
	5		
	6		
	Further comments:		

Informed Consent for Exercise Rehabilitation of Patients with Known or Suspected Heart Disease

Name _____

1. Purpose and Explanation of Procedure

In order to improve my physical capacity and generally aid in my medical treatment for heart disease, I hereby consent to enter a cardiac rehabilitation program that will include cardiovascular monitoring, physical exercise, dietary counseling, smoking cessation, stress reduction, and health education activities. The levels of exercise that I will perform will be based on the condition of my heart and circulation as determined by my physician. I will be given exact instructions regarding the amount and kind of exercise I should do. I agree to participate three times per week in the rehabilitation program. Professionally trained clinical personnel will provide leadership to direct my activities and monitor my electrocardiogram and blood pressure to be certain that I am exercising at the prescribed level. I understand that I am expected to attend every session and to follow physician and staff instructions with regard to any medications that may have been prescribed, exercise, diet, stress management, and smoking cessation. If I am taking prescribed medication, I have already so informed the program staff and further agree to so inform them promptly of any changes my doctor or I have made with regard to use of these.

I have been informed that in the course of my participation in exercise, I will be asked to complete the activities unless such symptoms as fatigue, shortness of breath, chest discomfort, or similar occurrences appear. At that point I have been advised that it is my complete right to stop exercise and that it is my obligation to inform the program personnel of my symptoms. I recognize and hereby state that I have been advised that I should immediately upon experiencing any such symptoms inform the program personnel of my symptoms.

I understand that during the performance of exercise, a trained observer will periodically monitor my performance and perhaps take my electrocardiogram, pulse, blood pressure, or make other observations for the purpose of monitoring my progress and/or condition. I also understand that the observer may reduce or stop my exercise program when findings indicate that this should be done for my safety and benefit.

2. Risks

It is my understanding, and I have been informed, that there exists the possibility during exercise of adverse changes including abnormal blood pressure; fainting; disorders of heart rhythm; and very rare instances of heart attack, stroke, or even death. Every effort, I have been told, will be made to minimize these occurrences by proper staff assessment of my condition before each exercise session, staff supervision during exercise, and my own careful control of exercise effort. I have also been informed that emergency equipment and personnel are readily available to deal with unusual situations should these occur. I understand that there is a risk of injury, heart attack, stroke, or even death as a result of my exercise, but knowing those risks, it is my desire to proceed to participate as herein indicated.

3. Benefits to Be Expected and Alternatives Available

I understand that this medical treatment may or may not benefit my health status or physical fitness. Generally, participation will help determine what recreational and occupational activities I can safely and comfortably perform. Many individuals in such programs also show improvements in their capacity

From *Guidelines for Cardiac Rehabilitation and Secondary Prevention Programs, Fourth Edition,* by American Association of Cardiovascular and Pulmonary Rehabilitation, 2003, Human Kinetics, Champaign, IL.

for physical work. For those who are overweight and able to follow the physician's and dietitian's recommended dietary plan, this program may also aid in achieving appropriate weight education and control.

4. Confidentiality and Use of Information

I have been informed that the information obtained from this rehabilitation program will be treated as privileged and confidential and will consequently not be released or revealed to any person without my express written consent. I do, however, agree to the use of any information for research and statistical purposes as long as same does not identify my person or provide facts that could lead to my identification. Any other information obtained, however, will be used only by the program staff in the course of prescribing exercise for me, planning my rehabilitation program, or advising my personal physician of my progress.

5. Inquiries and Freedom of Consent

I have been given an opportunity to ask certain questions as to the procedures of this program.

I further understand that there are remote risks other than those previously described that may be associated with this program. Despite the fact that a complete accounting of all remote risks is not entirely possible, I am satisfied with the review of these risks that was provided to me, and it is still my desire to participate.

I acknowledge that I have read this document in its entirety or that it has been read to me if I have been unable to read same.

I consent to the rendition of all services and procedures as explained herein by all program personnel.

_____ _____

Patient's Signature   Date

_____ _____

Witness's Signature   Date

_____ _____

Program Staff's Signature   Date

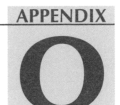

Example of Alternative Clauses to Be Considered for Possible Addition to Informed Consent Forms or Preparticipation Forms

Anxious Patient—Additional Spousal Consent

I have been informed by _____ that a full disclosure of all known risks associated with the procedure to be performed by my spouse has not been given to my spouse because in the professional opinion and judgment of _____ such a disclosure would have adverse consequences to my spouse and would expose my spouse to an increased risk while undergoing the procedure due to his/her anxiety and nervousness as to the procedure itself and the risks involved with treatment procedures. Consequently, I have been informed by _____ of the following risks which were not disclosed to my spouse:

_____

_____

_____

It is my agreement and consent that despite these risks, and the lack of full communication of same to my spouse, the procedure be carried out as to my spouse inasmuch as _____ has explained to me that the following benefits may be derived from the procedure:

_____

_____

_____

I agree with the assessment of _____ that further explanations as to the details of the test would undoubtedly cause increased anxiety and stress in my spouse, and as a consequence thereof, I believe that no further disclosure should be made to my spouse and that the test procedure should be performed as previously described.

From *Guidelines for Cardiac Rehabilitation and Secondary Prevention Programs, Fourth Edition,* by American Association of Cardiovascular and Pulmonary Rehabilitation, 2003, Human Kinetics, Champaign, IL.

Example of Outpatient Rehabilitation Standing Orders

1. Initiate monitored exercise program per outpatient CR policies and procedures.

2. Target HR is determined by sign- or symptom-limited graded exercise test (GXT) or sign- or symptom-limited responses to submaximal exercise.

3. Begin with a training duration of up to 30 min to tolerance one to three times a week.

4. Gradually increase duration of training exercise if the patient's cardiovascular responses are acceptable. Do not exceed 50 min of training duration.

5. Observe participant for signs of exercise intolerance and adapt or stop exercise as indicated in outpatient cardiovascular rehabilitation policies and procedures.

6. Lipid profile 6 weeks postevent.

7. May administer nitroglycerin 0.3 or 0.4 mg sublingually at 5 minutes × 3 as needed for angina/ischemia.

8. Contact the physician periodically to report on the patient's progress, unless the patient's condition indicates earlier contact. Send copies of reports to the patient's personal physician.

9. Initiate teaching/counseling sessions as the patient's needs indicate.

10. The patient's personal physician (who may not be on staff at this hospital) may be consulted regarding case-management orders. Orders will be the responsibility of CR supervising physician.

11. The CR dietitian may designate appropriate diet orders for each participant.

12. The patient may enter a non-ECG-monitored maintenance program upon completion of early outpatient CR program.

_____

Physician's Signature

_____

Date

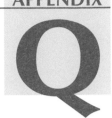

Example of Outpatient Rehabilitation Standing Orders*

Table of Contents

I. Code 99

A. Establish unresponsiveness and attempt to arouse the patient ("shake and shout").

B. Call for help.

1. If no one responds to assist, perform CPR for one minute, then go to the nearest phone and dial 4-911. Resume CPR after the operator is notified. If no other staff member is available, direct a rehabilitation participant to call 4-911 (or 9-911 before 8 a.m. and after 4:30 p.m.). Specific directions are posted beside each phone.

2. If someone does respond to assist, that person should go to the nearest phone and dial 4-911 (or 9-911 before 8 a.m. and after 4:30 p.m.). Specific directions are posted beside each phone.

3. When the call is answered, state "Code 99."

4. Identify the area or room the patient is in. Do not hang up until the operator repeats the information to verify location.

5. The operator will announce "Code 99" and the location over the intercom system.

6. The assigned code team will proceed immediately to that area.

7. The operator will then call 911 to initiate paramedical assistance and transport. He or she must report to 911 the appropriate entrance to use.

8. The operator will page each member of the Code 99 team (see Code 99 team schedule) so that 99 appears on their pagers. The code team personnel will call the operator for location information (if the overhead page is not heard).

9. The operator will also call the hospital emergency department and notify the charge nurse of the Code 99 situation and impending transfer of the patient.

10. A runner from the communication center will be dispatched to the appropriate entrance to direct the paramedic team to the Code 99 area.

First Nurse

a. If the cardiac arrest is witnessed, give a precordial thump.

b. Begin BLS.

Second Nurse

a. Take crash cart to the patient. (See Emergency on Track or Emergency in Locker Room for these areas).

b. Place patient on defibrillator monitor and assess cardiac rhythm.

c. Follow appropriate algorithm according to ACLS guidelines.

Third Responder if Available

a. Call cardiology who in turn will contact a staff cardiologist.

*Appendix Q should be used only as an example of Standing Orders which might be considered and adopted for use in freestanding outpatient or community-based programs.

From *Guidelines for Cardiac Rehabilitation and Secondary Prevention Programs, Fourth Edition,* by American Association of Cardiovascular and Pulmonary Rehabilitation, 2003, Human Kinetics, Champaign, IL.

b. Direct remaining patients to another area and dismiss class.

c. Direct and control incoming traffic.

d. Obtain extra supplies and equipment as needed.

e. Act as the recorder of events until the Code team arrives.

Emergency on Track

a. First responder will remove the backpack, defibrillator, and portable suction from the crash cart and take them to the track.

b. Initiate standard Code 99 procedure.

Emergency in Locker Rooms

a. Remove patient from locker room to a dry area when appropriate.

b. Appropriately dry patient with bath towels.

c. Initiate standard Code 99 procedure.

II. Chest Pain

A. If a patient develops chest pain while in the exercise area, the patient should immediately discontinue exercise.

B. The following protocol should be followed by the cardiac rehabilitation nurse:

1. Check pulse, blood pressure, and cardiac rhythm (attach telemetry monitor if not already monitored).

2. If no relief with one to three minutes of rest, give one NTG 1/150 gr SL.

3. Obtain 12-lead ECG and call a cardiology fellow.

C. If pain is relieved:

1. If this angina is of new onset, the patient should be evaluated by the cardiology fellow. The cardiology fellow should inform the patient's primary physician of the results of his/her evaluations and recommended treatment, if any.

2. If the patient experiences chronic stable angina, he/she will stop exercising until the angina is relieved. Patient may resume the exercise at a lower workload dependent on the clinical judgment of the professional staff. This patient should be observed closely for recurrent angina.

OR

The patient may be sent home and instructed to report any increase in frequency or severity of angina episodes to his/her primary physician.

D. If pain is not relieved:

1. Monitor pulse, blood pressure, and cardiac rhythm closely.

2. Repeat NTG 1/150 gr SL after five minutes.

3. Give a third NTG after another five minutes.

4. Place on oxygen at 2 to 4 liters per nasal prongs.

5. The cardiology fellow should evaluate the patient and consult the primary physician to determine the course of action.

III. Hypoglycemia

A. Be alert to signs and symptoms of hypoglycemia, which may include

1. Headache, weakness, diaphoresis, nervousness, and shakiness

2. Faintness, numbness or tingling of tongue and lips, blurred or double vision, and unsteady gait

3. Tachycardia, pallor, or chilling

4. Confusion, aggressive or erratic behavior

5. Convulsions or unconsciousness

B. If patient displays any of the above symptoms:

1. Obtain Accucheck to assess blood sugar level if possible.

2. If Accucheck results are below 70 mg/dL, or if patient remains symptomatic, give some form of glucose orally—orange juice.

3. If patient is uncooperative or unconscious, call cardiology fellow, start an IV of D5W, and give 50 cc (1 amp) 50% dextrose solution IV.

IV. Hyperglycemia

A. A participant with a blood sugar of greater than 250 mg/dL may not exercise. In situations in which a patient's referring physician and rehabilitation medical director have given their permission, this policy may be superseded.

From *Guidelines for Cardiac Rehabilitation and Secondary Prevention Programs, Fourth Edition,* by American Association of Cardiovascular and Pulmonary Rehabilitation, 2003, Human Kinetics, Champaign, IL.

B. Participants who have demonstrated reliable home blood sugar evaluations will have occasional blood sugar evaluations by the professional staff.

C. Participants who are found to be unreliable with home blood sugar evaluations may need their blood sugar levels evaluated more frequently by the rehabilitation staff.

D. The cardiac rehabilitation staff may request a blood sugar evaluation on any patient based on suspected signs and symptoms of hyperglycemia.

V. Hypotension

A. Remove the patient from the exercise area if possible.

B. Place patient in a supine position.

C. Attach a telemetry monitor if not already monitored.

D. Check blood pressure, pulse, and cardiac rhythm.

E. If no response to position change (SBP remains < 90 mmHg and/or patient remains symptomatic), call cardiology fellow.

   If the patient's condition continues to deteriorate, becomes progressively symptomatic, and/or BP continues to drop, start an IV of NS at 100 ml/hour and call the cardiology fellow to the exercise area STAT. After his/her evaluation and treatment of the patient, the cardiology fellow should notify the patient's primary physician of the hypotensive episode and discuss any further treatment if necessary.

F. If patient does respond to the supine position, keep supine until BP is greater than 100 systolic, then gradually assist to sitting position. Continue to carefully monitor BP, pulse, and rhythm. Encourage fluids. Notify the patient's primary physician of the episode.

VI. Hypertension

A. Check every patient's blood pressure prior to exercising and compare with previous recordings.

B. If the systolic reading is greater then 170 mmHg, have the patient sit and recheck the blood pressure in five minutes.

C. If the blood pressure remains elevated, do not exercise and refer the patient to his/her physician when appropriate.

D. Investigate whether patient is complying with taking medications, following diet, etc.

VII. Premature Ventricular Contractions (PCVs)

A. Observe for the following:

   1. Number per minute

   2. Whether multiform or uniform in origin

   3. Pairs or runs

   4. Signs or symptoms

   5. Palpate pulse to evaluate for peripheral perfusion

B. Document any new arrhythmias or increase in severity with a rhythm strip and make notation on chart.

C. Decrease workloads for frequent single PVCs (>10 min) and discontinue exercise if PVCs are new event, and/or if they develop into bigeminy or pairs, or if the patient becomes symptomatic. Contact patients' referring physician regarding new PVCs or a change in the severity of PVCs.

D. If the patient's condition deteriorates and becomes symptomatic, call the cardiology fellow, place oxygen at 2–4 L/NP, start an IV of D5W, and follow algorithm for ventricular ectopy: acute suppressive therapy.

E. Chronic Asymptomatic PVCs

   1. If the patient's primary physician has been consulted to evaluate frequent PVCs or pairs, and if they are determined to be benign, the patient may continue to exercise unless the patient becomes symptomatic.

VIII. Responsible Physician

A. 8:00 a.m. to 4:30 p.m.

   The cardiology fellow assigned to the clinic is responsible for responding to the cardiac rehabilitation area for nonemergent and emergent problems.

   The cardiology fellow assigned to the non-invasive area is responsible for completing initial evaluations.

The fellow may be reached by calling the appropriate pager number.

B. Before 8:00 a.m.

The cardiology fellow on-call from the previous day will cover the 6:00 a.m. exercise class.

Call his/her home phone number first, then call pager number

If a cardiology fellow on-call list is unavailable, call the coronary care unit (phone number) to obtain the name and number of the fellow on-call.

C. If unable to reach the cardiology fellow, contact the program medical director.

List appropriate phone numbers.

IX. Placement of Intravenous Line

Purpose: To provide immediate access to administer emergency medication and intravenous fluids.

A. An attempt will be made to notify the supervising physician.

B. Place a heparin lock or IV of D5W at TKO in participants when one or more of the following apply:

1. Chest pain protocol has been followed and chest pain persists.

2. ECG, vital signs, or participant appears to be clinically unstable.

3. Physician directs the placement of IV line.

4. Hypotension occurs.

X. Patient Transportation

The cardiac rehabilitation program has contracted with ambulance service to provide emergency transportation to the hospital. Their personnel include trained medical technicians. The ambulance service phone number is posted at each phone extension.

Ambulance Emergency Transportation:
Notify ambulance service personnel as above and instruct them to use the front entrance at the facility's address.

Nonemergency Transportation:
In the event the patient is stable but needs transportation to the hospital for a procedure or nonemergent admission, the program's shuttle van will be used. A nurse from the cardiac rehabilitation area will accompany the patient to the hospital to assure safety.

The physician will be called prior to transfer to see which method of transportation is required. Document physician's decision (if it is to transfer in shuttle van). Cardiac rehabilitation nursing personnel will document patient's condition prior to, during, and at the time of transfer to the hospital.

XI. Protocols for Nonemergent Symptomatic Patients in the Cardiac Rehabilitation Area

A. The cardiac rehabilitation program is not to be used as a patient care clinic or as an emergency room.

1. Patients scheduled to be seen in the cardiac rehabilitation program will be evaluated, and established protocols will be followed.

2. Symptomatic patients should use their primary care physician, closest emergency room, or the 911 emergency system as their primary source of care.

3. Symptomatic, unscheduled patients who arrive at the cardiac rehabilitation program may, in some cases, receive evaluation dependent on physician availability. When physician availability is limited or nonexistent and immediate evaluation is required, the 911 emergency system will be alerted.

B. Early morning (6:00 a.m.) program.

1. Patients participating in the early morning program will not be seen prior to 6:00 a.m.

2. After 6:00 a.m., and dependent on immediate physician availability, patients may be seen by a physician or the 911 emergency system will be alerted.

Cardiac Rehabilitation Department Emergency Procedures and Standing Orders Were Reviewed and Approved

_____

Physician's Name

_____

Signature

_____

Date of most recent review

Documentation of Emergency or Other Medical Intervention*

Patient name: _____   Date: _____

Summary of event: _____

_____

_____

_____

_____

Dispensation of patient (i.e., hospital/clinic/home): _____

_____

_____

_____

_____

Follow-up of outcome: _____

_____

_____

_____

_____

Staff signature: _____

*Attach appropriate physiological data such as 12-lead ECG, blood pressure measurement, code form, etc., to this form.

All notes should be made a permanent part of the participant's record with the appropriate incident form filled out as per usual community standard.

From *Guidelines for Cardiac Rehabilitation and Secondary Prevention Programs, Fourth Edition,* by American Association of Cardiovascular and Pulmonary Rehabilitation, 2003, Human Kinetics, Champaign, IL.

Standard Reporting of In-Hospital Cardiopulmonary Resuscitation

1 Date of event ___ / ___ / ___
Mo   Day   Year

2 Location
☐ CCU ☐ PAR
☐ ICU ☐ OR
☐ ED ☐ General care
☐ Outpatient
☐ Diagnostic & intervention
☐ Other _____

3 Witnessed?
☐ Yes ☐ No ☐ Unknown
Monitored? ☐ Yes ☐ No

4 ACLS intervention at time of event *(check all that apply)*
☐ None
☐ IV access
☐ IV medications
☐ ECG monitor
☐ Intubation
☐ Mechanical ventilation
☐ Implantable cardioverter defibrillator
☐ Intra-arterial catheter

Name [   ]

Date of birth ☐☐ ☐☐ ☐☐
Mo   Day   Year

Age ☐☐☐

M ☐   F ☐   Unknown ☐

Admit date ☐☐ ☐☐ ☐☐
Mo   Day   Year

ID# ☐☐☐☐☐☐☐

Event Variables

5 Immediate cause *(check one)*
☐ Lethal arrhythmias
☐ Hypotension
☐ Respiratory depression
☐ Metabolic
☐ MI or ischemia
☐ Unknown
☐ Other _____

6 Resuscitation attempted?
☐ Yes *(check all used)*
   ☐ Chest compressions
   ☐ Defibrillation
   ☐ Airway
☐ No *(check one)*
   ☐ Found dead
   ☐ Considered futile
   ☐ DNAR

7 Initial condition
Conscious? ☐ Yes ☐ No
Breathing? ☐ Yes ☐ No
Pulse? ☐ Yes ☐ No

8 Initial rhythm
☐ VF ☐ Bradycardia
☐ VT ☐ Asystole
☐ PEA ☐ Perfusing rhythm

CPR stopped _____

Why?
☐ ROSC ☐ Futile
☐ Death ☐ DNAR
Spontaneous circulation

☐ Returned *(if yes, time of ROSC)*
_____
☐ Never achieved
☐ Unsustained ROSC
   ☐ 20 min
   ☐ >20 min but 24 hours

9 Event times

(shaded times are required to calculate the AHA and ERC in-hospital chain-of-survival intervals)

Collapse/Onset ___:___
CPR team called ___:___
CPR team arrived ___:___
Arrest confirmed ___:___
CPR started ___:___ = ___min
1st defib shock ___:___ = ___min
Airway achieved ___:___ = ___min
1st dose EPI ___:___ = ___min

Outcome Variables

10 Time of awakening
Time _____ Date ___ / ___ / ___

11 In-hospital event outcome *(check one)*
☐ Hospital discharge medical **Date** ___ / ___ / ___
Discharge destination: other hospital ___ home ___
Chronic care facility _____ other_____
CPC at discharge = _____
Total GCS = _____ (eye _____ verbal _____ motor _____)
☐ In hospital death *(ROSC > 24 hours)* **Date** ___ / ___ / ___

From *Guidelines for Cardiac Rehabilitation and Secondary Prevention Programs, Fourth Edition,* by American Association of Cardiovascular and Pulmonary Rehabilitation, 2003, Human Kinetics, Champaign, IL.

12 Alive at six months?
☐ Yes *(CPC)* = _____
☐ No (Date of death) ___/___/___
☐ Unknown

13 Alive at one year?
☐ Yes *(CPC)* = _____
☐ No (Date of death) ___/___/___
☐ Unknown

☐ Medical records
☐ Death certificate
☐ Personal physician
☐ Autopsy ☐ Other

14 If died, principal cause of death
☐ CAD ☐ Trauma
☐ Cancer ☐ Other

15 ICD-CM code
☐☐☐☐☐☐

Abbreviations: **CPC** (Cerebral Performance Category) 1 = good, 2 = moderate, 3 = severe, 4 = comatose, 5 = brain death; **DNAR** (do not attempt resuscitation); **GCS** (Glasgow Coma Score) eye 1-4, verbal 1-5, motor 1-6; **ROSC** (return of spontaneous circulation)

Additional Information

Name ☐

16 Provider of CPR
☐ Nurse ☐ Respiratory therapist
☐ Physician ☐ Clinical assistant ☐ Other

Admit date ☐☐ ☐☐ ☐☐
Mo   Day   Year

ID# ☐☐☐☐☐☐☐

17 ET intubation time ___:___

18 Treatments during event *(below)*

Time	Comments	Vitals	Rhythm	Defib(J)	Medications	Dose/route

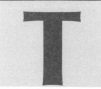
Emergency Code Chart

Cardiopulmonary Resuscitation Report

(Addressograph stamp)

Date: _____ Time discovered: _____

Physicians responding: _____ Time of arrival: _____

Patient's diagnosis: _____

Status prior to arrest: _____

Assessment at time of arrest: _____

Pupils: normal _____ constricted _____ dilated _____

Pulses: absent _____ present _____

Time cardiac massage begun: _____ Time ended: _____

Vital signs: BP _____ heart rate _____ respiratory rate _____

Patient's status at end of arrest: _____

Time of intubation: _____ Size _____ respiratory sounds present _____

Patient transferred to: _____ Time expired: _____

Time	Cardiac rhythm	Defibrillation watt/sec	Amiodarone/ Lidocaine	Epinephrine	Other medications	Ventilated with bag/mask	Document O₂ flow	Other treatments, invasive procedures, diagnostics, ABCs	Response to treatment, lab values, and comments

Date: _____ Time: _____
MD signature (code team leader)

Date: _____ Time: _____
RN signature

Adapted, by permission, from Stanford Center for Research in Disease Prevention Emergency Code Chart.

From *Guidelines for Cardiac Rehabilitation and Secondary Prevention Programs, Fourth Edition,* by American Association of Cardiovascular and Pulmonary Rehabilitation, 2003, Human Kinetics, Champaign, IL.

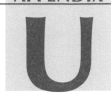
Daily Emergency Cart Checklist

Month____/Year____

1. Defibrillator discharges appropriate joules (unplugged)

1	2	3	4	5	6	7	8	9	10	11	12	13	14	15	16	17	18	19	20	21	22	23	24	25	26	27	28	29	30	31

2. Defibrillator plugged in

1	2	3	4	5	6	7	8	9	10	11	12	13	14	15	16	17	18	19	20	21	22	23	24	25	26	27	28	29	30	31

3. Defibrillator battery registers full capacity

1	2	3	4	5	6	7	8	9	10	11	12	13	14	15	16	17	18	19	20	21	22	23	24	25	26	27	28	29	30	31

4. Monitor display records ECG accurately (extra roll of paper available)

1	2	3	4	5	6	7	8	9	10	11	12	13	14	15	16	17	18	19	20	21	22	23	24	25	26	27	28	29	30	31

5. Electrode patches/gel pads and fast patches available

1	2	3	4	5	6	7	8	9	10	11	12	13	14	15	16	17	18	19	20	21	22	23	24	25	26	27	28	29	30	31

(continued)

From *Guidelines for Cardiac Rehabilitation and Secondary Prevention Programs, Fourth Edition,* by American Association of Cardiovascular and Pulmonary Rehabilitation, 2003, Human Kinetics, Champaign, IL.

(continued)

6. O₂ tank registers full capacity

1	2	3	4	5	6	7	8	9	10	11	12	13	14	15	16	17	18	19	20	21	22	23	24	25	26	27	28	29	30	31

7. Ambubag, oral airway, O₂ mask/cannula available

1	2	3	4	5	6	7	8	9	10	11	12	13	14	15	16	17	18	19	20	21	22	23	24	25	26	27	28	29	30	31

8. Suction machine functions with appropriate suction capacity

1	2	3	4	5	6	7	8	9	10	11	12	13	14	15	16	17	18	19	20	21	22	23	24	25	26	27	28	29	30	31

9. Suction canister, tubing, Yankauer suction tip available

1	2	3	4	5	6	7	8	9	10	11	12	13	14	15	16	17	18	19	20	21	22	23	24	25	26	27	28	29	30	31

10. Emergency code documentation sheets available

1	2	3	4	5	6	7	8	9	10	11	12	13	14	15	16	17	18	19	20	21	22	23	24	25	26	27	28	29	30	31

11. Sharps container present

1	2	3	4	5	6	7	8	9	10	11	12	13	14	15	16	17	18	19	20	21	22	23	24	25	26	27	28	29	30	31

12. Personal protective equipment available (gloves, eye/face shield)

1	2	3	4	5	6	7	8	9	10	11	12	13	14	15	16	17	18	19	20	21	22	23	24	25	26	27	28	29	30	31

13. Signature of reviewer (Name):

1	2	3	4	5	6	7	8	9	10	11	12	13	14	15	16	17	18	19	20	21	22	23	24	25	26	27	28	29	30	31

Monthly Emergency Cart Checklist

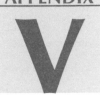

1. The entire emergency cart is to be checked monthly and following any cardiac arrest.
2. The defibrillator, monitoring equipment, and oxygen equipment are to be checked by an RN prior to the first exercise session of the day. (See daily emergency cart checklist.)
3. If there is any problem with the equipment, the RN checking it is responsible for calling the appropriate office and seeing that the equipment is restored to full function as soon as possible.

	Quantity	Jan	Feb	Mar	Apr	May	Jun	Jul	Aug	Sep	Oct	Nov	Dec
Date checklist completed													
Top of cart													
Defibrillator	1												
Extra rolls ECG paper	2												
ECG cable and fast patch cable	1												
Electrode sets and fast patches	2												
Adult oral airways (small/medium/large)	3												
ACLS algorithms	1												
Clipboard, pen, resuscitation documentation form	1												
Gel defib pads or NS pads	2												
Pocket face mask	1												
O_2 nasal prongs	2												
Oxygen mask/tubing	1												
Sterile tongue depressor	1												
Oxygen extension tubing	1												
Box of gloves	1												
Face shields	4												
Sharps/contaminated box	1												
Drawer #1													
Pharmacy drugs													
Adenosine 6 mg/2 ml	2												

(continued)

From *Guidelines for Cardiac Rehabilitation and Secondary Prevention Programs, Fourth Edition,* by American Association of Cardiovascular and Pulmonary Rehabilitation, 2003, Human Kinetics, Champaign, IL.

(continued)

Amiodarone 150 mg/3 ml	2															
Atropine sulfate 1 mg/10 ml	4															
Calcium chloride 1 g/10 ml	2															
Dextrose 50%, 25 g/50 ml	1															
Digoxin 0.5 mg/2 ml	2															
Diphenhydramine 50 mg/1 ml	2															
Epinephrine (1:1000) 1 mg/ml	1															
Epinephrine HCL (1:10,000) 1 mg/10 ml	6															
Esmolol 2.5 g/10 ml	2															
Flumazenil 1 mg/10 ml	2															
Isoproterenol 1 mg/1 ml	3															
Lidocaine HCL 100 mg/5 ml	3															
Magnesium sulfate 5 g	1															
Metoprolol 5 mg/5 ml	3															
Naloxone HCL .4 mg/1 ml	2															
Nitroglycerin 0.4 mg SL tablets or spray	1															
Phenylephrine 10 mg/1 ml	2															
Phenytoin sodium 100 mg/2ml	2															
Procainamide HCL 100 mg/10 ml	1															
Propranolol 1 mg/1 ml	4															
Sodium bicarbonate 50 mEq/ 50 ml	4															
Solumedrol 125 mg/2 ml	2															
Vasopressin 20 u/1ml	2															
Verapamil 5 mg/2 ml	2															
Drawer #2																
General supplies																
Latex-free tourniquets	2															
IV start kits	4															
#16 g. IV catheter	2															
#18 g. IV catheter	2															
#20 g. IV catheter	2															
Medium intracath	2															

From *Guidelines for Cardiac Rehabilitation and Secondary Prevention Programs, Fourth Edition,* by American Association of Cardiovascular and Pulmonary Rehabilitation, 2003, Human Kinetics, Champaign, IL.

Large intracath	2														
10 cc syringes	5														
5 cc syringes	10														
3 cc syringes	10														
50 cc syringes	2														
50 cc toomey syringe	1														
#18 needles	5														
#19 needles	5														
#22 needles	5														
Plastic anti-stick needle/ connectors	1														
Normal saline 20 ml vials	4														
Silk suture 3-0	2														
Scissors (pair)	1														
Alcohol wipes	30														
1-inch tape (roll)	1														
2-inch tape (roll)	1														
#18 salem sump tube	1														
Sterile alligator clamp	1														
2 × 2's (packages)	2														
4 × 4's (packages)	2														
Spinal needle #18 (3 1/2 in. long)	2														
Sterile gloves: sizes 6, 6 1/2, 7, 7 1/2, 8 (2 of each size)	10														
Suture set	1														
Disposable razor	1														
Drawer #3															
IV supplies															
Macrodrip IV tubing	3														
Minidrip IV tubing	3														
Infusion pump tubing	2														
Normal saline 1000 cc	2														
D5W 1000 cc	1														

(continued)

(continued)

Lactated ringers 1000 cc	1															
D5W 250 cc	4															
D5W 500 cc/20 mg Lidocaine	1															
D5W 250 cc/400 mg Dopamine	1															
IV extension tubing	2															
3-way stop cocks	2															
Cut-down tray	1															
Arrow introducers	2															
Triple lumen catheters	2															
Respiratory drawer																
Goggles/shield	1															
ABG kits	2															
1-inch tape	1															
Laryngoscope handle	1															
#2 Miller laryngoscope blade	1															
#3 Miller laryngoscope blade	1															
#2 McIntosh blade	1															
#4 McIntosh blade	1															
#80 cm oral airway	1															
#90 cm oral airway	1															
#100 cm oral airway	1															
M #7.0 cm nasal airway	1															
#14 suction catheter	2															
Afrin bottle	1															
Extra bulbs	2															
Stylette	1															
Flow meter with nipple attacher	1															
Hand ventilator bag and mask	1															
#6.5 cm endotracheal tube	1															
#7.0 cm endotracheal tube	1															
#7.5 cm endotracheal tube	1															
#8.0 cm endotracheal tube	1															
#8.5 cm endotracheal tube	1															
12 ml syringe	1															

From *Guidelines for Cardiac Rehabilitation and Secondary Prevention Programs, Fourth Edition,* by American Association of Cardiovascular and Pulmonary Rehabilitation, 2003, Human Kinetics, Champaign, IL.

Angiocath	1														
Lubafax	1														
Ameracaine spray	1														
Extra batteries	2														
Magill forceps	1														
Yankauer suction tip	1														
CO_2 detector	1														
Bottom drawer															
Sterile water or normal saline 1,000 cc	1														
Blood pressure cuff	1														
Stethoscope	1														
Flashlight	1														
Blanket	1														
Side of cart															
Oxygen tank	1														
Resuscitation bag/mask with O_2 tubing	1														
Portable suction machine	1														
Disposable suction canister	1														
Suction tubing	1														
Yankauer suction tip	1														
Back board	1														
Electrical extension cord	1														
Signature of reviewer															

From *Guidelines for Cardiac Rehabilitation and Secondary Prevention Programs, Fourth Edition,* by American Association of Cardiovascular and Pulmonary Rehabilitation, 2003, Human Kinetics, Champaign, IL.

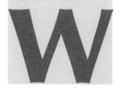

Maintenance and Calibration of Equipment Log

	Date of most recent maintenance check	Date due for next maintenance check
1. Defibrillator		
• Defibrillator batteries replaced		
2. Electrocardiographic monitor	_____	_____
3. Electrocardiographic output	_____	_____
4. Oxygen tank	_____	_____
5. Suction apparatus	_____	_____

Maintenance problems noted: Date corrected

1. _____   _____

2. _____   _____

3. _____   _____

etc. _____   _____

Program director notified (yes/no)   Date corrected

1. _____   _____

2. _____   _____

3. _____   _____

etc. _____   _____

From *Guidelines for Cardiac Rehabilitation and Secondary Prevention Programs, Fourth Edition,* by American Association of Cardiovascular and Pulmonary Rehabilitation, 2003, Human Kinetics, Champaign, IL.

Mock Code and Emergency Inservice Log

Brief description of activity: _____

_____

_____

_____

_____

Who attended the inservice?	Understood the required knowledge:	Needs further training and review:
_____	_____	_____
_____	_____	_____
_____	_____	_____
_____	_____	_____
_____	_____	_____
_____	_____	_____
_____	_____	_____
_____	_____	_____
_____	_____	_____
_____	_____	_____
_____	_____	_____
_____	_____	_____
_____	_____	_____

References

1. Ades PA, Ballor DL, Ashikaga T, et al. Weight training improves walking endurance in the healthy elderly. *Annals Intern Med* 1996;124:568-572.

2. Ades PA, Hanson JS, Gunther JGS, Tonino RP. Exercise conditioning in the elderly coronary patient. *J Am Geriatr Soc* 1987;35:121-124.

3. Ades PA, Gunvald MH. Cardiopulmonary exercise testing before and after conditioning in older coronary patients. *Am Heart J* 1990;120:585-589.

4. Ades P, Maloney A, Savage P, Carhart Jr. R. Physical function in coronary patients: Effect of cardiac rehabilitation. *Arch Intern Med* 1999;159:2357-2360.

5. Ades PA, Pashkow FJ, Fletcher G, et al. A controlled trial of cardiac rehabilitation in the home setting using electrocardiographic and voice transtelephonic monitoring. *Am Heart J* 2000;139:543-548.

6. Ades PA, Waldmann ML, McCann W, Weaver SO. Predictors of cardiac rehabilitation participation in older coronary patients. *Arch Intern Med* 1992;152:1033-1035.

7. Ades PA, Waldmann ML, Peohlman ET, et al. Exercise conditioning in older coronary patients: Submaximal lactate response and endurance capacity. *Circulation* 1993;88:572-577.

8. Ades PA, Waldmann ML, Polk D, Coflesky JT. Referral patterns and exercise response in the rehabilitation of female coronary patients aged ≥62 years. *Am J Cardiol* 1992;69:1422-1425.

9. Adler AJ, Holub BJ. Effect of garlic and fish-oil supplementation on serum lipid and lipoprotein concentrations in hypercholesterolemic men. *Am J Clin Nutr* 1997;65:445-450.

10. Ainsworth BE, Haskell WL, Leon AS, et al. Compendium of physical activities: Classification of energy costs of human physical activities. In: *ACSM's resource manual for guidelines for exercise testing and prescription*, 4th ed. JL Roitman, et al. (eds.). Philadelphia: Lippincott Williams & Wilkins, 2001. pp. 673-686.

11. Albanes D, Heinonen OP, Taylor PR, et al. Alpha-tocopherol and beta-carotene supplements and lung cancer incidence in the alpha-tocopherol, beta-carotene cancer prevention study: Effects of base-line characteristics and study compliance. *J Natl Cancer Inst* 1996;88:1560-1570.

12. Albert MA, Ridker PM. The role of C-reactive protein in cardiovascular disease risk. *Curr Cardiol Rep* 1999;1:99-104.

13. Albright AL. Diabetes. In: *ACSM's exercise management for persons with chronic diseases and disabilities*. Durstine JL (ed.). Champaign, IL: Human Kinetics, 1997. pp. 94-100.

14. Alexander RW, Dzau VJ. Vascular biology: The past 50 years. *Circulation* 2000;102:IV112-IV116.

15. Allan R, Scheidt S. *Heart and mind: The practice of cardiac psychology*. Washington, DC: American Psychological Association, 1996.

16. Allen JK, Blumenthal RS. Coronary risk factors in women six months after coronary artery bypass grafting. *Am J Cardiol* 1995;75:1092-1095.

17. Allen JP, Eckardt MJ, Wallen J. Screening for alcoholism: Techniques and issues. *Public Health Reports* 1988;10:586-592.

18. Allison JJ, Kiefe CI, Centor RM, et al. Racial differences in the medical treatment of elderly Medicare patients with acute myocardial infarction. *J Gen Intern Med* 1996; 11:736-743.

19. Allison TG, Williams DE, Miller TD, et al. Medical and economic costs of psychologic distress in patients with coronary artery disease. *Mayo Clinic Proceedings* 1995;70:734-742.

20. The Alpha-Tocopherol, Beta Carotene Cancer Prevention Study Group. The effect of vitamin E and beta carotene on the incidence of lung cancer and other cancers in male smokers. *N Engl J Med* 1994;330:1029-1035.

21. American Association of Critical Care Nurses. *Clinical practice protocol for cardiac rehabilitation for the acute care nurse*. Aliso Viejo, CA: American Association of Critical Care Nurses, 2001.

22. American College of Cardiology/American Heart Association. Guidelines for the evaluation and management of chronic heart failure in the adult: Executive summary. *J Am Coll Cardiol* 2001;38:2102-2112.

23. American College of Cardiology/American Heart Association. Guidelines for the management of patients with acute myocardial infarction. *J Am Coll Cardiol* 1996;28:1328-1428.

24. American College of Cardiology/American Heart Association. 2002 guideline update for the management of patients with chronic stable angina: Summary article. *Circulation* 2003;107:149-158.

25. American College of Sports Medicine/American Diabetes Association: Diabetes mellitus and exercise. *Med Sci Sports Exerc* 1997;29(12);i-vi.

26. American Diabetes Association. Clinical practice recommendations: Diabetes mellitus and exercise. *Diabetes Care* 1999;22.(Suppl 1);549-553.

27. American Diabetes Association. Clinical practice recommendations: Summary of revisions for the 2001 clinical practice recommendations. *Diabetes Care* 2001:24(suppl 1).

28. American Diabetes Association. Evidence-based nutrition principles and recommendations for the treatment and prevention of diabetes and related complications. *Diabetes Care* 2002;25(Suppl 1):S50-S60.

29. American Diabetes Association. Standards of medical care for patients with diabetes mellitus. *Diabetes Care* 2002;25: 213-229.

30. American Heart Association. *Fundamentals of BCLS for healthcare providers*. American Heart Association, Dallas, TX, 2001.

31. American Heart Association. *Heart disease and stroke statistical-update*. Dallas: American Heart Association, 2003.

32. American Heart Association. *ACLS provider manual*. Dallas: American Heart Association, 2001.

33. American Heart Association Nutrition Committee. Dietary guidelines for healthy American adults. A statement for physicians and health professionals. *Circulation* 1988;77: 721A-724A.

34. American Nursing Credentialing Center. *Cardiac/Vascular nurse*. http://nursingworld.org/ancc/index.htm. 2002.

35. American Physical Therapy Association. Minimum eligibility criteria for cardiovascular and pulmonary physical therapy. http://www.apta.org/Education/specialist/ABPTSCert/minimum_eligibility/cert_cardio. 2003.

36. Anderson J, Davidson M, Blonde L, et al. Long-term cholesterol-lowering effects of psyllium as an adjunct to diet therapy in the treatment of hypercholesterolemia. *Am J Clin Nutr* 2000;71:1433-1438.

37. Anderson JW, Johnstone BM, Cook-Newell ME. Meta-analysis of the effects of soy protein intake on serum lipids. *N Engl J Med* 1995;333:276-282.

38. Anderson UK. The person participating in inpatient and outpatient cardiac rehabilitation. In: *Cardiovascular nursing holistic practice*. CE Guzzetta, BM Dossey (eds.). St. Louis: Mosby Yearbook, 1992.

39. Angell M, Kassirer J. Alternative medicine—the risks of untested and unregulated remedies. *N Engl J Med* 1998;339: 839-841.

40. Angerer P, Siebert U, Kothny W, et al. Impact of social support, cynical hostility and anger expression on progression of coronary atherosclerosis. *J Am Coll Cardiol* 2000;136:1781-1788.

41. Ansell BJ, Watson KE, Fogelman AM. An evidence-based assessment of the NCEP Adult Treatment Panel II Guidelines. *JAMA* 1999;282:2051-2057.

42. Anthony MS, Clarkson TB, Bullock BC, Wagner JD. Soy protein versus soy phytoestrogens in the prevention of diet-induced coronary artery atherosclerosis of male cynomolgus monkeys. *Arterioscler Thromb Vasc Biol* 1997;17:2524-2531.

43. Anthony MS, Clarkson TB, Hughes CL Jr., et al. Soybean isoflavones improve cardiovascular risk factors without affecting the reproductive system of peripubertal rhesus monkeys. *J Nutr* 1996;126:43-50.

44. Anthony MS, Clarkson TB, Williams JK. Effects of soy isoflavones on atherosclerosis: Potential mechanisms. *Am J Clin Nutr* 1998;68(Suppl 6):1390S-1393S.

45. Appel LJ, Moore TJ, Obarzanek E, et al. A clinical trial of the effects of dietary patterns on blood pressure. DASH Collaborative Research Group. *N Engl J Med* 1997;336:1117-1124.

46. Arena R, Humphrey R, McCall R. Altered exercise pulmonary function after left ventricular assist device implantation. *J Cardiopulm Rehabil* 1999;19:344-346.

47. Ariyo AA, Haan M, Tangen CM, et al. Depressive symptoms and risks of coronary heart disease and mortality in elderly Americans. *Circulation* 2000;102:1773-1779.

48. Armstrong W, Marcovitz PA. Stress echocardiography. In: *Heart disease updates*. Braunwald E (ed.). Philadelphia: WB Saunders, 1993. pp. 1-10.

49. Arntz HR, Agrawal R, Wunderlich W, et al. Beneficial effects of pravastatin (± cholestyramine/niacin) initiated immediately after a coronary event (the randomized lipid-coronary artery disease [L-CAD] study). *Am J Cardiol* 2000;86:1293-1298.

50. Austin M, Hokanson J, Edwards K. Hypertriglyceridemia as a cardiovascular risk factor. *Am J Cardiol* 1998;81(4A): 7B-12B.

51. Badenhop DT, Dunn CB, Eldridge S, et al. Monitoring and management of cardiac rehabilitation patients with Type 2 diabetes. *Clin Exercise Physiol* 2001;3:71-77.

52. Bader D, Maguire T, Spahn C, et al. Clinical profile and outcome of obese patients in cardiac rehabilitation as stratified according to NHLBI criteria. *J Cardiopulm Rehabil* 2001;21: 210-217.

53. Bader D, McInnis K, Maguire T., et al. Accuracy of a pre-test questionnaire in exercise test protocol selection. *Am J Cardiol* 2000;85:767-770.

54. Bailey L. New standard for dietary folate intake in pregnant women. *Am J Clin Nutr* 2000;71:1304S-1307S.

55. Balady GJ, Ades PA, Comoss PM, et al. Core components of cardiac rehabilitation/secondary prevention programs. *Circulation* 2000;102:1069-1073.

56. Balady GJ, Chaitman B, Driscoll D., et al. Recommendations for cardiovascular screening, staffing and emergency policies at health/fitness facilities. *Circulation* 1998;97:2283-2293.

57. Balady GJ, Chaitman B, Foster C, et al. Automated external defibrillators in health/fitness facilities. *Circulation* 2002;105: 1147-1150.

58. Balady GJ, Fletcher BJ, Froelicher ES, et al. Cardiac rehabilitation programs: A statement for healthcare professionals from the American Heart Association. *Circulation* 1994;90: 1602-1610.

59. Bandura A. *Social learning theory*. Englewood Cliffs, NJ: Prentice Hall, 1977.

60. Bandura A. Self-efficacy: Toward a unifying theory of behavioral change. *Psychology Review* 1977;85:191-215.

61. Bandura A. *Social foundations of thought and action: A social cognitive theory*. Englewood Cliffs, NJ: Prentice Hall, 1986.

62. Barefoot JC, Helms MJ, Mark DM. Depression and long-term mortality risk in patients with coronary artery disease. *Am J Cardiol* 1996;78:489-495.

63. Barlow CE, Kohl HW III, Gibbons LW, Blair SN. Physical fitness, mortality, and obesity. *Int J Obesity* 1995;19(S4):S41-S44.

64. Barlow CW, Quayyum MS, Davey PP, et al. Effect of physical training on exercise-induced hyperkalemia in chronic heart failure. Relation with ventilation and catecholamines. *Circulation* 1994;89:1144-1152.

65. Barnard J. Effects of life-style modification on serum lipids. *Arch Intern Med* 1991;151:1389-1394.

66. Barnason S, Zimmerman L. A comparison of patient teaching outcomes among postoperative coronary artery bypass graft patients. *Prog Cardiovasc Nursing* 1995;10:11-20.

67. Barzilay JI, Kronmal RA, Bittner V, et al. Coronary artery disease and coronary artery bypass grafting in diabetic patients aged ≥65 years (reports from the Coronary Artery Surgery Study, CASS, Registry). *Am J Cardiol* 1994;74:334-339.

68. Baum JA, Teng H, Erdman JW Jr., et al. Long-term intake of soy protein improves blood lipid profiles and increases mononuclear cell low-density-lipoprotein receptor messenger RNA in hypercholesterolemic, postmenopausal women. *Am J Clin Nutr* 1998;68:545-551.

69. Beck AT, Steer RA, Brown GK. *BDI-II manual*. San Antonio, TX: The Psychological Corporation, 1996.

70. Begs VAL, Willis SB, Mails EL, et al. Patient education for discharge after coronary bypass surgery in the 1990s: Are patients adequately prepared? *J Cardiovasc Nurs* 1998;12:72-86.

71. Belardinelli R, Georgiou D, Cianci G, et al. Exercise training improves left ventricular diastolic filling in patients with dilated cardiomyopathy: Clinical and prognostic implications. *Circulation* 1995;91:2775-2784.

72. Belardinelli R, Georgiou D, Cianci G, Purcaro A. Randomized, controlled trial of long-term moderate exercise training in chronic heart failure: Effects on functional capacity, quality of life, and clinical outcome. *Circulation* 1999;99:1173-1182.

73. Belardinelli R, Georgiou D, Scocco V, et al. Low intensity exercise training in patients with chronic heart failure. *J Am Coll Cardiol* 1995;26:975-982.

74. Bellosta S, Ferri N, Arnaboldi L, et al. Pleiotropic effects of statins in atherosclerosis and diabetes. *Diabetes Care* 2000;23(Suppl 2):B72-B78.

75. Ben-Ari E. Rehabilitation of the cardiac patient during hospitalization: Inpatient programs. In: *Heart disease and rehabilitation*, 3d ed. ML Pollock, DH Schmidt (eds.). Champaign, IL: Human Kinetics, 1995.

76. Benowitz NL, Gourlay SG. Cardiovascular toxicity of nicotine: Implications for nicotine replacement therapy. *J Am Coll Cardiol* 1997;29:1422-1431.

77. Bergholm R, Makimattila S, Valkonen M, et al. Intense physical training decreases circulating antioxidants and endothelium-dependent vasodilatation in vivo. *Atherosclerosis* 1999;145:341-349.

78. Bernard TE. Environmental considerations: Heat and cold. In: ACSM's *resource manual for guidelines for exercise testing and prescription*, 4th ed. JL Roitman, et al. (eds.). Baltimore: Williams & Wilkins, 2001. pp. 209-216.

79. Bernardi L, Spadacini G, Bellwon J, et al. Effect of breathing rate on oxygen saturation and exercise performance in chronic heart failure. *Lancet* 1998;351:1308-1311.

80. Bin Aris I, Wagie AAE, Bin Mariun NB, Jamma ABE. An internet-based blood pressure monitoring system for patients. *J Telemedicine Telecare* 2001;7:51-53.

80a. Bin J-P, Le E, Pelberg RA, et al. Mechanism of inducible regional dysfunction during dipyridamole stress. *Circulation* 2002;106:112-117.

81. Black HR. Isolated systolic hypertension in the elderly: From clinical trials and future directions. *J Hypertension* 1999;17(suppl 5):550-554.

82. Blair SN, Kampert JB, Kohl HW 3d, et al. Influences of cardiorespiratory fitness and other precursors on cardiovascular disease and all-cause mortality in men and women. *JAMA* 1996;276:205-210.

83. Blair SN, Kohl HW III, Paffenbarger RS Jr, et al. Physical fitness and all-cause mortality: A prospective study of healthy men and women. *JAMA* 1989;262:2395-2401.

84. Blazer DG. Alcohol and drug problems. In: *Textbook of geriatric psychiatry*, 2d ed. EW Busse, DG Blazer (eds.). Washington, DC: American Psychiatry Press, 1996. pp. 341-356.

85. Block G, Clifford C, Naughton M, et al. A brief dietary screen for high fat intake. *J Nutrition Education* 1989;21:199-207.

86. Blumenthal M, Busse W, Goldberg A, et al. *The complete German Commission E monographs. Therapeutic guide to herbal medicines*. Austin, TX: American Botanical Council, 1998.

87. Bor M, Cevik C, Uslu I, et al. Selenium levels and glutathione peroxidase activities in patients with acute myocardial infarction. *Acta Cardiol* 1999;54:271-276.

88. Boushey CJ, Beresford SAA, Omenn GS, Motulsky AG. A quantitative assessment of plasma homocysteine as a risk factor for vascular disease: Probable benefits of increasing folic acid intakes. *JAMA* 1995;274:1049-1057.

89. Bowles DK, Woodman CR, Laughlin MH. Coronary smooth muscle and endothelial adaptations to exercise training. *Exerc Sports Sci Rev* 2000;28:57-62.

90. Braith RW, Clapp L, Brown T, et al. Rate-responsive pacing improves exercise tolerance in heart transplant recipients: A pilot study. *J Cardiopulm Rehabil* 2000; 20:377-382.

91. Braith RW, Limacher MC, Mills RM, et al. Exercise-induced hypoxemia in heart transplant recipients. *J Am Coll Cardiol* 1993;22:768-776.

92. Braith RW, Mills RM, Welsch MA, et al. Resistance exercise training restores bone mineral density in heart transplant recipients. *J Am Coll Cardiol* 1996;28:1471-1477.

93. Branch KR, Dembitsky WP, Peterson KL, et al. Physiology of the native heart and Thermo Cardiosystems left ventricular assist device complex at rest and during exercise: Implications for chronic support. *J Heart Lung Transplant* 1994;13:641-651.

94. Brent NJ. Cardiac rehabilitation in the home. *Home Health Nurse* 1995;13:8-9.

95. Brezinka V, Kittel F. Psychosocial factors of coronary heart disease in women: A review. *Social Sci Med* 1996;42:1351-1365.

96. Brezynskie H, Pendon E, Lindsay P, Adam M. Identification of the perceived learning needs of balloon angioplasty patients. *J Cardiovasc Nursing* 1998;9:8-14.

97. Brochu M, Poehlman EP, Savage PD, et al. Coronary risk profiles in male coronary patients: Effects of body composition, fat distribution, age and fitness. *Coronary Artery Dis* 2000;1:137-144.

98. Brook R, Ware J, Davies-Avery A, et al. Overview of validity and the index of well-being. *Health Services Res* 1976;11: 478-507.

99. Brooks TR. Pitfalls in communication with Hispanic and African American patients: Do translators help or harm? *J Nat Med Assoc* 1992;84:941-947.

100. Brouwer IA, van Dusseldorp M, West CE, et al. Dietary folate from vegetables and citrus fruit decreases plasma homocysteine concentrations in humans in a dietary controlled trial. *J Nutr* 1999;129:1135-1139.

101. Brown WV. Cholesterol lowering in atherosclerosis. *Am J Cardiol* 2000;86:29H-34H.

102. Brubaker PH, Brozena SC, Morley DL, et al. Exercise-induced ventilatory abnormalities in orthotopic heart transplant patients. *J Heart Lung Transplant* 1997;16:1011-1017.

103. Burell G. Group psychotherapy in Project New Life: Treatment of coronary-prone behaviors for patients who have had coronary artery bypass graft surgery. In: *Heart and mind: The practice of cardiac psychology.* R Allan, S Scheidt (eds.). Washington, DC: American Psychological Association, 1996.

104. Butler TG, Yanowitz FG. Obesity I. *Cardiovasc Review Rep* 1994;June:31-54.

105. Cahalin LP. Exercise training in heart failure: Inpatient and outpatient considerations. *AACN Clinical Issues* 1998;9:225-243.

106. Cahalin LP. Heart failure. *Phys Ther* 1996;76:516-533.

106a. Cahalin LP. Cardiac muscle dysfunction. In: *Essentials of cardiopulmonary physical therapy.* E. Hillegas and H. Sadowsky (eds.) Philadelpoia: WB Saunders, 1995.

107. Campbell NC, Grimshaw JM, Ritchie LD, Rawles JM. Outpatient cardiac rehabilitation: Are the potential benefits being realized? *J R Coll Physicians Lond* 1996;30:514-519.

108. Cannistra L, O'Malley CJ, Balady GJ. Comparison of outcome of cardiac rehabilitation in black women and white women. *Amer J Cardiol* 1995;75:890-893.

109. Cannistra LB, Balady GJ, O'Malley CJ, et al. Comparison of the clinical profile and outcome of women and men in cardiac rehabilitation. *Am J Cardiol* 1992;69:1274-1279.

110. Carbone LM. An interdisciplinary approach to the rehabilitation of open-heart surgical patients. *Rehabil Nurs* 1999;24: 55-61.

110a. Cardiovascular Credentialing International, Virginia Beach, VA 2002. http://www.cci-online.org.

111. Carhart RL Jr, Ades PA. Gender differences in cardiac rehabilitation. *Cardiol Clin* 1998;16:37-43.

112. Carter W, Bobbitt R, Bergner M, Gibson B. Validation of an interval scaling: The sickness impact profile. *Health Services Res* 1976;11:516-528.

113. Case RB, Moss AJ, Case N, et al. Living alone after myocardial infarction: Impact of prognosis. *JAMA* 1992;117: 1003-1009.

114. Caulin-Glaser T. Gender differences in referral to cardiac rehabilitation programs after revascularization. *J Cardiopulm Rehabil* 2001;21:24-30.

115. Chait A, Brunzell JD, Denke MA, et al. Rationale of the diet-heart statement of the American Heart Association. Report of the Nutrition Committee. *Circulation* 1993;88:3008-3029.

116. Chambers JC, Seddon MD, Shah S, Kooner JS. Homocysteine—a novel risk factor for vascular disease. *J Royal Soc Med* 2001;94:1-3.

116a. Chan AW, Bhatt DL, Chew DP, et al. Early and sustained survival benefit associated with statin therapy at the time of percutaneous coronary intervention. *Circulation* 2002;105: 691-696.

117. Chetlin MD, Alpert JS, Armstrong WF, et al. ACC/AHA guidelines for the clinical application of echocardiography: A report of the ACC/AHA Task Force on Practice Guidelines (Committee on Clinical Application of Echocardiography). *J Am Coll Cardiol* 1997;29:862-879.

118. Cheung DG, Weber MA. Hypertension in the elderly. In: *Cardiovascular disease in the elderly patients.* DD Tresch, WS Aronow (eds). New York: Marcel Dekker, 1994. pp. 149-181.

119. Coats AJS, Adamoupoulos S, Radaelli A, et al. Controlled trial of physical training in chronic heart failure: Exercise performance, hemodynamics, ventilation, and autonomic function. *Circulation* 1992;85:2119-2131.

120. Commission on Accreditation of Rehabilitation Facilities. Medical rehabilitation. 2002. http://www.carf.org/CARF/MedicalRehab.htm.

121. Comoss PM. Education of the coronary patient and family: Principles and practice. In: *Rehabilitation of the coronary patient.* 3rd ed. NK Wenger, HK Hellerstein (eds.). New York: Churchill Livingstone, 1992. pp. 439-60.

122. Comoss PM. Optimizing patient recovery—inpatient cardiac rehabilitation. In: *Critical care nursing.* JM Clochesy, et al. (eds.). Philadelphia: WB Saunders, 1993.

123. Comoss PM. The new infrastructure for cardiac rehabilitation practice. In: *Cardiac rehabilitation: A guide to practice in the 21st century.* NK Wenger, et al. (eds.). New York:Marcel Dekker, 1999. pp. 315-326.

124. Connor S, Gustafson J, Sexton G, et al. The diet habit survey: A new method of dietary assessment that relates to plasma cholesterol changes. *J Am Dietetics Assoc* 1992;92:41-47.

125. Consoli SM, Ben SM, Jean J, et al. Benefits of a computer-assisted education program for hypertensive patients compared with standard education tools. *Patient Education Counseling* 1995;26:343-347.

126. Cooke JP, Tsao PS. Arginine: A new therapy for atherosclerosis? *Circulation* 1997;95:311-312.

127. Cormier WH, Cormier LS. *Interviewing strategies for helpers: Fundamental skills and cognitive behavioral interventions.* Pacific Grove, CA: Brooks/Cole, 1993.

128. CorSolutions. Our program. http://www.ralinmed.com/ourprogramscad.html June 2001.

129. Cress ME, Buchner DM, Questad KA, et al. Continuous-scale physical functional performance in a broad range of older adults: A validation study. *Arch Phys Med Rehabil* 1996;7: 1243-1250.

130. Criqui MH, Langer RD, Fronek A, et al. Mortality over a period of 10 years in patients with peripheral arterial disease. *N Engl J Med* 1992;326:381-386.

131. Crouse JR 3d, Morgan T, Terry JG, et al. A randomized trial comparing the effect of casein with that of soy protein containing varying amounts of isoflavones on plasma concentrations of lipids and lipoproteins. *Arch Intern Med* 1999;159:2070-2076.

132. Crummer MB, Carter V. Critical pathways—the pivotal tool. *J Cardiovasc Nurs* 1993;7:30-37.

133. Cummins RO, Chamberlain D, Hazinski MF, et al. Recommended guidelines for reviewing, reporting, and conducting

research on in-hospital resuscitation: The in-hospital 'Utstein Style.' *Circulation* 1997;95:2213-2239.

134. Cummins RO, Sanders A, Mancini E, Hazinski MF. In-hospital resuscitation. A statement for healthcare professionals from the American Heart Association Emergency Cardiac Care Committee and the Advanced Life Support, Basic Life Support, Pediatric Resuscitation, and Program Administration Subcommittees. *Circulation* 1997;95:2211-2212.

135. Cupples SA. Inpatient cardiac rehabilitation: Patient education implementation and documentation. *J Cardiopulm Rehabil* 1995;15:412-417.

136. D'Agostino RB, Russell MW, Huse DM, et al. Primary and subsequent coronary risk appraisal: New results from the Framingham Study. *Am Heart J* 2000;139:272-281.

137. Daida H, Squires RW, Allison TG, et al. Sequential assessment of exercise tolerance in heart transplantation compared with coronary artery bypass surgery after phase II cardiac rehabilitation. *Am J Cardiol* 1996;77:696-700.

138. Davey P, Meyer TE, Coats AJS, et al. Ventilation in chronic heart failure: Effects of physical training. *Br Heart J* 1992;68: 474-477.

138a. Daviglus ML, Stamler J, Orencia AJ, et al. Fish consumption and the 30-year risk of fatal myocardial infarction. *N Engl J Med* 1997;336:1046-1053.

139. Day JC. Population projections of the United States by age, sex, race and origins 1995 to 2050 (Current Population Reports, P251130). Washington, DC: US Government Printing Office.

140. DeBusk RF, Miller NH, Superko HR, et al. A case-management system for coronary risk factor modification after acute myocardial infarction. *Ann Intern Med* 1994;120:721-729.

141. DeBusk RF. A new approach to risk factor modification. *Cardiol Clinics* 1996;14:143-157.

142. Delagardelle C, Feiereisen P, Krecke R, et al. Objective effects of a 6 months endurance and strength training program in outpatients with congestive heart failure. *Med Sci Sports Exerc* 1999;31:1102-1107.

143. deLorgeril M, Salen P, Martin JL, et al. Mediterranean diet, traditional risk factors and the rate of cardiovascular complications after myocardial infarction. *Circulation* 1999;99: 779-785.

144. de Lorgeril M, Salen P, Martin JL, et al. Mediterranean dietary pattern in a randomized trial: Prolonged survival and possible reduced cancer rate. *Arch Intern Med* 1998;158: 1181-1187.

145. Deming WE. *Quality productivity and competitive position.* Cambridge, MA: Massachusetts Institute of Technology, Center for Advanced Engineering Study, 1996.

146. Demopoulos L, Bijou R, Fergus I, et al. Exercise training in patients with severe congestive heart failure: Enhancing peak aerobic capacity while minimizing the increase in ventricular wall stress. *J Am Coll Cardiol* 1997;29:597-603.

147. Dennis LI, Blue CL, Stahl SM, et al. The relationship between hospital readmission of Medicare beneficiaries with chronic illness and home care nursing interventions. *Home Healthcare Nurse* 1996;14:303-309.

148. Depre C, Wijns W, Robert AM, et al. Pathology of unstable plaque: Correlation with clinical severity of acute coronary syndromes. *J Am Coll Cardiol* 1997;30:694-702.

149. Derogatis LR. *SCL-90-R: Administration, scoring and procedure manual.* Baltimore: Clinical Psychometric Research, 1983.

150. DeSouza CA, Shapiro LF, Clevenger CM, et al. Regular aerobic exercise prevents and restores age-related endothelium-dependent vasodilation in healthy men. *Circulation* 2000;102: 1351-1357.

151. Diabetes Control and Complications Trial Research Group. The effect of intensive treatment of diabetes on the development and progression of long-term complications in insulin-dependent diabetes mellitus. *N Engl J Med* 1993;329: 977-986.

152. Diabetes Prevention Program Research Group. Reduction in incidence of Type 2 diabetes with lifestyle intervention or metformin. *N Engl J Med* 2002;346:393-403.

152a. Diamond GA. Reverend Bayes' silent majority. An alternative factor affecting sensitivity and specificity of exercise electrocardiography. *Am J Cardiol* 1986;57:1175-1180.

153. Diaz MN, Frei B, Vita JA, Keaney JF. Antioxidants and atherosclerotic heart disease. *N Engl J Med* 1997;337:408-416.

154. Digenio AG, Noakes TD, Cantor A, et al. Predictors of exercise capacity and adaptability to training in patients with coronary artery disease. *J Cardiopulm Rehabil* 1997;17: 110-120.

155. Doran K, Sampson B, Status R, et al. Clinical pathways across tertiary and community care after an interventional cardiology procedure. *J Cardiovasc Nurs* 1997;11:2:1-14.

156. Douard H, Parrens E, Billes MA, et al. Predictive factors of maximal aerobic capacity after cardiac transplantation. *Eur Heart J* 1997;18:1823-1828.

157. Dracup K, Bryan-Brown CW. An open door policy in ICU. *Am J Critical Care* 1992;2:16-18.

158. Dunne M. Wizard and the design of trials for secondary prevention of atherosclerosis with antibiotics. *Am Heart J* 1999;138:S542-S544.

159. Dylewics P, Przywarska I, Szczesniak L, et al. The influence of short-term endurance training on the insulin blood level, binding, and degradation of 125I-insulin by erythrocyte receptors in patients after myocardial infarction. *J Cardiopulm Rehabil* 1999;19:98-105.

160. Eagle KA, Guyton RA, Davidoff R, et al. ACC/AHA guidelines for coronary artery bypass graft surgery: Executive summary and recommendations. *Circulation* 1999;100:1464-1480.

161. Eckel RH. Obesity and heart disease: A statement for health care professionals from the Nutrition Committee, American Heart Association. *Circulation* 1997;96:3248-3250.

162. Edwards FH, Carey JS, Grover FL, et al. Impact of gender on coronary bypass operative mortality. *Ann Thorac Surg* 1998;66:125-131.

163. Edwardson SR. The consequences and opportunities of shortened lengths of stay for cardiovascular patients. *J Cardiovasc Nursing* 1999;14:1-11.

164. Eikelboom J, Lonn E, Genest J, et al. Homocyst(e)ine and cardiovascular disease: A critical review of the epidemiologic evidence. *Ann Intern Med* 1999;131:363-375.

165. Eisenberg DM, Davis RB, Ettner SL, et al. Trends in alternative medicine use in the United States, 1990-1997: Results of a follow-up national survey. *JAMA* 1998;280:1569-1575.

166. Ekers MA, Hirsch AT. Vascular medicine and vascular rehabilitation. In: *Vascular nursing*, 3d ed. VA Fahey (ed.). Philadelphia: WB Saunders, 1999.

167. Elhendy A, Sozzi FB, van Domburg RT, et al. Relation among exercise-induced ventricular arrhythmias, myocardial

ischemia, and viability late after acute myocardial infarction. *Am J Cardiol* 2000;86:723-729.

168. ENRICHD Investigators. Enhancing recovery in coronary heart disease patients (ENRICHD): Study design and methods. *Am Heart J* 2000;139:1-9.

169. Ernst E, Resch KL. Fibrinogen as a cardiovascular risk factor: A meta-analysis and review of the literature. *Annals Intern Med* 1993;118:956-963.

170. ESHA Research, Inc. The food processor: Nutrition analysis & fitness software, version 7.6, 2001. http://www.esha.com.

171. European Heart Failure Training Group. Experience from controlled trials of physical training in chronic heart failure—protocol and patient factors in effectiveness in the improvement in exercise tolerance. *Eur Heart J* 1998;19: 466-475.

172. Evenson KR, Rosamond WD, Luepker RV. Predictors of outpatient cardiac rehabilitation utilization: The Minnesota Heart Surgery Registry. *J Cardiopulm Rehabil* 1998;18: 192-198.

173. Everson SA, Godberg DE, Kaplan GA, et al. Hopelessness and risk of mortality and incidence of myocardial infarction and cancer. *Psychosomatic Med* 1996;58:113-121.

174. Ewing JA. Detecting alcoholism: The CAGE Questionnaire. *JAMA* 1984;252:1905-1907.

175. Expert Committee on the Diagnosis and Classification of Diabetes Mellitus. Report of the Expert Committee on the Diagnosis and Classification of Diabetes Mellitus. *Diabetes Care* 1997;20:1183-1197.

176. Expert Panel on the Identification, Evaluation, and Treatment of Overweight and Obesity in Adults. Executive summary of the Clinical Guidelines on the Identification, Evaluation, and Treatment of Overweight and Obesity in Adults. *Arch Internal Med* 1998;158:1855-1867.

177. Falk E, Shah PK, Fuster V. Coronary plaque disruption. *Circulation* 1995;92:657-671.

178. Falk E, Fuster V. Angina pectoris and disease progression. *Circulation* 1995;92:2033-2035.

179. Fardy PS, White RE, Haltiwanger-Schmitz K, et al. Coronary disease risk factor reduction and behavior modification in minority adolescents: The PATH Program. *J Adolesc Health* 1996;18:247-253.

180. Feigenbaum MS, Pollock ML. Strength training: Rationale for current guidelines for adult fitness programs. *Physician Sportsmed* 1997;25(2):44-63.

181. Ferguson JA, Tierney WM, Westmoreland GR, et al. Examination of racial differences in management of cardiovascular disease. *J Am Coll Cardiol* 1997;30:1707-1713.

182. Ferguson JA, Adams TA, Weinberger M. Examining racial differences in cardiac catheterization utilization and appropriateness. *Am J Med Sci* 1998;315:302-306.

183. Ferguson JA, Weinberger M, Westmoreland GR, et al. Racial disparity in cardiac decision making: Results from patient focus groups. *Arch Intern Med* 1998;158:1450-1453.

184. Fiedler RC, Granger CV, Ottenbacher KJ. The uniform data system for medical rehabilitation: Report of first admissions from 1994. *Am J Phys Med Rehab* 1996;75:125-129.

185. Fiore MC, Bailey WC, Cohen SJ, et al. A clinical practice guideline for treating tobacco use and dependence. A US Public Health Service Report. *JAMA* 2000;283:3244-3254.

186. Fix AJ, Daughton DM. *Human activity profile*. Tampa, FL: Psychological Assessment Resources, 1997.

187. Fletcher GF. Rehabilitation exercise for the cardiac patient. *Cardiol Clinics* 1993;11:267-275.

188. Fletcher GF, Balady G, Amsterdam EA, et al. Exercise standards for testing and training. A statement for healthcare professionals from the American Heart Association. *Circulation* 2001;104:1694-1740.

189. Fletcher GF, Balady G, Froelicher VF, et al. Exercise standards, a statement for health professionals from the American Heart Association. AHA Medical/Scientific Statement. *Circulation* 1995;91:580-615.

190. Fonarow GC, Stevenson LW, Walden JA, et al. Impact of a comprehensive heart failure management program on hospital readmission and functional status of patients with advanced heart failure. *J Am Coll Cardiol* 1997;30:725.

191. Fonarow GC, WJ French, LS Parsons, et al. Use of lipid-lowering medications at discharge in patients with acute myocardial infarction: Data from the National Registry of Myocardial Infarction. *Circulation* 2001;103:38-44.

192. Fong IW. Emerging relations between infectious disease and coronary artery disease and atherosclerosis. *Canadian Med Assoc J* 2000;163:49-56.

193. Foss-Campbell B, Sheldahl L, Wilke N, et al. Effects of upper extremity load distribution on weight carrying in men with ischemic heart disease. *J Cardiopulm Rehabil* 1993;13:37-42.

194. Frank E, Bendrich A, Denniston M. Use of vitamin-mineral supplements by female physicians in the United States. *Am J Clin Nutr* 2000;72:969-975.

195. Franklin, BA (ed.). *ACSM's guidelines for graded exercise testing and prescription*, 6th ed. Baltimore: Williams & Wilkins, 2000.

196. Franklin BA, Bonzheim K, Gordon S, et al. Snow shoveling: A trigger for acute myocardial infarction and sudden coronary death. *Am J Cardiol* 1996;77:855-858.

197. Franklin BA, Bonzheim K, Gordon S, Timmis GC. Safety of medically supervised outpatient cardiac rehabilitation exercise therapy: A 16-year follow-up. *Chest* 1998;114:902-906.

198. Franklin BA, Hogan P, Bonzheim K, et al. Cardiac demands of heavy snow shoveling. *JAMA* 1995;273:880-882.

199. Frantz A. Cardiac recovery in the home: Improving quality of care while reducing costs. *The Remington Report* Oct-Nov 1993.

200. Frasure-Smith N, Lesperance F, Taljic M. Depression and 18-month prognosis after myocardial infarction. *Circulation* 1995;91:999-1005.

201. Frazier OH, Duncan JM, Radovancevic B, et al. Successful bridge to heart transplantation with a new left ventricular assist device. *J Heart Lung Transplant* 1992;11:530-537.

202. Frazier OH, Macris MP, Myers TJ, et al. Improved survival after extended bridge to cardiac transplantation. *Annals Thoracic Surgery* 1994;57:1416-1422.

203. Freeman DJ, Norrie J, Sattar N, et al. Pravastatin and the development of diabetes mellitus: Evidence for a protective treatment effect in the West of Scotland Coronary Prevention Study. *Circulation* 2001;103:357-362.

204. Fried LP, Kronmal RA, Newman AB, et al. Risk factors for 5-year mortality in older adults. *JAMA* 1998;279:585-592.

204a. Froelicher VF, Lehmann KG, Thomas R, et al. The electro-cardiographic exercise test in a population with reduced workup bias: Diagnostic performance, computerized interpretation, and multivariable prediction. *Annals Internal Med* 1998;128:965-974.

205. Froelicher VF, Myers JN. *Exercise and the heart*, 4th ed. Philadelphia: WB Saunders, 2000. pp. 353-354.

205a. Frolkis JP, Pothier CE, Blackstone EH, Lauer MS. Frequent ventricular ectopy after exercise as a predictor of death. *N Engl J Med* 2003;348:781-790.

206. Frost P, Havel R. Rationale for use of non-high-density lipoprotein cholesterol rather than low-density lipoprotein cholesterol as a tool for lipoprotein cholesterol screening and assessment of risk and therapy. *Am J Cardiol* 1998;81(4A): 26B-31B.

207. Furberg CD, Psaty BM, Meyer JV. Nifedipine-dose related increase in mortality in patients with coronary heart disease. *Circulation* 1995;92:1326-1331.

208. Fuster V, Fayad ZA, Badimon JJ. Acute coronary syndromes. *Lancet* 1999;353(suppl I):5-9.

209. Fuster V, Gotto AM. Risk reduction. *Circulation* 2000;102: IV94-IV102.

210. Fuster V, Pearson TA. Matching the intensity of risk factor management with the hazard for coronary disease events. *J Am Coll Cardiol* 1996;27:957-1047.

211. Gallagher-Thompson D, Thompson LW. Bereavement and adjustment disorders. In: *Textbook of geriatric psychiatry*, 2d ed. EW Busse, DG Blazer (eds.). Washington, DC: American Psychiatry Press, 1996. pp. 313-328.

212. Ganz DA, Kuntz KM, Jacobson GA, Avorn J. Cost-effectiveness of 3-hydroxy-3-methylglutaryl coenzyme A reductase inhibitor therapy in older patients with myocardial infarction. *Ann Intern Med* 2000;132:780-787.

213. Gao SZ, Hunt SA, Schroeder JS, et al. Early development of accelerated graft coronary artery disease: Risk factors and course. *J Am Coll Cardiol* 1996;28:673-679.

214. Gardner AW. The effect of cigarette smoking on exercise capacity in patients with intermittent claudication. *Vascular Med* 1996;1:181-186.

215. Gardner C, Fortmann S, Krauss R. Association of small low-density lipoprotein particles with the incidence of coronary artery disease in men and women. *JAMA* 1996;276:875-881.

216. Gardner CD, Chatterjee LM, Carlson JJ. The effect of a garlic preparation on plasma lipid levels in moderately hypercholesterolemic adults. *Atherosclerosis* 2001;154:213-220.

217. Gardner CD, Newell KA, Cherin R, Haskell WL. The effect of soy protein with or without isoflavones relative to milk protein on plasma lipids in hypercholesterolemic postmenopausal women. *Am J Clin Nutr* 2001;73:728-735.

217a. Gauri AJ, Raxwal VK, Roux L, et al. Effects of chronotropic incompetence and beta-blocker use on the treadmill test in men. *Am Heart J* 2001;142:136-141.

218. Gaziano JM, Manson JE, Branch LG, et al. A prospective study of consumption of carotenoids in fruits and vegetables and decreased cardiovascular mortality in the elderly. *Ann Epidemiol* 1995;5:255-260.

219. Geelen G, Greenleaf JE. Orthostatis: Exercise and exercise training. In: *Exercise and sports sciences seviews*. JO Holloszy (ed.). Baltimore: Williams & Wilkins, 1993.

220. Geissler EM. *Cultural assessment: Pocket guide*. St. Louis: Mosby-Year Book, 1994.

221. Getz GS. Report on the workshop on diabetes and mechanisms of atherogenesis. *Arteriolscler and Thromb* 1993;13: 459-464.

222. Ghiadoni L, Donald AE, Cropley M, et al. Mental stress induces transient endothelial dysfunction in humans. *Circulation* 2000;102:2473-2478.

223. Gibbons RA, Balady GJ, Bricker JT, et al. ACC/AHA 2002 update for exercise testing. *J Am Coll Cardiol* 2002;40:1531-1540.

224. Gilson BS, Gilson JS, Bergner M, et al. The sickness impact profile: Development of an outcome measure of health care. *Annals Internal Med* 1975;65:1304-1310.

225. Girdano DA, Dusek DE. *Changing health behavior*. Scottsdale, AZ: Gorsuch Scarisbrick, 1988.

226. GISSI-Prevenzione Trial. Dietary supplementation with n-3 polyunsaturated fatty acids and vitamin E after myocardial infarction. *Lancet* 1999;354;447-455.

227. Glover ED (ed.). Nicotine addiction, smoking cessation, and nicotine replacement therapy. *Am J Health Behavior* 1993;17: 12-79.

228. Golberg KC, Hartz AJ, Jacobson SJ, et al. Racial and community factors influencing coronary artery bypass graft surgery rates for all 1986 Medicare patients. *JAMA* 1992; 267:1473-1477.

229. Goldman L, Hashimoto B, Cook EF, Loscalzo A. Comparative reproducibility and validity of systems for assessing cardiovascular functional class: Advantages of a new Specific Activity Scale. *Circulation* 1981;64:1227-1234.

230. Gordon A, Tyni Lenne R, Jansson E, et al. Beneficial effects of exercise training in heart failure patients with low cardiac output response to exercise—a comparison of two training models. *J Intern Med* 1999;246:175-182.

231. Gordon NF. Exercise guidelines for patients with NIDDM: An update. *J Cardiopulm Rehab* 1994;14:217-220.

232. Gordon NF. The exercise prescription. In: *The health professional's guide to diabetes and exercise*. Alexandria, VA: American Diabetes Association, 1995. pp. 70-82.

233. Gordon NF, English CD, Contractor AS, et al. Effectiveness of three models from comprehensive cardiovascular risk reduction. *Am J Cardiol* 2002;89:1263-1268.

234. Gottlieb SS, Fisher ML, Freudenberger R, et al. Effects of exercise training on peak performance and quality of life in congestive heart failure patients. *J Cardiac Failure* 1999;5: 188-194.

235. Gotto AM, Grundy SC. Lowering LDL cholesterol: Questions from recent meta-analyses and subset analyses of clinical trial data issues from the Interdisciplinary Council on Reducing the Risk for Coronary Heart Disease, Ninth Council Meeting. *Circulation* 1999;99:1-7.

236. Gotto AM. Lipid lowering, regression, and coronary events. *Circulation* 1995;92:646-656.

237. Gould KL, Ornish D, Shcerwitz L, et al. Changes in myocardial perfusion abnormalities by positron emission tomography after long-term intense risk factor modification. *JAMA* 1995;274:1402-1403.

238. Grayston JT. Does chlamydia pneumoniae cause atherosclerosis? *Arch Surg* 1999:134:930-934.

239. Grayston JT. Secondary prevention antibiotic treatment trials for coronary artery disease. *Circulation* 2000;102:1742-1743.

240. Grayston JT, Jackson LA, Kennedy WJ, et al. Secondary prevention trials for coronary artery disease with antibiotic treatment for Chlamydia pneumoniae: Design issues. *Am Heart J* 1999;138:S545-S549.

241. Greaves KA, Parks JS, Williams JK, Wagner JD. Intact dietary soy protein, but not adding an isoflavone-rich soy extract to casein, improves plasma lipids in ovariectomized cynomolgus monkeys. *J Nutr* 1999;129:1585-1592.

242. Green CP, Porter CB, Bresnahan DR, Spertus JA. Development and evaluation of the Kansas City Cardiomyopathy Questionnaire: A new health status measure for heart failure. *J Am Coll Cardiol* 2000;35:1245-1255.

243. Green K, Lydon S. Home health cardiac rehabilitation. *Home Healthcare Nurse* 1995;13:29-39.

244. Grillo CM, Brownell KD. Interventions for weight management. In: *ACSM's resource manual for exercise testing and prescription,* 4th ed. JL Roitman, et al. (eds.). Baltimore: Lippincott Williams & Wilkins, 2001. pp. 584-591.

245. Grundy S, Balady GJ, Criquie M, et al. When to start cholesterol lowering therapy in patients with coronary heart disease. *Circulation* 1997;9:1683-1685.

246. Gruppo Italiano per lo Studio della Sopravvivenza nell'Infarto miocardico. Dietary supplementation with n-3 polyunsaturated fatty acids and vitamin E after myocardial infarction: Results of the GISSI-Prevenzione trial. *Lancet* 1999;354:447-455.

246a. Guallar E, Hennekens CH, Sacks FM, et al. A prospective study of plasma fish oil levels and incidence of myocardial infarction in U.S. male physicians. *J Am Coll Cardiol* 1995;25:387-394.

247. Gueyffier F, Bulpit C, Boissel J-P, et al. Antihypertensive treatment in very old people: A sub-group meta analysis of randomized controlled trials. *Lancet* 1999;353:793-796.

248. Gundling K, Ernst E. Complementary and alternative medicine in cardiovascular disease: What is the evidence it works? *West J Med* 1999;171:191-194.

249. Guralnik JM, Ferruci L, Simonsick EM, et al. Lower-extremity function in persons over the age of 70 years as a predictor of subsequent disability. *N Engl J Med* 1996;332:556-561.

250. Gurwitz JH, McLaughlin TJ, Willison DJ, et al. Delayed hospital presentation in patients who have had acute myocardial infarction. *Ann Intern Med* 1997;126:593-599.

251. GUSTO Angiographic Investigators. The effects of tissue plasminogen activator, streptokinase, or both on coronary artery patency, ventricular function, and survival after acute myocardial infarction. *N Engl J Med* 1993;329:1615-1622.

252. Guyatt GH. Measurement of health-related quality of life in heart failure. *J Am Coll Cardiol* 1993;4:185A-191A.

253. Guyton JR, Blazing MA, Hagar J, et al. Extended-release niacin vs gemfibrozil for treatment of low levels of high density lipoprotein cholesterol. *Arch Intern Med* 2000;160:1177-1184.

254. Gylling H, Radhakrishnan R, Miettinen TA. Reduction of serum cholesterol in postmenopausal women with previous myocardial infarction and cholesterol malabsorption induced by dietary sitostanol ester margarine: Women and dietary sitostanol. *Circulation* 1997;96:4226-4231.

255. Hakim AA, Petrovitch H, Burchfiel CM, et al. Effects of walking on mortality among nonsmoking retired men. *N Engl J Med* 1998;338:94-99.

256. Halm MA. Collaborative care: Improving patient outcomes in cardiovascular surgery. *Prog Cardiovasc Nurs* 1997;2:15-23.

257. Hambrecht R, Hilbrich L, Erbs, et al. Correction of endothelial dysfunction in chronic heart failure: Additional effects of exercise training and L-larginine supplementation. *J Am Coll Cardiol* 2000;35:706-713.

258. Hambrecht R, Niebauer J, Fiehn E, et al. Physical training in patients with stable chronic heart failure: Effects on cardiorespiratory fitness and ultrastructural abnormalities of leg muscles. *J Am Coll Cardiol* 1995;25:1239-1249.

259. Hanumanthu S, Butler J, Chomsky D, et al. Effect of a heart failure program on hospitalization frequency and exercise tolerance. *Circulation* 1997;96:2842-2848.

260. Hare DL, Ryan TM, Selig SE, et al. Resistance exercise training increases muscle strength, endurance, and blood flow in patients with chronic heart failure. *Am J Cardiol* 1999;83:1674-1677.

261. Haskell W. The efficacy and safety of exercise programs in cardiac rehabilitation. *Med Sci Sports Exerc* 1994;26:815-823.

262. Haskell WL. Cardiovascular complications during exercise training of cardiac patients. *Circulation* 1978;57:920-924.

263. Haskell WL, Alderman EL, Fair JM, et al. Effects of intensive multiple risk factor reduction on coronary atherosclerosis and clinical cardiac events in men and women with coronary artery disease. The Stanford Coronary Risk Intervention Project (SCRIP). *Circulation* 1994;89:975-990.

264. Health Care Financing Administration. Health care financing administration. http://www.hcfa.gov/quality/3q2.htm June 2001.

265. HeartLinks. https://www.heartlinks.net/hlinfo.htm June 2001.

266. Heber D, Yip I, Asheley J, et al. Cholesterol-lowering effects of a proprietary Chinese red-yeast-rice dietary supplement. *Am J Clin Nutr* 1999;69:231-236.

266a. Heeschen C, Hamm CW, Laufs U, et al. Withdrawal of statins increases event rates in patients with acute coronary syndromes. *Circulation* 2002;15:1446-1452.

267. Heffner JE, Barbieri C. End-of-life care preferences of patients enrolled in cardiovascular rehabilitation programs. *Chest* 2000;117:1474-1481.

268. Heffner JE, Barbiere C. Involvement of cardiovascular rehabilitation programs in advance directive education. *Arch Internal Med* 1996;156:1746-1751.

269. Hennekens CH, Buring JE, Manson JE, et al. Lack of effect of long-term supplementation with beta carotene on the incidence of malignant neoplasms and cardiovascular disease. *N Engl J Med* 1996;334:1145-1149.

270. Herbert DL, Herbert WG. Medicolegal aspects of rehabilitation of the coronary patient. In: *Rehabilitation of the coronary patient.* NK Wenger, HK Hellerstein (eds.). New York: Livingstone, 1995.

271. Hercberg S, Preziosi P, Briancon S, et al. A primary prevention trial using nutritional doses of antioxidant vitamins and minerals in cardiovascular disease and cancers in a general

population: The SU.VI.MAX study—design, methods, and participant characteristics. SUpplementation en VItamines et Mineraux AntioXydants. *Control Clin Trials* 1998;19:336-351.

272. Hermann J, Lerman A. The endothelium: Dysfunction and beyond. *J Nuclear Cardiol* 2001;8:197-206.

273. Hertog MG, Kromhout D, Aravanis C, et al. Flavonoid intake and long-term risk of coronary heart disease and cancer in the seven countries study. *Arch Intern Med* 1995;155:381-386.

274. Hiatt WR, Hirsch AT, Regensteiner JG, Brass EP. Clinical trials for claudication: Assessment of exercise performance, functional status and clinical end points. *Circulation* 1995; 92:614-621.

275. Hlatky MA, Boineau RE, Higginbotham MB, et al. A brief self-administered questionnaire to determine functional capacity: The Duke Activity Status Index. *Am J Cardiol* 1989;64:651-654.

276. Hoffmeister A, Rothenbacher D, Bazner U, et al. Role of novel markers of inflammation in patients with stable coronary artery disease. *Am J Cardiol* 2001;87:262-266.

277. Holubarsch C, Colucci W, Meinertz T, et al. Survival and prognosis: Investigation of crataegus extract WS 1442 in congestive heart failure (SPICE)—rationale, study design and study protocol. *Eur J Heart Fail* 2000;2:431-437.

278. Homocysteine Lowering Trialists' Collaboration. Lowering blood homocysteine with folic acid based supplements: Meta-analysis of randomised trials. *BMJ* 1998;316:894-898.

279. Honore EK, Williams JK, Anthony MS, Clarkson TB. Soy isoflavones enhance coronary vascular reactivity in atherosclerotic female macaques. *Fertil Steril* 1997;67:148-154.

280. Hornig B, Maier V, Drexler H. Physical training improves endothelial function in patients with chronic heart failure. *Circulation* 1996;93:210-214.

281. Hosenpud JD, Bennett LE, Keck BM, et al. The registry of the International Society for Heart and Lung Transplantation: Seventeenth official report-2000. *J Heart Lung Transplant* 2000;19:909-931.

282. Hu FB, Rimm EB, Stampfer MJ, et al. Prospective study of major dietary patterns and risk of coronary heart disease in men. *Am J Clin Nutr* 2000;72:912-921.

283. Hu FB, Stampfer MJ, Manson JE, et al. Frequent nut consumption and risk of coronary heart disease in women: Prospective cohort study. *Br Med J* 1998;317:1341-1345.

284. Huggins GS, Pasternak RC, Alpert NM, et al. Effects of short-term treatment of hyperlipidemia on coronary vasodilator function and myocardial perfusion in regions having a substantial impairment of baseline dilator reserve. *Circulation* 1998;98:1291-1296.

285. Hughes SJ. Novel risk factors for coronary heart disease: Emerging connections. *Cardiovasc Nurs* 2000;14:91-103.

286. Humphrey R. Exercise physiology in patients with left ventricular assist devices. *J Cardiopulm Rehabil* 1997;17:73-75.

287. Hunt ME, O'Malley PG, Vernalis MN, et al. C-reactive protein is not associated with the presence or extent of calcified subclinical atherosclerosis. *Am Heart J* 2001;141:206-210.

288. Hunt S, McEwen J, McKenna S. A quantitative approach to perceived health. *J Epidemiol Community Health* 1980;34: 281-295.

289. Intervent USA. Implementation of an innovative, community-based cardiovascular risk reduction program.

http://www.interventusa.com/research_usa.html June 2001.

290. Isaacsohn JL, Moser M, Stein EA, et al. Garlic powder and plasma lipids and lipoproteins: A multicenter, randomized, placebo-controlled trial. *Arch Intern Med* 1998;158: 1189-1194.

291. Iso H, Rexrode KM, Stampfer MJ, et al. Intake of fish and omega-3 fatty acids and risk of stroke in women. *JAMA* 2001;285:304-312.

292. Jacobs DR Jr., Meyer KA, Kushi LH, Folsom AR. Whole-grain intake may reduce the risk of ischemic heart disease death in postmenopausal women: The Iowa Women's Health Study. *Am J Clin Nutr* 1998;68:248-257.

293. Jaski BE, Kelley RB, Adamson R, et al. Exercise hemodynamics during long-term implantation of a left ventricular assist device in patients awaiting heart transplantation. *J Am Coll Cardiol* 1993;22:1574-1580.

294. Jenkins GH, Grieve LA, Yacoub MH, Singer DRJ. Effect of simvastatin on ejection fraction in cardiac transplant recipients. *Am J Cardiol* 1996;78:1453-1456.

295. Jette AM, Davies AR, Cleary PD, et al. The Functional Status Questionnaire: Reliability and validity when used in primary care. *J General Intern Med* 1986;1:143-149.

296. Jialal I, Fuller CJ, Huet BA. The effect of alpha-tocopherol supplementation on LDL oxidation. A dose-response study. *Arterioscler Thromb* 1995;15:190-198.

297. Jialal I, Stein D, Balis D, et al. Effect of hydroxymethyl glutaryl coenzyme A reductase inhibitor therapy on high sensitive c-reactive protein levels. *Circulation* 2001;103:1933-1935.

298. Johansson AG, Forslund A, Sjodin A, Ljunghall S. Determination of body composition. A comparison of dual energy x-ray absorptiometry and hydrodensitometry. *Am J Clin Nutrition* 1993;57:323-326.

299. Johnson PA, Lee TH, Cook EF, et al. Effect of race on the presentation and management of patients with acute chest pain. *Ann Intern Med* 1993;118:593-601.

300. Johnson PH, Cowley AJ, Kinnear WJM. A randomized controlled trial of inspiratory muscle training in stable chronic heart failure. *Eur Heart J* 1998;19:1249-1253.

301. Joint Commission on Accreditation of Healthcare Organizations. Management of Human Resources. *Hospital Accreditation Standards*. Oakbrook Terrace, IL: Joint Commission Resources, 2001. pp. 221-226.

302. Joint Commission on Accreditation of Healthcare Organizations. *Hospital*. 2002. http://www.jcaho.org/htba/hospital/index.htm.

303. Joint Commission on Accreditation of Healthcare Organizations. *Ambulatory Care*. 2002. http://www.jcaho.org/htba/ambulatory+care/index.htm.

304. Joint National Committee on Prevention, Detection, Evaluation, and Treatment of High Blood Pressure. Seventh report of Joint National Committee on Prevention, Detection, Evaluation, and Treatment of High Blood Pressure. *JAMA* 2003; 289:2560-2572.

305. Joseph AM, Norman SM, Ferry LH, et al. The safety of transdermal nicotine as an aid to smoking cessation in patients with cardiac disease. *N Engl J Med* 1996;335:1792-1798.

306. Jourven X, Zureik M, Desnos M, et al. Long-term outcome in asymptomatic men with exercise-induced premature ventricular depolarizations. *N Engl J Med* 2000;243:826-833.

307. Kaiser Permanente National Diversity Council. *A provider's handbook on culturally competent care*. 1996. Author: Oakland, CA.

308. Kao AC, Van Trigt P, Shaeffer-McCall GS, et al. Central and peripheral limitations to upright exercise in untrained cardiac transplant recipients. *Circulation* 1994;89:2605-2615.

309. Kaski JC, Valenzuela Garcia LF. Therapeutic options for the management of patients with cardiac syndrome "X". *Eur Heart J* 2001;22:283-293.

310. Katan MB, Grundy SM, Willett WC. Should a low-fat, high-carbohydrate diet be recommended for everyone? Beyond low-fat diets. *N Engl J Med* 1997;337:563-567.

311. Katzel LI, Coon PJ, Dengel J, Goldberg AP. Effects of an American Heart Association step I diet and weight loss on lipoprotein lipid levels in obese men with silent myocardial ischemia and reduced high-density lipoprotein cholesterol. *Metabolism* 1995;44:307-314.

312. Kauffman HM, McBride MA, Shield CF, et al. Determinants of waiting time for heart transplants in the United States. *J Heart Lung Transplant* 1999;18:414-419.

313. Kavanagh T, Myers MG, Baigrie RS, et al. Quality of life and cardiorespiratory function in chronic heart failure: Effects of 12 months' aerobic training. *Heart* 1996;76:42-49.

314. Kavanagh T. Physical training in heart transplant recipients. *J Cardiovasc Risk* 1996;3:154-159.

315. Kavanagh T, Yacoub MH, Kennedy J, Austin PC. Return to work after heart transplantation: 12-year follow-up. *J Heart Lung Transplant* 1999;18:846-851.

316. Kaye DM, Esler M, Kingwell B, et al. Functional and neuro-chemical evidence for partial cardiac sympathetic reinnervation after cardiac transplantation in humans. *Circulation* 1993;88:1110-1118.

317. Kelly TM. Exercise testing and training of patients with malignant ventricular arrhythmias. *Med Sci Sports Exer* 1996;28:53-61.

318. Keteyian SJ, Brawner C. Cardiac transplant. In: *American College of Sports Medicine. ACSM's exercise management for persons with chronic diseases and disabilities*. JL Durstine, et al. (eds.). Champaign, IL: Human Kinetics, 1997. pp. 54-58.

319. Keteyian SJ, Brawner CA, Schairer JR, et al. Effects of exercise training on chronotropic incompetence in patients with heart failure. *Am Heart J* 1999;138:233-240.

320. Keteyian SJ, Mellett PA, Fedel JF, et al. Electrocardiographic monitoring during cardiac rehabilitation. *Chest* 1995;107:1242-1246.

321. Kimble LP. Impact of cardiac symptoms on self-reported household task performance in women with coronary artery disease. *J Cardiopulm Rehabil* 2001;21:18-23.

322. King G, Bendel RA. A statistical model estimating the number of African American physicians in the United States. *J Natl Med Assoc* 1994;86:264-272.

323. Kirwan JP, Kohrt WM, Wojta DM, et al. Endurance exercise training reduces glucose-stimulated insulin levels in 60- to 70-year-old men and women. *J Gerontol* 1993;48:M84-M90.

324. Klatsky AL, Armstrong MA, Friedman GD. Alcohol and mortality. *Annals Intern Med* 1992;177:646-654.

325. Kloeck W, Cummins RO, Chamberlain D, et al. Early defibrillation: An advisory statement from the Advanced Life Support Working Group of the International Liaison Committee on Resuscitation. *Circulation* 1997;95:2183-2184.

326. Kobashigawa JA, Katznelson S, Laks H, et al. Effect of pravastatin on outcomes after cardiac transplantation. *N Engl J Med* 1995;333:621-627.

327. Koch H, Lawson L. (eds). *Garlic: The science and therapeutic application of allium sativum L. and related species*. Philadelphia: Williams & Wilkins; 1996.

328. Kong K, Kevorkian G, Rossi CD. Functional outcomes of patients on a rehabilitation unit after open heart surgery. *J Cardiopulm Rehabil* 1996;16:413-418.

329. Kornowski R, Seeli D, Averbuch M, et al. Intensive home care surveillance prevents hospitalization and improves morbidity rates among elderly patients with severe congestive heart failure. *Am Heart J* 1995;129:762.

330. Kovaleski JE, Gurchiek LR, Pearsall AW. Musculoskeletal injuries: Risks, prevention and care. In: *ACSM's resource manual for guidelines for exercise testing and prescription*, 4th ed. JL Roitman, et al. (eds.). Baltimore: Williams and Wilkins, 2001.

331. Krauss RM, Eckel RH, Howard B, et al. AHA Dietary Guidelines: Revision 2000: A statement for healthcare professionals from the Nutrition Committee of the American Heart Association. *Circulation* 2000;102:2284-2299.

332. Kris-Etherton PM, Daniels SR, Eckel RH, et al. Summary of the scientific conference on dietary fatty acids and cardiovascular health: Conference summary from the Nutrition Committee of the American Heart Association. *Circulation* 2001;103:1034-1039.

333. Kris-Etherton PM, Eckel RH, Howard BV, et al. Lyon Diet Heart Study: Benefit of a Mediterranean-style, National Cholesterol Education Program/American Heart Association Step 1 dietary pattern on cardiovascular disease. *Circulation* 2001;103:1823-1825.

334. Kriska AM, Casperson CJ (eds.). A collection of physical activity questionnaires for health related research. *Med Sci Sports Exerc* 1997;29(6):S1-S205.

335. Krumholz HM, Butler J, Miller J, et al. Prognostic importance of emotional support for elderly patients hospitalized with heart failure. *Circulation* 1998;97:958-964.

336. Kulavuori K, Toivonen L, Naveri H, Leinonen H. Reversal of autonomic derangements by physical training in chronic heart failure. *Eur Heart J* 1995;16:490-495.

337. Kushi LH, Fee RM, Folsom AR, et al. Physical activity and mortality in postmenopausal women. *JAMA* 1997;277:1287-1292.

338. LaFontaine TP, Gordon NF. Comprehensive cardiovascular risk reduction in patients with coronary artery disease. In: JL Roitman, et al. (eds.) *ACSM's resource manual for guidelines for exercise testing and prescription*, 4th ed. Philadelphia: Lippincott Williams & Wilkins 2001. pp. 263-273.

339. Lampert E, Mettauer B, Hoppeler H, et al. Structure of skeletal muscle in heart transplant recipients. *J Am Coll Cardiol* 1996;28:980-984.

340. Lampert E, Mettauer B, Hoppeler H, et al. Skeletal muscle response to short endurance training in heart transplant recipients. *J Am Coll Cardiol* 1998;32:420-426.

341. Lasater M. The effect of a nurse-managed CHF clinic on patient readmission and length of stay. *Home Healthcare Nurse* 1996;14:351.

341a. Lauer MS, Francis GS, Okin P, et al. Impaired chronotropic response to exercise stress testing as a predicator of mortality. *JAMA* 1999; 281: 524-529.

342. Lavie C, Milani R. Effects of cardiac rehabilitation, exercise training, and weight reduction on exercise capacity, coronary risk factors, behavior characteristics, and quality of life in obese coronary patients. *Am J Cardiol* 1997;79:397-401.

343. Lavie CJ, Milani RV. Effects of cardiac rehabilitation programs on exercise capacity, coronary risk factors, behavioral characteristics, and quality of life in a large elderly cohort. *Am J Cardiol* 1995;76:177-179.

344. Lavie CJ, Milani RV, Littman AB. Benefits of cardiac rehabilitation and exercise training in secondary coronary prevention in the elderly. *J Am Coll Cardiol* 1993;22:678-683.

345. Lawson DL, Wang ZJ. Allicin release from garlic supplements: A major problem due to the sensitivities of allinease activity. *J Agric Food Chem* 2001;49:2592-2599.

346. Lawson LD. Garlic powder for hyperlipidemia: Analysis of recent negative results. *Quarterly Review Natural Med* 1998;Fall:187-189.

346a. Lefer DJ. Statins as potent anti-inflammatory drugs. *Circulation* 2002;106:2041-2042.

347. Levin, ME. The diabetic foot. In: *The health professional's guide to diabetes and exercise.* Alexandria, VA: American Diabetes Association, 1995. pp.136-142.

348. Lewis SJ, Moye LA, Sacks FM, et al. Effect of pravastatin on cardiovascular events in older patients with myocardial infarction and cholesterol levels in the average range. Results of the Cholesterol and Recurrent Events (CARE) trial. *Ann Intern Med* 1998;129:681-689.

349. Libby P, Ridker PM. Novel inflammatory markers of coronary risk. *Circulation* 1999;11:1148-1150.

350. Linden W, Stossel C, Maurice J. Psychosocial interventions for patients with coronary artery disease: A meta-analysis. *Arch Intern Med* 1996;156:745-752.

351. Lipson JG, Dibble SL, Minarik PA. *Culture and nursing care: A pocket guide.* San Francisco: UCSF Nursing Press, 1996

352. Liu S, Manson JE, Lee IM, et al. Fruit and vegetable intake and risk of cardiovascular disease: The Women's Health Study. *Am J Clin Nutr* 2000;72:922-928.

353. Lo R, Lo B, Wells E, et al. The development and evaluation of a computer-aided diabetes education program. *Australian J Advanced Nursing* 1996;13:19-27.

354. Ma J, Folsom AR, Melnick SL, et al. Associations of serum and dietary magnesium with cardiovascular disease, hypertension, diabetes, insulin, and carotid arterial wall thickness: The ARIC study. Atherosclerosis Risk in Communities Study. *J Clin Epidemiol* 1995;48:927-940.

355. MacMahon S, Rodger A. The effects of blood pressure reduction in older patients: An overview of five randomized controlled trials in elderly hypertensives. *J Clin Exp Hypertension* 1993;15:967-978.

356. Maddahi J, Rodrigues E, Berman DS, et al. State of the art myocardial perfusion imaging. In: *Nuclearcardiology: state of the art.* MS Verani (ed.). Philadelphia: Saunders, 1994. pp. 199-202.

357. Magnusson G, Gordon A, Kaijser L, et al. High intensity knee extensor training in patients with chronic heart failure: Major skeletal muscle improvement. *Eur Heart J* 1996;17: 1048-1055.

358. Mahler D, Weinberg D, Wells C, Feinstein A. The measurement of dyspnea. *Chest* 1984;6:751-758.

359. Mahmarian JJ, Moye LA, Nasser GA, et al. Nicotine patch therapy in smoking cessation reduces the extent of exercise-induced myocardial ischemia. *J Am Coll Cardiol* 1997;30: 125-130.

359a. Mahon NG, Blackstone EH, Francis GS, et al. The prognostic value of estimated creatine clearance alongside functional capacity in ambulatory patients with chronic congestive heart failure. *J Am Coll Cardiol* 203;40:1106-1113.

360. Maiorana A, O'Driscoll G, Cheetham C, et al. Combined aerobic and resistance exercise training improves functional capacity and strength in CHF. *J Appl Physiol* 2000;88:1565-1570.

361. Malinow MR, Bostom AG, Krauss RM. Homocysteine, diet, and cardiovascular dieases. *Circulation* 1999;99:178-182.

362. Malloy MJ, Kane JP. Aggressive medical therapy for the prevention and treatment of coronary artery disease. *Disease-a-Month* 1998;44:5-40.

363. Malmberg K, Yusuf S, Gerstein HC, et al. Impact of diabetes on long-term prognosis in patients with unstable angina and non-Q wave myocardial infarction: Results of the OASIS registry. *Circulation* 2000;102:1014-1019.

364. Mancini DM, Henson D, La Manca J, et al. Benefit of selective respiratory muscle training on exercise capacity in patients with chronic congestive heart failure. *Circulation* 1995;91: 320-329.

365. Martens KH, Mellor SD. A study of the relationship between home care services and hospital readmission of patients with congestive heart failure. *Home Healthcare Nurse* 1997;15:123-129.

366. Marz W, Schnaragl J, Abletshauser C, et al. Fluvastatin lowers atherogenic dense low-density lipoproteins in postmenopausal women with the atherogenic lipoprotein phenotype. *Circulation* 2001;103:1942-1948.

367. Matano RA, Bronstone AB. Assessment, intervention, and referral of patients suffering from alcoholism. *J Cardiopulm Rehabil* 1994;14:27-29.

368. Mayer E, Jacobsen D, Robinson K. Homocysteine and coronary atherosclerosis. *J Am Coll Cardiol* 1996;27:517-527.

369. Mayer-Davis E, D'Agostino R, Karter A, et al. Intensity and amount of physical activity in relation to insulin sensitivity. *JAMA* 1998;279:669-674.

370. McConnell TR. Exercise prescription: When the guidelines do not work. *J Cardiopulm Rehabil* 1996;16:34-37.

371. McDaniel AM. Assessing the feasibility of a clinical practice guideline for inpatient smoking cessation intervention. *Clinical Nurse Specialist* 1999;13:228-235.

372. McGregor CGA. Cardiac transplantation: Surgical considerations and early postoperative management. *Mayo Clin Proc* 1992;67:577-585.

373. McNair D, Lorr M, Dropplemann L. *Profile of mood states.* San Diego: Educational and Industrial Testing Service, 1971.

374. Mensink RP, Katan MB. Effect of dietary fatty acids on serum lipids and lipoproteins. A meta-analysis of 27 trials. *Arterioscler Thromb* 1992;12:911-919.

375. Mertens DJ, Kavanagh T, Campbell RB, Shephard RJ. Exercise without dietary restriction as a means to long-term fat loss in the obese cardiac patient. *J Sports Med Phys Fitness* 1998;38:310-316.

376. Merz-Demlow BE, Duncan AM, Wangen KE, et al. Soy isoflavones improve plasma lipids in normocholesterolemic, premenopausal women. *Am J Clin Nutr* 2000;71:1462-1469.

377. Mettauer B, Zhao QM, Epailly E, et al. VO2 kinetics reveal a central limitation at the outset of subthreshold exercise in heart transplant recipients. *J Appl Physiol* 2000;88:1228-1238.

378. Meyer, GC. Reimbursement issues. In: *Developing and managing cardiac rehabilitation programs.* LK Hall (ed.). Champaign, IL: Human Kinetics, 1993.

379. Meyer JW, Feingold MG. Using standard treatment protocols to manage costs and quality of hospital services. *Hospital Technology Special Report* 1993;12:1-23.

380. Meyer K, Gornandt L, Schwaibold M, et al. Predictors of response to exercise training in severe chronic congestive heart failure. *Am J Cardiol* 1997;80:56-61.

381. Meyer K, Hajric R, Westbrook, et al. Hemodynamic responses during leg press exercise in patients with chronic congestive heart failure. *Am J Cardiol* 1999;83:1537-1543.

382. Meyer K, Samek L, Samek L, et al. Interval training in patients with severe chronic heart failure: Analysis and recommendations for exercise procedures. *Med Sci Sports Exerc* 1997;29:306-312.

383. Meyer K, Schwaibold M, Westbrook S, et al. Effects of exercise training and activity restriction on 6-minute walking test performance in patients with chronic heart failure. *Am Heart J* 1997;133:447-453.

384. Midgley JP, Matthew AG, Greenwood CM, Logan AG. Effect of reduced dietary sodium on blood pressure: A meta-analysis of randomized controlled trials. *JAMA* 1996;275:1590-1597.

385. Miettinen TA, Puska P, Gylling H, et al. Reduction of serum cholesterol with sitostanol-ester margarine in a mildly hypercholesterolemic population. *N Engl J Med* 1995;333:1308-1312.

386. Miettinen TA, Pyorala K, Olsson AG, et al. Cholesterol-lowering therapy in women and elderly patients with myocardial infarction or angina pectoris: Findings from the Scandinavian Simvastatin Survival Study (4S). *Circulation* 1997;96:4211-4218.

387. Miller FA, Rajamannan N, Grogan M, Murphy JG. Prosthetic heart valves. In: *Mayo Clinic cardiology review.* JD Murphy (ed.). Philadelphia: Lippincott Williams & Wilkins, 2000. pp. 337-352.

388. Miller NH, Smith PM, DeBusk RF, et al. Smoking cessation and hospitalized patients: Results of a randomized trial. *Arch Intern Med* 1997;157:409-415.

389. Miller NH, Smith PM. Smoking cessation. In: American College of Sports Medicine: *Resource manual for guidelines for exercise testing and prescription,* 3d ed. J Roitman, et al. (eds.). Baltimore: Williams & Wilkins, 1998.

390. Miller NH, Taylor CB. *Lifestyle management for patients with coronary heart disease.* Champaign, IL: Human Kinetics, 1995.

391. Miller NH, Warren D, Myers D. Home-based cardiac rehabilitation and lifestyle modification: The MULTIFIT model. *J Cardiovasc Nursing* 1996;11:76-87.

391a. Miller TD, Hodge DO, Christian TF, et al. Effects of adjustment for referral bias on the sensitivity of single photon emission computed tomography for the diagnosis of coronary artery disease. *Am J Med* 2002;112:290-297.

392. Mittleman MA, Maclure N, Tofler GH, et al. Triggering of acute MI by heavy physical exertion: Protection against triggering by regular physical exertion. *N Engl J Med* 1993;329:1677-1683.

393. Moghadasian MH, McManus BM, Frohlich JJ. Homocysteine and coronary artery disease: Clinical evidence and genetic and metabolic background. *Arch Internal Med* 1997;157:2299-2308.

394. Money SR, Herd JA, Issacsohn JL, et al. Effect of cilostazol on walking distances in patients with intermittent claudication caused by peripheral vascular disease. *J Vascular Surgery* 1998;27:267-275.

395. Morgan GD, Noll EL, Orleans BK, et al. Reaching midlife and older smokers: Tailored interventions for routine medical care. *Prev Med* 1996;25:346-354.

396. Morrone TM, Buck LA. Rehabilitation of the ventricular assist device recipient. In: *Cardiac assist devices.* DJ Goldstein, MC Oz (eds.). Armonk, NY: Futura, 2000. pp. 167-176.

397. Morrone TM, Buck LA, Catanese KA, et al. Early progressive mobilization of patients with left ventricular assist devices is safe and optimizes recovery before heart transplantation. *J Heart Lung Transplant* 1996;14:423-429.

397a. Morshedi-Meibod A, Larson MG, Levy D, et al. Heart rate recovery after treadmill exercise testing and risk of cardiovascular disease events (the Framingham Heart Study). *Am J Cardiol* 2002;90:848-852.

398. Motwani JG, Topol EJ. Aortocoronary saphenous vein graft disease: Pathogenesis, predisposition, and prevention. *Circulation* 1998;97:916-931.

399. Murray CJ, Lopez AD. Alternative projection of mortality and disability by cause 1990-2020: Global Burden of Disease Study. *Lancet* 1997;349:1498-1504.

400. Myers J, Buchanan N, Smith D, et al. Individualized ramp treadmill, observations on a new protocol. *Chest* 1992;101:236S-241S.

401. Myers J, Dat D, Herbert W, et al. A nomogram to predict exercise capacity from a specific activity questionnaire and clinical data. *Am J Cardiol* 1994;73:591-596.

402. Myers J, Manish P, Froelicher V, et al. Exercise capacity and mortality among men referred for exercise testing. *N Engl J Med* 2002;346:793-801.

403. National Cholesterol Education Program (NCEP). Executive summary of the third report of the Expert Panel on Detection, Evaluation and Treatment of High Blood Cholesterol in Adults (Adult Treatment Panel III). *JAMA* 2001;285:2486-2497.

404. National Committee for Quality Assurance. *Health plan employer data and information set (HEDIS).* http://www.ncqa.org, 2003.

405. National Heart Lung and Blood Institute. *Congestive heart failure in the United States: A new epidemic.* Bethesda, MD: US Department of Health and Human Services, 1996.

406. National High Blood Pressure Education Program Working Group. Report on primary prevention of hypertension. *Arch Intern Med* 1993;153:186-208.

407. Nestel PJ, Yamashita T, Sasahara T, et al. Soy isoflavones improve systemic arterial compliance but not plasma lipids in menopausal and perimenopausal women. *Arterioscler Thromb* 1997;17:3392-3398.

408. Newman AB, Siscovick DS, Manolio TA, et al. Ankle-arm index as a marker of atherosclerosis in the Cardiovascular Health Study. *Circulation* 1993;88:837-845.

409. National Health and Nutrition Examination Survey (NHANES). Atlanta: Centers for Disease Control, 2001. http://www.cdc.gov/nchs/nhanes.htm.

410. Niset G, Preumont N. Determinants of peak aerobic capacity after heart transplantation. *Eur Heart J* 1997;18:1692-1693.

411. Nohria A, Vaccarino V, Krumholz HM. Gender differences in mortality after myocardial infarction. *Cardiol Clin* 1998;16: 45-57.

412. Obarzanek E, Sacks FM, Vollmer WM, et al. Effects on blood lipids of a blood pressure-lowering diet: The Dietary Approaches to Stop Hypertension (DASH) Trial. *Am J Clin Nutr* 2001;74:80-89.

413. Ockene J, Kristeller J, Goldberg R, et al. Smoking cessation and severity of disease: The coronary artery smoking intervention study. *Health Psychology* 1992;11:119-126.

414. O'Connor G, Buring Y, Yusuf S, et al. An overview of randomized trials of rehabilitation with exercise after myocardial infarction. *Circulation* 1989;80:234-244.

415. Oden KE, Kevorkian CG, Levy JK. Rehabilitation of the post-cardiac surgery stroke patient: Analysis of cognitive and functional assessment. *Arch Phys Med Rehabil* 1998;79: 67-71.

416. O'Keefe JH Jr, Sutton MB, McCallister BD, et al. Coronary angioplasty versus bypass surgery in patients >70 years old matched for ventricular function. *J Am Coll Cardiol* 1994;24: 425-430.

417. Oldridge NB, Furlong W, Feeny D, et al. Economic evaluation of cardiac rehabilitation after acute myocardial infarction. *Am J Cardiol* 1993;72:154-161.

418. Oldridge NB, Guyatt G, Fischer M, Rimm A. Cardiac rehabilitation after myocardial infarction: Combined experience of randomized clinical trials. *JAMA* 1988;260:945-950.

419. Oldridge NB, Pashkow FJ. Compliance and motivation in cardiac rehabilitation. In: *Clinical rehabilitation: A cardiologist's guide.* FJ Pashkow, WA Dafoe (eds.). Baltimore: Williams & Wilkins, 1993. pp. 335-348.

420. Omenn GS, Goodman GE, Thornquist MD, et al. Effects of a combination of beta carotene and vitamin A on lung cancer and cardiovascular disease. *N Engl J Med* 1996;334: 1150-1155.

421. Ornish D, Scherwitz L, Billings JH, et al. Intensive lifestyle changes for reversal of coronary heart disease. *JAMA* 1998;280:2001-2007.

422. Ottenbacher KJ, Hsu Y, Granger CV, Fiedler RC: The reality of the functional independence measure: A quantitative review. *Arch Phys Med Rehabil* 1996;77:1226-1232.

423. Owen PM, Porter KA, Frost CG, et al. The determination of the readability of education materials for patients with cardiac disease. *J Cardiopulmon Rehabil* 1993;3:20-24.

424. Oxman T, Freeman D, Manheimer E. Lack of social participation or religious strength and comfort as risk factors for death after cardiac surgery in the elderly. *Psychosomatic Med* 1995;57:5-15.

425. Paffenbarger RS, Hyde RT, Wing AL, Hsich CC. Physical activity, all-cause mortality, and longevity of college alumni. *N Engl J Med* 1986;314:605-614.

426. Paffenbarger RS, Kampert JB, Lee IM, et al. Changes in physical activity and other lifeway patterns influencing longevity. *Med Sci Sports Exerc* 1994;26:857-865.

427. Pashkow FJ. Issues in contemporary cardiac rehabilitation: A historical perspective. *J Am Coll Cardiol* 1993;21:822-834.

428. Pashkow FJ, Schweikert RA, Wilkoff BL. Exercise testing and training in patients with malignant arrhythmias. In: *Exercise and sport sciences review*, vol. 25. J Holloszy (ed.). Baltimore: Williams & Wilkins, 1997.

429. Pashkow P, Ades PA, Emery CF, et al. Outcomes measurement in cardiac and pulmonary rehabilitation. *J Cardiopulm Rehabil* 1995;15:394-405.

430. Pashkow P, Emery CF, Frid DJ, et al. *AACVPR outcomes tools resource guide.* Middleton, WI: American Association of Cardiovascular and Pulmonary Rehabilitation, 1996.

431. Paul SD, O'Gara PT, Mahjoub ZA, et al. Geriatric patients with acute myocardial infarction: Cardiac risk factor profiles, presentation, thrombolysis, coronary interventions, and prognosis. *Am Heart J* 1996;131:710-715.

432. Pauwels RA, Buist AS, Calverley PMA, et al. Global strategy for the diagnosis, management, and prevention of chronic obstructive pulmonary disease. *Am J Respir Crit Care Med* 2001;163:1256-1276.

433. Pearson TA, Fuster V. 27th Bethesda Conference: Matching the intensity of risk factor management with the hazard for coronary disease event. Executive summary. *J Am Coll Cardiol* 1996;27:961-963.

434. Pearson T, Rapaport E, Criqui M, et al. Optimal risk factor management in the patient after coronary revascularization: A statement from the AHA for healthcare professionals. *Circulation* 1994;90:3125-3133.

435. Penson MG, Winter WE, Fricker FJ, et al. Tacrolimus-based triple-drug immunosuppression minimizes serum lipid elevations in pediatric cardiac transplant recipients. *J Heart Lung Transplant* 1999;18:707-713.

436. Perez-Jimenez F, Castro P, Lopez-Miranda J, et al. Circulating levels of endothelial function are modulated by dietary monounsaturated fat. *Atherosclerosis* 1999;145:351-358.

437. Perry M, Kannel S. Barriers to health coverage for hispanic workers: Focus group findings. The Commonwealth Fund, 2002. www.cmwf.org.

438. Peterson ED, Cowper PA, Jollis JG, et al. Outcome of coronary artery bypass graft surgery in 24,461 patients aged 80 years or older. *Circulation* 1995;92(suppl II):85-91.

439. Peterson ED, Wright SM, Daley J, et al. Racial variation in cardiac procedure use and survival following acute myocardial infarction in the Department of Veterans Affairs. *JAMA* 1994;271:1175-1180.

439a. Piña IL, Apstein CS, Balady EJ, et al. Exercise and heart failure. *Circulation* 2003;107:1210-1225.

440. Piña IL, Balady GF, Nason P, et al. Guidelines for clinical exercise testing laboratories. A statement for healthcare professionals from the Committee on Exercise and Cardiac Rehabilitation, American Heart Association. *Circulation* 1995;91:912-921.

441. Pittler M, Ernst E. Gingko biloba extract for the treatment of intermittent claudication: A meta-analysis of randomized trials. *Am J Med* 2000;108:276-281.

442. Plotnick GD, Corretti MC, Vogel RA. Effect of antioxidant vitamins on the transient impairment of endothelium-dependent brachial artery vasoactivity following a single high-fat meal. *JAMA* 1997;278:1682-1686.

443. Poehlman ET, Toth MJ, Gardner AW. Changes in energy balance and body composition at menopause: A controlled, longitudinal study. *Annals Internal Med* 1995;123: 673-675.

444. Poldermans D, Fioretti PM, Forster T, et al. Dobutamine stress echocardiography for assessment of perioperative cardiac risk in patients undergoing major vascular surgery. *Circulation* 1993;87:1506.

445. Pollock ML, Evans WJ. Resistance training for health and disease. *Med Sci Sports Exerc* 1999;31:10-11.

446. Pollock ML, Franklin BA, Balady GJ, et al. Resistance training in individuals with and without cardiovascular disease: Benefits, rationale, safety, and prescription. *Circulation* 2000;101: 828-833.

447. Pollock ML, Gaesser GA, Butcher JD, et al. The recommended quantity and quality of exercise for developing and maintaining cardiorespiratory and muscular fitness in healthy adults. *Med Sci Sports Exer* 1998;30:975-991.

448. Prochaska JO, DiClemente CC, Norcross JC. In search of how people change: Applications to addictive behaviors. *Am Psychologist* 1992;47:1102-1114.

449. Prochaska JO, Norcross JC, DiClemente CC. *Changing for good*. New York: Avon, 1994.

450. Protas EJ. Flexibility and range of motion. In: *ACSM's resource manual for guidelines for exercise testing and prescription*, 4th ed. JL Roitman, et al. (eds.). Baltimore: Williams & Wilkins, 2001. pp. 381-390.

450a. Pruefer D, Makowski J, Schnell M, et al. Simvastatin inhibits inflammatory properties of staphylococcus aureus alpha-toxin. *Circulation* 2002;106:2104-2110.

451. Pryor WA, Stahl W, Rock CL. Beta carotene: From biochemistry to clinical trials. *Nutr Rev* 2000;58(2 Pt 1):39-53.

452. Pu CT, Johnson MT, Forman DE, et al. Randomized trial of progressive resistance training to counteract the myopathy of chronic heart failure. *J Appl Physiol* 2001;90:2341-2350.

453. Pyörälä M, Miettinen H, Laakso M, Pyörälä K. Hyperinsulinemia predicts coronary heart disease risks in healthy middle-aged men: The 22-year follow-up results of the Helsinki policeman study. *Circulation* 1998;98:398-404.

454. Quaglietti SE, Atwood JE, Ackerman L, Froelicher V. Management of the patient with congestive heart failure using outpatient, home, and palliative care. *Prog Cardiovasc* 2000;43:259-274.

455. Quittan M, Sochor A, Wiesinger GF, et al. Strength improvement of knee extensor muscles in patients with chronic heart failure by neuromuscular electrical stimulation. *Artif Organs* 1999;23(5):432.

456. Quittan M, Sturm B, Wiesinger GF, et al. Quality of life in patients with chronic heart failure: A randomized controlled trial of changes induced by a regular exercise program. *Scand J Rehab Med* 1999;31:223-228.

457. Radloff L. The C.E.S.-D Scale: A self-report depression scale for research in the general population. *Applied Psychological Measurement* 1977;1:385-401.

458. Reardon JZ, DeMartinis J. AACVPR racial and cultural diversity questionaire: Results. *News and Views*, Spring 1999.

459. Reaven G. Pathophysiology of insulin resistance in human disease. *Physiol Rev* 1995;75:473-486.

460. Reaven GM. Role of insulin resistance in human disease. *Diabetes* 1998;37:1595-1607.

461. Rector TS, Kubo SH, Cohn JN. Patients' self-assessment of their congestive heart failure. Part 2: Content, reliability and validity of a new measure, The Minnesota Living with Heart Failure Questionnaire. *Heart Failure* 1987;3:198-209.

462. Reinhart SL. Uncomplicated acute myocardial infarction: A critical path. *J Cardiovasc Nurs* 1995;31:1-7.

463. Ren XS, Amick BC, Williams DR. Racial/ethnic disparities in health: The interplay between discrimination and socio-economic status. *Ethn Dis* 1999;9:151-165.

464. Reuben DB, Siu AL. An objective measure of physical function of elderly outpatients. The physical performance test. *J Am Geriatric Soc* 1990;38:1105-1111.

465. Ribisl PM, Shumaker SA. Enhancing social support and group dynamics. In: *ACSM's resource manual for guidelines for exercise testing and prescription*, 4th ed. JL Roitman, et al. (eds.). Baltimore: Williams & Wilkins, 2001.

466. Rich MW, Beckham V, Wittenberg C, et al. A multidisciplinary intervention to prevent the readmission of elderly patients with congestive heart failure. *N Engl J Med* 1995;333: 1190-1195.

467. Richardson LA, Buckenmeyer PJ, Bauman BD, et al. Contemporary cardiac rehabilitation: Patient characteristics and temporal trends over the past decade. *J Cardiopulm Rehabil* 2000;20:57-64.

468. Riddell LJ, Chisholm A, Williams S, Mann JI. Dietary strategies for lowering homocysteine concentrations. *Am J Clin Nutr* 2000;71:1448-1454.

469. Ridker PM, Cushman M, Stampfer MJ, et al. Inflammation, aspirin, and the risk of cardiovascular disease in apparently healthy men. *N Engl J Med* 1997;336:973-979.

470. Ridker PM, Hennekens CH, Buring JE, Rifai N. C-reactive protein and other markers of inflammation in the prediction of cardiovascular disease in women. *N Engl J Med* 2000;342: 836-843.

470a. Ridker PM, Rifai N, Pfeffer M, et al. Long term effects of pravastatin on plasma concentration of C-reactive protein. *Circulation* 1999;100:230-235.

471. Ridker PM. Novel risk factors and markers for coronary disease. *Adv Intern Med* 2000;45:391-418.

472. Riegel B, Gates DM, Gocka I, et al. Effectiveness of a program of early hospital discharge of cardiac surgery patients. *J Cardiovasc Nursing* 1996;11:63-75.

473. Rigotti NA, McKool KM, Shiffman S. Predictors of smoking cessation after coronary bypass graft surgery: Results of a randomized trial with 5-year follow-up. *Annals Intern Med* 1994;120:287-293.

474. Rihal CS, Smith HC. Percutaneous transluminal coronary angioplasty and bypass surgery in coronary artery disease. In: *Mayo Clinic cardiology review*. JD Murphy (ed.). Philadelphia: Lippincott Williams & Wilkins, 2000. pp. 145-158.

475. Rimm EB, Willett WC, Hu FB, et al. Folate and vitamin B6 from diet and supplements in relation to risk of coronary heart disease among women. *JAMA* 1998;279:359-364.

476. Ritchie DE, Froelicher ES: Exercise and activity. In: *Cardiac nursing*, 3d ed. SL Woods, ES Froelicher, CJ Halpenny, SU Motzer (eds.). Philadelphia: Lippincott, 1995.

476a. Roger VL, Pellikka PA, Bell MR, et al. Sex and text verification bias: Impact on the diagnostic value of exercise echocardiography. *Circulation* 1997;95:405-410.

477. Rodgers G, Ayanian K, Balady G, et al. American College of Cardiology/American Heart Association Clinical Competence statement on exercise testing. *Circulation* 2000;102;1726-1738.

478. Rogutski S, Berra K, Haskell W. Home-based cardiac rehabilitation: Variations on a theme. In: *Cardiac rehabilitation: A guide to practice in the 21st century*. NK Wenger, et al. (eds). New York: Marcel Dekker, 1999. pp. 343-360.

479. Roitman JL, LaFontaine T, Drimmer AM. A new model for risk stratification and delivery of cardiovascular rehabilitation services in the long-term clinical management of patients with coronary artery disease. *J Cardiopulm Rehabil* 1998;18:113-123.

480. Rose MI, Robbins B. Psychosocial recovery issues and strategies in cardiac rehabilitation. In: *Clinical rehabilitation: A cardiologist's guide*. FJ Pashkow, WA Dafoe (eds.). Baltimore: Williams & Wilkins, 1993. pp. 248-262.

480a. Ross R. Atherosclerosis: An inflammatory disease. *N Engl J Med* 1999;340:115-126.

481. Rouleau JC, Talajic M, Sussex B, et al. Myocardial infarction in the 1990's. Their risk factors, stratification, and survival in Canada: The Canadian Assessment of Myocardial Infarction (CAMI) study. *J Am Coll Cardiol* 1996;27:1119-1127.

482. Rozanski A, Blumenthal JA, Kaplan J. Impact of psychological factors on the pathogenesis of cardiovascular disease and implications for therapy. *Circulation* 1999;99:2192-2217.

483. Ruderman N, Devlin JT (eds.). *The health professional's guide to diabetes and exercise*. Alexandria, VA: American Diabetes Association, 1995.

484. Ruderman NB, Schneider SH. Diabetes, exercise and atherosclerosis. *Diabetes Care* 1992;15(Suppl. 4):1787-1793.

485. Ryder KM, Benjamin EJ. Epidemiology and significance of atrial fibrillation. *Am J Cardiol* 1999;84:131R-138R.

486. Sacks FM. Lipid-lowering therapy in acute coronary syndromes. *JAMA* 2001;285:1758-1760.

487. Sacks FM, Pfeffer MA, Moye LA, et al. The effect of pravastatin on coronary events after myocardial infarction with average cholesterol levels. Cholesterol and Recurrent Events trial investigations. *N Engl J Med* 1996;335:1001-1009.

488. Sacks FM, Tonkin AM, Shepherd J, et al. Effect of pravastatin on coronary disease events in subgroups defined by coronary risk factors: The Prospective Pravastatin Pooling Project. *Circulation* 2000;102:1893-1900.

489. Sandra CA. Inpatient cardiac rehabilitation. *J Cardiopulm Rehabil* 1995;15:412-417.

490. Savage PD, Brochu M, Scott P, Ades PA. Low caloric expenditure in cardiac rehabilitation. *Am Heart J* 2000;140:527-533.

491. Scanu AM. Lipoprotein(a): A genetic risk factor for premature coronary heart disease. *JAMA* 1992;267:3326-3329.

492. Schaefer EJ, Lamon-Fava S, Jenner JL, et al. Lipoprotein(a) levels and risk of coronary heart disease in men. The Lipid Research Clinics Coronary Primary Prevention Trial. *JAMA* 1994;271:999-1003.

493. Schmeieder RE, Weihprecht H, Schobel H, et al. Is endothelial function of the radial artery altered in human essential hypertension? *Am J Hypertension* 1997;10(Part 1):323-331.

494. Schneider SH, Khachadurian AK, Amorosa LF, et al. Ten-year experience with an exercise-based outpatient life-style modification program in the treatment of diabetes mellitus. *Diabetes Care* 1992;15:1800-1810.

494a. Schnyder G, Roffi M, Pin R, et al. Decreased rate of coronary restenosis after lowering of plasma homocysteine levels. *N Engl J Med* 2001:345:1593-1600.

495. Schuler G, Hambretch R, Schlief G, et al. Regular physical exercise and low-fat diet: Effects on progression of coronary artery disease. *Circulation* 1992;86:1-17.

496. Schurgin S, Rich S, Mazzone T. Increased prevalence of significant coronary artery calcification in patients with diabetes. *Diabetes Care* 2001;24:335-338.

497. Schwartz GG, Olsson AG, Ezekowitz MD, et al. Effects of atorvastatin on early recurrent ischemic events in acute coronary syndromes (the MIRACL study): A randomized controlled trial. *JAMA* 2001;285:1711-1718.

498. Scott CD, Dark JH, McComb JM. Evolution of the chronotropic response to exercise after cardiac transplantation. *Am J Cardiol* 1995;76:1292-1296.

499. Scott JP, Higenbottam TW, Large S, Wallwork J. Cyclosporine in heart transplant recipients. An exercise study of vasopressor effects. *Eur Heart J* 1992;13:531-534.

500. Seche LA. The Themo Cardiosystems implantable left ventricular device as a bridge to cardiac transplantation. *Heart Lung* 1992;21:112-114.

501. Seman LJ, McNamara JR, Schaeler EJ. Lipoprotein(a), homocysteine, and remnant-like particles: Emerging risk factors. *Curr Opin Cardiol* 1999;14:186-191.

502. Serxner S, Miyaji M, Jeffords J. Congestive heart failure disease management study: A patient education intervention. *Congestive Heart Fail* 1998;4:23-28.

503. Shah NB, Der E, Ruggerio C, et al. Prevention of hospitalizations for heart failure with an interactive home monitoring program. *Am Heart J* 1998;135:373-378.

504. Sigurdsson G, Baldursdottir A, Sigvaldson H, et al. Predictive value of apolipoprotein in a prospective survey of coronary artery disease in men. *Am J Cardiol* 1992;69:1251-1254.

505. Silagy CA, Neil HA. A meta-analysis of the effect of garlic on blood pressure. *J Hypertens* 1994;12:463-468.

506. Silagy C, Neil A. Garlic as a lipid lowering agent: A meta-analysis. *J R Coll Physicians Lond* 1994;28:39-45.

507. Simon JA, Solkowitz SN, Carmody TP, Browner WS. Smoking cessation after surgery. *Arch Intern Med* 1997;157:1371-1376.

508. Simon JA. Vitamin C and cardiovascular disease: A review. *J Am Coll Nutr* 1992;11:107-125.

509. Simons LA, Balasubramaniam S, von Konigsmark M, et al. On the effect of garlic on plasma lipids and lipoproteins in mild hypercholestcrolaemia. *Atherosclerosis* 1995;113:219-225.

510. Simons LA, von Konigsmark M, Simons J, Celermajer DS. Phytoestrogens do not influence lipoprotein levels or endothelial function in healthy, postmenopausal women. *Am J Cardiol* 2000;85:1297-1301.

511. Simvastatin Survival Study Group. Randomised trial of cholesterol lowering in 4444 patients with coronary heart disease: The Scandinavian Simvastatin Survival Study (4S). *Lancet* 1994;344:1383-1389.

512. Singer M. Studying hidden and hard-to-reach populations. In: *Mapping networks, spatial data and hidden populations. Book 4. The ethnographer's toolkit*. Walnut Creek, CA: Altamira Press, 1999.

513. Singh RB, Rastogi SS, Verma R, et al. Randomised controlled trial of cardioprotective diet in patients with recent acute myocardial infarction: Results of one year follow up. *Br Med J* 1992;304:1015-1019.

514. Smith D, Gupta S, Kaski JC. Chronic infections and coronary heart disease. *Int J Clin Pract* 1999;53:460-466.

515. Smith LE, Fabbri SA, Pai R, et al. Symptomatic improvement and reduced hospitalization for patients attending a cardiomyopathy clinic. *Clin Cardiol* 1997;20:949-954.

516. Smith PM, Kraemer HC, Miller NH, et al. In-hospital smoking cessation programs: Who responds, who doesn't? *J Clinical Consult Psych* 1999;67:19-27.

517. Smith SC Jr, Blair SN, Bonow RO, et al. Guidelines for preventing heart attack and death in patients with atherosclerotic cardiovascular disease: 2001 update: A statement for healthcare professionals from the AHA/ACC. *Circulation* 2001;104:1577-1579.

518. Smith SC Jr. Risk-reduction therapy: The challenge to change. *Circulation* 1996;93:2205-2211.

519. Sotile WM. *Heart illness and intimacy: How caring relationships aid recovery.* Baltimore: Johns Hopkins University Press, 1992.

520. Sotile WM, Sotile MO, Ewen GS, Sotile LJ. Marriage and family factors relevant to effective cardiac rehabilitation: A review of risk factor literature. *Sports Med Training Rehabil* 1993;4:115-128.

521. Sotile WM, Sotile MO, Sotile LJ, Ewen GS. Marital and family factors relevant to cardiac rehabilitation: An integrative review of the psychosocial literature. *Sports Med Training Rehabil* 1993;4:217-236.

522. Sotile WM. *Psychosocial interventions for cardiopulmonary patients: A guide for health professionals.* Champaign, IL: Human Kinetics, 1996.

523. Sotile WM. The intimacy factor in cardiopulmonary rehabilitation: A practical model for structuring interventions. *J Cardiopulm Rehabil* 1993;13:237-242.

524. Southard DR, Certo C, Comoss P, et al. Core competencies for cardiac rehabilitation professionals. *J Cardiopulm Rehabil* 1994;14:87-92.

525. Sparks KE, Shaw DK, Eddy D, et al. Alternatives for cardiac rehabilitation patients unable to return to a hospital-based program. *Heart Lung* 1993;22:298-303.

526. Spector RE. *Cultural diversity in health and illness,* 4th ed. Stamford, CT: Appleton & Lange, 1995.

527. Spector RE. *Guide to heritage assessment and health traditions.* Stamford, CT: Appleton & Lange, 1996.

528. Spielberger C, Gorsuch R, Luschene R. *Manual for the State Trait Anxiety Inventory.* Palo Alto, CA: Consulting Psychologists Press, 1970.

529. Squires RW. Cardiac transplantation. In: *Clinical cardiac rehabilitation: A cardiologist's guide.* FJ Pashkow, WA Dafoe (eds.). Baltimore: Williams & Wilkins, 1993. pp. 155-163.

530. Squires RW. Transplant. In: *Clinical cardiac rehabilitation: A cardiologist's guide,* 2d ed. FJ Pashkow, WA Dafoe (eds.). Baltimore: Williams & Wilkins, 1999. pp. 175-191.

531. Squires RW, Hoffman CJ, James GA, et al. Arterial oxygen saturation during graded exercise testing after cardiac transplantation. *J Cardiopulm Rehabil* 1998;18:348.

532. Staessen JA, Fagard R, Thijs I, et al. Randomized double blind comparison of placebo and active treatment for older patients with isolated systolic hypertension. *Lancet* 1997;350: 575-764.

533. Stampfer M, Krauss R, Ma J, et al. A prospective study of triglyceride level, low-density lipoprotein particles diameter, and risk of myocardial infarction. *JAMA* 1996;276:882-888.

534. Stapleton DD, Mehra MR, Dumas D, et al. Lipid-lowering therapy and long-term survival in heart transplantation. *Am J Cardiol* 1997;80:802-804.

535. Steele B. The six-minute walk. *AACVPR proceedings, 9th annual meeting,* Portland, OR, October 1994. Middleton, WI: American Association of Cardiovascular and Pulmonary Rehabilitation. pp. 383-388.

536. Stefanick M, Mackey S, Sheehan M, et al. Effects of diet and exercise in men and postmenopausal women with low levels of HDL-cholesterol and high levels of LDL-cholesterol. *N Engl J Med* 1998;339:12-20.

537. Steiner G. Lipid intervention trials in diabetes. *Diab Care* 2000;23(suppl 2):B49-B53.

538. Stenestrand U, Wallentin L. Early statin treatment following acute myocardial infarction and 1-year survival. *JAMA* 2001;285:430-436.

539. Stephens NG, Parsons A, Schofield PM, et al. Randomised controlled trial of vitamin E in patients with coronary disease: Cambridge Heart Antioxidant Study (CHAOS). *Lancet* 1996;347:781-786.

540. Stevinson C, Pittler M, Ernst E. Garlic for treating hypercholesterolemia. A meta-analysis of randomized clinical trials. *Ann Intern Med* 2000;133:420-429.

541. Stewart S, Pearson S, Horrowitz JD. Effects of a home-based intervention among patients with congestive heart failure discharged from acute hospital care. *Arch Intern Med* 1998;158:1067-1072.

542. St. Jeor ST, Brownell KD, Atkinson RL, et al. Obesity. Workshop III. American Heart Association Prevention Conference III. Behavior change and compliance: Keys to improving cardiovascular health. *Circulation* 1993;88:1391-1396.

543. Stratton JR, Kemp GJ, Daly RC, et al. Effects of cardiac transplantation on bioenergetic abnormalities of skeletal muscle in congestive heart failure. *Circulation* 1994;89:1624-1631.

544. Suadicani P, Hein H, Gyntelberg F. Serum selenium concentration and risk of ischaemic heart disease in a prospective cohort study of 3000 males. *Atherosclerosis* 1992;96:33-42.

545. Sumida H, Watanabe H, Kugiyama K, et al. Does passive smoking impair endothelium-dependent coronary artery dilation in women? *Am J Cardiol* 1998;31:811-815.

546. Superko H, Krauss R. Garlic powder, effect on plasma lipids, postprandial lipidemia, low-density lipoprotein particle size, high-density lipoprotein subclass distribution and lipoprotein(a). *J Am Coll Cardiol* 2000;35:321-326.

547. Svetkey LP, Simons-Morton D, Vollmer WM, et al. Effects of dietary patterns on blood pressure: Subgroup analysis of the Dietary Approaches to Stop Hypertension (DASH) randomized clinical trial. *Arch Intern Med* 1999;159:285-293.

548. Swenson JR, Abbey SE. Management of depression and anxiety disorders in the cardiac patient. In: *Clinical rehabilitation: A cardiologist's guide.* FJ Pashkow, WA Dafoe (eds.). Baltimore: Williams & Wilkins, 1993. pp. 263-286.

549. Tagusari O, Kormos RL, Kawai A, et al. Native heart complications after heterotopic heart transplantation: Insight into the potential risk of left ventricular assist device. *J Heart Lung Transplant* 1999;18:1111-1119.

550. Tauchert M, Gildor A, Lipinski J. High-dose Crataegus extract WS 1442 in the treatment of NYHA stage II heart failure. *Herz* 1999;24:465-467.

551. Taunton, JE, McCargar L. Managing activity in patients who have diabetes. *Phys Sportsmed* 1995;23:41-52.

552. Taylor CB, Miller NH. Pyschopathology. In: *ACSM's resource manual for guidelines for exercise testing and prescription.* JL Roitman, et al. (eds.). Baltimore: Lippincott Williams & Wilkins, 2001.

553. Taylor CB, Miller NH. The behavioral approach. In: *Rehabilitation of the coronary patient,* 3d ed. NK Wenger, HK Hellerstein (eds.). New York: Churchill Livingstone, 1992. pp. 461-471.

554. Taylor CB, Miller NH, Herman S, et al. A nurse-managed smoking cessation program for hospitalized smokers. *Am J Public Health* 1996;86:1557-1560.

555. Taylor CB, Miller NH, Killen JD, et al. Smoking cessation after myocardial infarction: Effects of a nurse-managed intervention. *Annals Intern Med* 1990;113:118-123.

556. Taylor CB, Miller NH, Smith PM, DeBusk RF. The effect of a home-based, case-managed, multifactorial risk-reduction program on reducing psychological distress in patients with cardiovascular disease. *J Cardiopulm Rehabil* 1997;17: 157-162.

557. Tharrett SJ, Peterson JA. *ACSM's health/fitness facility standards and guidelines.* Champaign, IL: Human Kinetics, 1997.

558. Thomas RJ, Houston Miller N, Lamendola C, et al. National survey on gender differences in cardiac rehabilitation programs. *J Cardiopulm Rehabil* 1996;16:402-412.

559. Thomas S, Reading J, Shepard RJ. Revision of the Physical Activity Readiness Questionnaire (PAR-Q). *Canadian J Sport Science* 1992;17:338-345.

560. Thomas T, LaFontaine T. Exercise, nutritional strategies, and lipoproteins. In: *ACSM's resource manual for guidelines for exercise testing and prescription,* 4th ed. JL Roitman, et al. (eds.). Baltimore: Williams & Wilkins, 2001.

561. Thompson P. The safety of exercise testing and participation. In: *ACSM's resource manual for guidelines for exercise testing and prescription,* 2d ed. American College of Sports Medicine. Philadelphia: Lea & Febiger, 1993. pp. 359-363.

562. Thompson PD (ed). *Exercise and sports cardiology.* New York: McGraw Hill, 2001.

563. Tikkanen MJ, Adlercreutz H. Dietary soy-derived isoflavone phytoestrogens. Could they have a role in coronary heart disease prevention? *Biochem Pharmacol* 2000;60:1-5.

564. Tikkanen MJ, Wahala K, Ojala S, et al. Effect of soybean phytoestrogen intake on low density lipoprotein oxidation resistance. *Proc Natl Acad Sci USA* 1998;95:3106-3110.

565. Titler MG, Pettit DM. Discharge readiness assessment. *J Cardiovasc Nursing* 1995;9:64-74.

566. Tobacco use and dependence clinical practice guideline panel, staff, and consortium representatives. A clinical practice guideline for treating tobacco use and dependence. *JAMA* 2000;28:3244-3254.

567. Tokmakova M, Dobreva B, Kostianev S. Effects of short-term exercise training in patients with heart failure. *Folia Medica* 1999;41:68-71.

568. Tresch DD, Aronow WS. Recognition and diagnosis of coronary artery disease in the elderly. In: *Cardiovascular disease in the elderly patient.* DD Tresch, WS Aronow (eds.). New York: Marcel Dekker, 1999. pp. 197-212.

569. Tresch DD, Brady WJ, Aufderheide TP, et al. Comparison of elderly and younger patients with out-of-hospital chest pain. Clinical characteristics, acute myocardial infarction, therapy, and outcomes. *Arch Internal Med* 1996;156:1089-1093.

570. Turcato E, Bosello O, Francesco VD, et al. Waist circumference and abdominal sagittal diameter as surrogates of body fat distribution in the elderly: Their relation with cardiovascular risk factors. *Int J Obes Relat Metab Disord* 2000;24: 1005-1010.

571. Tyni-Lenne R, Gordon A, Jansson E, et al. Skeletal muscle endurance training improves peripheral oxidative capacity, exercise tolerance, and health-related quality of life in women with chronic congestive heart failure secondary to either ischemic cardiomyopathy or idiopathic dilated cardiomyopathy. *Am J Cardiol* 1997;80:1025-1029.

572. Tyni-Lenne R, Gordon A, Sylven C. Improved quality of life in chronic heart failure patients following local endurance training with leg muscles. *J Cardiac Failure* 1996;2:111-117.

573. Unger BT, Warren DA. Case management in cardiac rehabilitation. In: *Cardiac rehabilitation: A guide to practice in the 21st century.* NK Wenger, et al (eds.). New York: Marcel Dekker, 1999. pp. 327-341.

574. United States Department of Health and Human Services. *Depression is a treatable illness: A patient's guide.* Rockville, MD: USDHHS publication AHCPR 93-0553, 1993.

575. United States Department of Health and Human Services, Centers for Disease Control and Prevention. *Physical activity and health: A report of the Surgeon General.* Atlanta: National Center for Chronic Disease Prevention and Health Promotion, 1996.

576. United States Department of Health and Human Services, Health Care Financing Administration. Payment for services furnished to patients in hospital based and free standing cardiac rehabilitation clinics. *Federal Register* 1982;41:934.

577. United States Department of Health and Human Services, Health Care Financing Administration. Health care financing administration. http://www.hcfa.gov/quality/3q2.htm June, 2001.

578. United States Department of Health and Human Services, Public Health Service, Agency for Health Care Policy and Research, and the National Heart, Lung, and Blood Institute. *Diagnosing and managing unstable angina.* AHCPR Publication No. 96-0602. Rockville, MD.

579. United States Department of Health and Human Services, Public Health Service, Agency for Health Care Policy and Research, and the National Heart, Lung, and Blood Institute. *Guide for smoking cessation specialists.* AHCPR Publication No. 96-0693. Rockville, MD, April 1996.

580. Van Camp SP, Peterson RA. Cardiovascular complications of outpatient cardiac rehabilitation programs. *JAMA* 1986;256: 1160-1163.

581. Van Horn L. Fiber, lipids, and coronary heart disease. A statement for healthcare professionals from the Nutrition

Committee, American Heart Association. *Circulation* 1997;95: 2701-2704.

582. Vangvanich P, Paul-Labrador MJ, Bairey Merz CN. Safety of medically supervised exercise in a cardiac rehabilitation center. *Am J Cardiol* 1996;77:1383-1385.

583. Veatch RM (ed.). *Cross-cultural perspectives in medical ethics*, 2d ed. Boston: Jones & Bartlett, 2000.

584. Verani MS, Mahmarian JJ. Nonexercise stress testing. In: *American Journal of Cardiology, Continuing Education Series, Myocardial Perfusion Imaging.* AS Iskandrian (ed.). 1993;4: 10.

585. Verbrugge L, Jette A. The disablement process. *Soc Sci Med* 1994;38:114.

586. Verrill D, Ashley R, Witt K, Forkner T. Recommended guidelines for monitoring and supervision of North Carolina Phase II/III cardiac rehabilitation programs: A position paper by the North Carolina Cardiopulmonary Rehabilitation Association. *J Cardiopulm Rehabil* 1996;16:9-24.

587. Verrill D, Shoup E, Boice L, et al. Recommended guidelines: Body composition assessment in cardiac rehabilitation. *J Cardiopulm Rehabil* 1994;14:104-121.

588. Vogel RA, Corretti MC, Plotnick GD. Post-prandial effect of components of the Mediterranean diet on endothelial function. *J Am Coll Cardiol* 2000;36:1455-1460.

589. Vokonas PS, Kannel WB. Diabetes mellitus and coronary heart disease in the elderly. *Clin Geriatr Med* 1996;2:69-78.

590. Vokonas PS, Kannel WB. Epidemiology of coronary heart disease in the elderly. In: *Cardiovascular disease in the elderly patient.* DD Tresch, WS Aronow (eds.). New York: Marcel Dekker, 1994. pp. 91-123.

591. von Eckardstein A, Schulte H, Cullen P, Assman G. Lipoprotein(a) further increases risk of coronary events in men with high global cardiovascular risk. *J Am Coll Cardiol* 2001;37:434-439.

592. von Shakey C. n-3 fatty acids and the prevention of coronary atherosclerosis. *Am J Clin Nutr* 2000;71:224S-227S.

593. Walberg-Henriksson H. Exercise and diabetes mellitus. In: *Exercise and sport sciences reviews*, vol. 20. JO Holloszy (ed.). Baltimore: Williams & Wilkins, 1992. pp. 339-368.

594. Walbroehl GS. Sexual concerns of the patient with pulmonary disease. *Postgrad Med* 1992;91:455-460.

595. Wang WWT. The educational needs of myocardial infarction patients. *Prog Cardiovasc Nurs* 1994;9:28-36.

596. Wannamethee SG, Shaper AG, Walker M. Physical activity and mortality in older men with diagnosed heart disease. *Circulation* 2000;102:1358-1363.

597. Ware JE, Sherbourne CD. The MOS 36-item short-form health survey (SF-36): Conceptual framework and item selection. *Med Care* 1992;30:473-485.

598. Warshafsky S, Kamer RS, Sivak SL. Effect of garlic on total serum cholesterol. A meta-analysis. *Ann Intern Med* 1993;119: 599-605.

599. Wassib J, Keller A, Rubenstrin L, et al. Benefits and obstacles of health status assessment in ambulatory settings: The clinician's point of view. *Medical Care* 1992;30(5):42-49.

600. Watts GF, Lewis B, Brunt JN, et al. Effects on coronary artery disease of lipid-lowering diet or diet plus cholestyramine in the St. Thomas Arteriosclerosis Regression Study. *Lancet* 1992;339:563-569.

601. Weiner P, Waizman J, Magadle R, et al. The effect of specific inspiratory muscle training on the sensation of dyspnea and exercise tolerance in patients with congestive heart failure. *Clin Cardiol* 1999;22:727.

602. Weis M, von Scheidt W. Cardiac allograft vasculopathy: A review. *Circulation* 1997; 96:2069-2077.

603. Welty FK. Cardiovascular disease and dyslipidemia in women. *Arch Int Med* 2001;161:514-522.

604. Wenger NK, Froelicher ES, Smith LK, et al. *Cardiac Rehabilitation.* Clinical Practice Guideline No. 17. Rockville, MD: US Department of Health and Human Services, Public Health Service, Agency for Health Care Policy and Research, and the National Heart, Lung, and Blood Institute. AHCPR Publication No. 96-0672. October 1995.

605. Wenger NK. In-hospital exercise rehabilitation after myocardial infarction and myocardial revascularization: Physiologic basis, methodology, and results. In: *Rehabilitation of the coronary patient*, 3d ed. NK Wenger, HK Hellerstein (eds.). New York: Churchill Livingstone, 1992.

606. Wenke K, Meiser B, Thiery J, et al. Simvastatin reduces graft vessel disease and mortality after heart transplantation: A four-year randomized trial. *Circulation* 1997;96:1398-1402.

607. West JA, Miller NH, Parker KM, et al. A comprehensive management system for heart failure improves clinical outcomes and reduces medical resource utilization. *Am J Cardiol* 1997;79:58-63.

608. Weststrate JA, Meijer GW. Plant sterol-enriched margarines and reduction of plasma total- and LDL-cholesterol concentrations in normocholesterolaemic and mildly hypercholesterolaemic subjects. *Eur J Clin Nutr* 1998;52:334-343.

609. Whelton PK, Appel LJ, Espeland MA, et al. Sodium reduction and weight loss in the treatment of hypertension in older persons. A randomized trial of non-pharmacologic interventions in the elderly (TONE). *JAMA* 1998;279:839-846.

610. Whittle J, Conigliario J, Good CB, Joswiak M. Do patient preferences contribute to racial differences in cardiovascular procedure use? *J Gen Intern Med* 1997;12:267-273.

611. Wielenga RP, Huisveld IA, Bol E, et al. Safety and effects of physical training in chronic heart failure. Results of the Chronic Heart Failure and Graded Exercise study (CHANGE). *Eur Heart J* 1999;20:872-879.

612. Wilke NA, Sheldahl LM, Dougherty SM, et al. Baltimore Therapeutic Equipment (BET) work simulator: Energy expenditure of work activities in cardiac patients. *Arch Phys Med Rehabil* 1993;74:419-424.

613. Willenheimer R, Erhardt L, Cline C, et al. Exercise training in heart failure improves quality of life and exercise capacity. *Eur Heart J* 1998;19:774-781.

614. Willett W, Reynolds R, Cottrell-Hoehner S, et al. Validation of a semi-quantitative food frequency questionnaire: Comparison with a 1-year diet record. *J Am Dietetics Assoc* 1987;87:43-47.

615. Willett W, Sampson L, Stampfer M, et al. Reproducibility and validity of a semi-quantitative food frequency questionnaire. *Am J Epidemiol* 1985;122:51-65.

616. Williams J. A structured guide for the Hamilton Depression Rating Scale. *Arch Gen Psychiatr* 1998;45:742-747.

617. Williams MA, Esterbrooks DJ, Sketch MH Sr. Limitations of Phase II exercise training in the "older" elderly cardiac patient. *Circulation* 1990;82:III-576.

618. Williams MA: *Exercise testing and training in the elderly cardiac patient*. Champaign, IL: Human Kinetics, 1994.

619. Williams MA. Exercise testing in cardiac rehabilitation: Exercise prescription and beyond. *Cardiology Clinics* 2001;19: 415-431.

620. Williams MA, Fleg JL, Ades PA, et al. Secondary prevention of coronary heart disease in the elderly (with emphasis on patients ≥75 years of age). *Circulation* 2002;105:1735-1743.

621. Williams MA, Maresh CM, Esterbrooks, DJ, et al. Early exercise training in patients older than age 65 years compared with that in younger patients after acute myocardial infarction or coronary artery bypass grafting. *Am J Cardiol* 1985;55:263-266.

622. Williams MA, Maresh CM, Esterbrooks DJ, Sketch MH Jr. Characteristics of exercise responses following short and long term aerobic training in elderly cardiac patients. *J Am Geriatr Soc* 1987;35:904.

623. Williams MA, Thalken LJ, Esterbrooks DJ, Sketch MH Sr. Effects of short-term and long-term exercise training in older elderly cardiac patients. *Circulation* 1992;86:I-670.

624. Williams RB, Barefoot, JC, Califf RM, et al. Prognostic importance of social and economic resources among medically treated patients with angiographically documented coronary artery disease. *JAMA* 1992;267:520-524.

625. Williams RB, Williams V. *Anger kills: Seventeen strategies for controlling the hostility that can harm your health*. New York: Times Books, 1993.

626. Willich SN, Lewis M, Lowel H, et al. Physical exertion as a trigger of acute myocardial infarction. *N Engl J Med* 1993;329: 1684-1690.

627. Wilson JR, Groves J, Rayos G. Circulatory status and response to cardiac rehabilitation in patients with heart failure. *Circulation* 1996;94:1567-1572.

628. Woo KS, Chook P, Leong HC, et al. The impact of heavy passive smoking on arterial endothelial function in modernized Chinese. *J Am Coll Cardiol* 2000;36:1228-1232.

629. Wood D. Prevention of coronary heart disease in clinical practice. *Eur Heart J* 1998;19:1434-1503.

630. Wood D. Established and emerging cardiovascular risk factors. *Am Heart J* 2001;141:S49-57.

631. World Health Organization Expert Committee. *Rehabilitation after cardiovascular diseases with special attention on developing countries*. Technical report series no. 831. Geneva: World Health Organization, 1993.

632. World Health Organization Society of Hypertension. Guidelines for the management of hypertension. *J Hypertension* 1999;17:151-183.

633. Young AJ, Young PM. Human acclimatization to high terrestrial altitude. In: *Human performance physiology and environmental medicine at terrestrial extremes*. KB Pandolph, MN Sawka, RR Gonzalez (eds.). Indianapolis: Benchmark, 1988. pp. 497-543.

634. Yusuf S, Dagenais G, Pogue J, et al. Vitamin E supplementation and cardiovascular events in high-risk patients. The Heart Outcomes Prevention Evaluation Study Investigators. *N Engl J Med* 2000;342:154-160.

635. Zarich S, Waxman S, Freeman R, et al. Effect of autonomic nervous system dysfunction on the circadian pattern of myocardial ischemia in diabetes mellitus. *J Am Coll Cardiol* 1994;24:956-962.

636. Zava DT, Duwe G. Estrogenic and antiproliferative properties of genistein and other flavonoids in human breast cancer cells in vitro. *Nutr Cancer* 1997;27:31-40.

637. Zavaroni I, Bonini L, Gasparini P, et al. Hyperinsulinemia in a normal population as a predictor of non-insulin dependent diabetes mellitus, hypertension, and coronary heart disease: The Barilla factory revisited. *Metabolism* 1999;48:989-994.

638. Zeni AI, Hoffman MD, Clifford PS. Energy expenditure with indoor exercise machines. *JAMA* 1998;275:1424-1427.

639. Zhao QM, Mettauer B, Epailly E, et al. Effect of exercise training on leukocyte subpopulations and clinical course in cardiac transplant patients. *Transplant Proceedings* 1998;30: 172-175.

Index

Note: The italicized *f* and *t* following page numbers refer to figures and tables, respectively.

high-density lipoprotein (HDL) 101, 102*f*, 108*f*
Hispanic Americans 142, 143, 144
Hispanic Health Council 144
HMG Co-A reductase inhibitors (statins) 107
HMOs. *See* health maintenance organizations
home care 48-49, 204, 205
homocysteine 26-27, 133
Human Activity Scale 84
human resources 193-196. *See also* staff
   core functions and 194-195
   program personnel 195-196
   staff education and performance review 196
hyperglycemia 200
hypertension 110-113
   assessment of 110, 200
   blood pressure classification 111*t*
   guideline for 111
   intervention 112-113
   lifestyle modifications of 112*f*
   management of 14*f*, 56*t*
   in older patients 138
   pharmacological therapy for 113
   plant-based diet and 23
   prevalence of 112-113
   risk assessment in secondary prevention 56*t*, 60
   risk stratification and treatment of 113*t*
   screening for 200
hypoglycemia 200
hypotension 200

I

ICDs. *See* implantable cardioverter defibrillators
imaging modalities 82-83
implantable cardioverter defibrillators 150-151
inactivity. *See* physical inactivity
independence, encouraging 87-88
inflammation, markers of 133-134
information management issues 188-191
   confidentiality 191
   documentation 188-191
   education and counseling 191
   patient rights 191
informed consent form 210-211, 225
   alternative clauses for 227
inpatient cardiac rehabilitation 31-51
   activities used in 37*t*, 37*f*
   challenges and opportunities in 9*t*
   clinical pathways in 43-44
   continuum of care and 8*t*
   discharge planning 42-43
   early assessment 32-36
   facilities and equipment 181-182
   intervention in 93, 126-127
   mobilization 36-38

process recommendations 51*f*
psychosocial concerns and 124-127
risk-factor management 38-42
service record 207
space and equipment 47
staffing for 45
structure recommendations for 50*f*
time requirements for services 46*t*
transitional programming 47-48
inpatient interventions 93
insulin resistance 105, 107*f*
insurance 191-193
   health insurance companies 191-192
   plan coverage 192
   reimbursement 192, 193*f*
International Classification of Disease (ICD-9 Code Book) 193
International Liaison Committee on Resuscitation (ILCOR) 201
Iowa Women's Health Study 23
ischemia, assessment and screening of 199
ischemic heart disease 3

J

Jackson Heart Study 144
JNC-VII. *See* Joint National Committee–VII
job-task simulation 84
Joint Commission on Accreditation of Healthcare Organizations (JCAHO) 5, 178, 184, 187, 196, 198
Joint National Committee–VII (JNC-VII) 110, 111*t*

K

Kansas City Cardiomyopathy Questionnaire 151

L

language of patients 94
LDL cholesterol. *See* low-density lipoprotein (LDL) cholesterol
leadership 178-180
left ventricular assist devices (LVADs) 157-159
   exercise training and 159
   heart failure and 156
   versions of 158
lifestyle changes, for lipid management 103-105
lipid management 13-14*f*, 58-59, 101-110
   CHD risk and 102
   elevated triglycerides and 105-107, 108*t*
   general treatment guidelines for 107
   guideline for 101
   insulin resistance and 105, 107*f*
   LDL and 102-104, 105*t*
   long-term follow-up for 109-110
   metabolic syndrome and 105
   with older patients 138

About the AACVPR

History and Purpose

Founded in 1985, the American Association of Cardiovascular and Pulmonary Rehabilitation (AACVPR) is dedicated to the professional development of its members through networking and educational opportunities. Central to the mission is improving the quality of life for patients and their families.

Mission Statement

To reduce morbidity, mortality, and disability from cardiovascular and pulmonary diseases through education, prevention, rehabilitation, research, and aggressive disease management.

Fast Facts

- Founded in 1985
- 2002 membership: 2,600 (and growing)
- Oversees the well-respected Program Certification for Cardiac and Pulmonary Rehabilitation programs
- Members are behavioral scientists, cardiovascular physicians, nutritionists/dieticians, cardiovascular nurses, cardiopulmonary physical therapists, exercise physiologists, pulmonary nurses, exercise rehabilitation specialists, pulmonary physicians, and respiratory therapists
- Headquarters: 401 N. Michigan Ave., Suite 2200, Chicago, IL 60611; 312-321-5146.
- Promotes advocacy for reimbursement issues in Washington, DC

Membership Benefits

Be part of a national network of professionals dedicated to the advancement of cardiovascular and pulmonary rehabilitation. Members receive the following:

Timely Information

- The bimonthly *Journal of Cardiopulmonary Rehabilitation*, a well-respected publication that features the most current research as well as clinical and practical information about the science of rehabilitation
- *Monthly News and Views*, AACVPR's e-mailed newsletter that provides the latest updates from the association and its affiliate societies, as well as practical information for daily practice
- Access to the members-only section of the AACVPR Web site
- E-mail updates of timely information regarding federal and state guidelines, reimbursement, and other issues of concern to professionals in the field

Influence

- Opportunities to join colleagues to promote the quality of patient care through efforts in Washington, DC, and to increase reimbursement for cardiac and pulmonary rehab services

Quality Education

- Members' discount to attend the AACVPR annual meeting

- Members' discount for new proposed distance-learning formats
- Members' discount on a wide variety of AACVPR publications and programs

Benchmarking and Standards of Care

- Members' discount for program certification and recertification applications
- Participation in a new AACVPR Mentorship program

Networking

- A complimentary copy of the membership directory, published annually
- Access to the members-only section of the Web site
- Opportunity to participate in the national network of professionals dedicated to the advancement of cardiac and pulmonary care

Professional Growth

- Access to the AACVPR career link—an on-line listing of nationwide job opportunities
- Invitation to submit articles to the *Journal of Cardiopulmonary Rehabilitation* and *News and Views* and to present your research at the annual meeting
- Opportunity to apply for AACVPR grants and scholarships
- Volunteer to serve on national committees with nationally recognized experts in the field

Publications

- *Journal of Cardiopulmonary Rehabilitation* (published bimonthly)
- *News and Views of AACVPR* (published quarterly)
- *Guidelines for Cardiac Rehabilitation and Secondary Prevention Programs*, third edition
- *Guidelines for Pulmonary Rehabilitation Programs*, second edition

- *How to Inform Payers and Influence Payment for Cardiac and Pulmonary Rehabilitation Services*
- Bibliography: *Outcomes of Pulmonary Rehabilitation*
- Bibliography: *Outcomes of Cardiac Rehabilitation*
- Annual membership and programs directory
- Outcomes tool resource guide
- Educational resource guide
- Annual meeting syllabus
- Agency for Health Care Policy and Research, *Clinical Practice Guideline for Cardiac Rehabilitation*
- Agency for Health Care Policy and Research, *Patient Guide: Recovering from Heart Problems Through Cardiac Rehabilitation*
- Fitness Products Council, *How to Buy Exercise Equipment for the Home*
- Agency for Health Care Policy and Research, *Cardiac Rehabilitation as Secondary Prevention: Quick Reference for Clinician*

It's Easy to Apply

To apply for membership, select one of these fast and easy methods:

- By mail: Complete the enclosed form and mail it to AACVPR headquarters.
- Online: Go to www.aacvpr.org and complete the online form or print out the form and mail it to AACVPR headquarters (address on application).

With either method of application, please include credit card information or a check for the dues amount in U.S. funds. If you wish to receive additional applications, or if you have any questions, please call headquarters at 312-321-5146, or send an e-mail to aacvpr@sba.com.

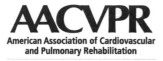

American Association of Cardiovascular and Pulmonary Rehabilitation
Membership Application

Name_____

Professional Degree _____
(Please list no more than two)

Job Title _____

Place of Employment_____

Mailing Address_____

City _____

State/Province_____

Zip Code/Postal Code _____

Country _____

This address is: ❑ Home   ❑ Business

(The above address will be used for mailings and will be listed in the Membership Directory.)

Email:_____

(Be sure to include your email address for frequent Regulatory Updates and the monthly News and Views. The AACVPR does not distribute email addresses to other groups).

Daytime Phone: (   )_____

Fax: (   ) _____

Are you a current member of your state/regional society?

❑ Yes   ❑ No

General Information

Where did you hear about the AACVPR?

❑ From an AACVPR Member

❑ Was a Previous Member—Year(s)

❑ Journal of Cardiopulmonary Rehabilitation

❑ Professional Colleague

❑ State/Regional Society

❑ University/School

❑ Other

What made you decide to join the AACVPR? _____

_____

Membership Categories

❑ Member
Membership Fee $150

Shall be any interested person of majority age who is a nurse, physician, medical scientist, allied health-care practitioner or educator, and who in his or her professional endeavors, is regularly involved in some aspect of cardiovascular and/or pulmonary rehabilitation. Members have AACVPR voting privileges.

Which of these categories best represents you?
Check only one:
❑ Behavioral Scientist
❑ Cardiopulmonary Physical Therapist
❑ Exercise Rehabilitation Specialist
❑ Cardiovascular Physician
❑ Exercise Physiologist
❑ Pulmonary Physician
❑ Nutritionist/Dietician
❑ Pulmonary Nurse
❑ Respiratory Therapist
❑ Cardiovascular Nurse
❑ Other _____

Are you certified by a professional association?
❑ Yes   ❑ No

Association Name _____

Certification _____

Does your current employer support individual AACVPR membership?
❑ Yes   ❑ No

❑ Student Member
Membership Fee $75

A Student Member shall be any interested undergraduate or graduate college student currently carrying the equivalent of at least one half of a full-time academic load for one year, as defined by the university or college of attendance. The area of study must be in a medical or allied health curriculum. Student Membership also applies to physicians-in-training, including residents and interns.

To qualify as a Student Member, one must submit a copy of his or her current student identification card along with this completed application.

Educational Institution _____

Major _____

Year Degree Expected_____

❑ Associate Member
Membership Fee $150

Shall be any person with an interest in cardiovascular and /or pulmonary rehabilitation, but not currently eligible for classification as a Member or Student Member. Dues are established by the Board of Directors and may be changed at its discretion. Associate Member privileges include a subscription to the AACVPR newsletter and placement on the Association mailing list.

Primary Occupation_____

Place of Employment_____

Current Program Involvement

In what area(s) do you spend the majority of your practice?

Check one:

❑ In-patient Cardiovascular/Pulmonary/Vascular

❑ Out-patient Cardiovascular/Pulmonary/Vascular

❑ In-patient & Out-patient Cardiovascular/Pulmonary/Vascular

Who is your employer?

❑ Hospital　　　　　　❑ Educational Institution

❑ Physician/Group practice　　❑ Other: _____

How many new out-patients would you estimate are seen in your program annually?

❑ Less than 100　　　❑ 101-200 patients

❑ 201-300 patients　　❑ Over 300 patients

How many new in-patients would you estimate are seen in your program annually?

❑ Less than 100　　　❑ 101-500 patients

❑ 501-1000 patients　❑ Over 1000 patients

❑ Does not apply

Which of the following best describes the emphasis of your work environment?

❑ 100% rehabilitation

❑ 75% rehabilitation/25% prevention

❑ 50% rehabilitation/50% prevention

❑ 25% rehabilitation/75% prevention

Membership Agreement

I certify that the above information is correct and I agree to abide by the Code of Ethical and Professional conduct of the American Association of Cardiovascular and Pulmonary Rehabilitation. Visit the AACVPR Web site for the code of ethics.

Signature _____ Date _____

Payment

Purchase orders are not accepted.
Payment must accompany application.

❑ Check (Payable to AACVPR; US Funds Only)

❑ MC/Visa/American Express—Exp. Date _____

Cardholder's Name _____

Card Number_____

Cardholder's City/State _____

Cardholder's Signature _____

Heart and Lung Foundation Contribution Opportunities

The Heart and Lung Foundation strives to assist the AACVPR in becoming the recognized leader in professional and public education for the field of cardiopulmonary rehabilitation through:

- **Education**
- **Service/Outreach**
- **Research**

All donations are tax deductible.

Yes, I want to do my part to advance my profession by pledging the following:

❑ $25 .... Foundation Supporter

❑ $50 .... Foundation Member

❑ $100 .... Foundation Partner

❑ $250 .... Foundation Sponsor

❑ $500 .... Foundation Patron

❑ $1,000 .... Foundation Benefactor

Foundation benefactors will be acknowledged on the AACVPR Web site.

AACVPR membership is effective
July through June 30. Membership is
not pro-rated; however, members joining
after march 1 will be deferred until July 1.
Membership dues are non-refundable, nor
deductible as a charitable contribution.
Membership dues may be deductible as an
ordinary and necessary business expense.
Consult your tax advisor for information.

Please send completed application to:

AACVPR National Office

401 N Michigan Avenue, Suite 2200

Chicago, IL 60611

Telephone: 312-321-5146

Email: aacvpr@sba.com

Web site: www.aacvpr.org

Credit Card Users may fax application to:

312-245-1085

Guidelines for Cardiac Rehabilitation and Secondary Prevention Programs

Fourth Edition

American Association of
Cardiovascular and Pulmonary
Rehabilitation

The AACVPR's *Guidelines for Cardiac Rehabilitation
and Secondary Prevention Programs, Fourth Edition,*
has been reviewed and endorsed by the
American Heart Association

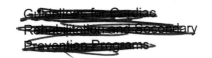

Library of Congress Cataloging-in-Publication Data

Guidelines for cardiac rehabilitation and secondary prevention programs /
American Association of Cardiovascular & Pulmonary Rehabilitation.--
4th ed.
   p. ; cm.
Includes bibliographical references and index.
  ISBN 0-7360-4864-2 (alk. paper)
  1. Heart--Diseases--Patients--Rehabilitation. 2.
Heart--Diseases--Prevention.
   [DNLM: 1. Heart Diseases--rehabilitation. 2. Heart
Diseases--prevention & control. WG 210 G946 2004] I. American
Association of Cardiovascular & Pulmonary Rehabilitation.
  RC682G76 2004
  616.1'203--dc21

        2003005444

ISBN: 0-7360-4864-2

This book is a revised edition of *Guidelines for Cardiac Rehabilitation Programs,* published in 1991, 1995, and 1999 by Human Kinetics Publishers, Inc.

The Web addresses cited in this text were current as of July 1, 2003, unless otherwise noted.

Acquisitions Editor: Loarn D. Robertson, PhD; **Developmental Editor:** Anne Rogers; **Assistant Editors:** Amanda S. Ewing and Sandra Merz Bott; **Copyeditor:** Barbara Walsh; **Proofreader:** Jim Burns; **Indexer:** Robert Howerton; **Permission Manager:** Dalene Reeder; **Graphic Designer:** Nancy Rasmus; **Graphic Artist:** Dawn Sills; **Photo Manager:** Kareema McLendon; **Cover Designer:** Fred Starbird; **Photographer (interior):** Tom Roberts; **Art Manager:** Kelly Hendren; **Illustrator:** Accurate Art; **Printer:** Custom Color Graphics

We thank The Cardiac Center of Creighton University in Omaha, Nebraska, for assistance in providing the location for the photo shoot for this book.

Printed in the United States of America   10 9 8 7 6 5 4 3 2 1

Human Kinetics
Web site: www.HumanKinetics.com

United States: Human Kinetics
P.O. Box 5076
Champaign, IL 61825-5076
800-747-4457
e-mail: humank@hkusa.com

Canada: Human Kinetics
475 Devonshire Road Unit 100
Windsor, ON N8Y 2L5
800-465-7301 (in Canada only)
e-mail: orders@hkcanada.com

Europe: Human Kinetics
107 Bradford Road
Stanningley
Leeds LS28 6AT, United Kingdom
+44 (0) 113 255 5665
e-mail: hk@hkeurope.com

Australia: Human Kinetics
57A Price Avenue
Lower Mitcham, South Australia 5062
08 8277 1555
e-mail: liahka@senet.com.au

New Zealand: Human Kinetics
P.O. Box 105-231, Auckland Central
09-523-3462
e-mail: hkp@ihug.co.nz